Sports Injuries

IN CHILDREN AND ADOLESCENTS

An Essential Guide for
DIAGNOSIS, TREATMENT AND MANAGEMENT

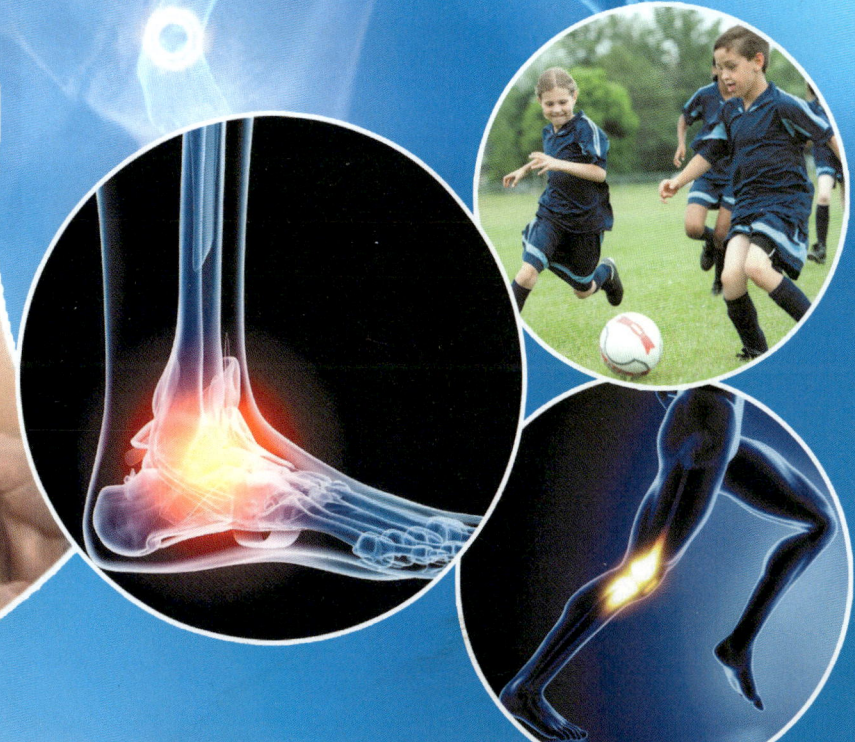

Dr Solomon Abrahams, PhD, MSc, BSc, MCSP, SRP

Copyright © 2013 by Dr Solomon Abrahams. 305947-ABRA
Library of Congress Control Number: 2013908613
ISBN: Softcover   978-1-4836-3974-1
           Hardcover   978-1-4836-3975-8
           Ebook   978-1-4836-3976-5

Rev. date: 07/17/2013

To order additional copies of this book, contact:
Xlibris LLC
0800-056-3182
www.xlibrispublishing.co.uk
Orders@ Xlibrispublishing.co.uk

Sports Injuries in Children and Adolescents: An Essential Guide

Author

Dr Solomon Abrahams, PhD, MSc, BSc, MCSP, SRP
Consultant Physiotherapist, Anatomie Physiotherapy (London, UK)
Specialist in paediatric and adolescent sports and orthopaedic injuries
Senior Clinical Fellow, School of Emergency Medicine, University of Hertfordshire
London, United Kingdom

Xlibris Publishing
A Penguin Company

Editor: Faye Triggs & Solomon Abrahams
Medical Illustrator: Isobel Kilbey
Photographer: Malcolm Hoppen

Contents

Dedication

I dedicate this book to my family, who allowed me the precious time to write this book and put up with my grumpiness. To my dear wife, Gem, and my gorgeous and precious daughters, Jessica and Amy. I love you all.

I also dedicate this book to all my respected colleagues, who have advised me and supported me.

Disclaimer Notice

The author wishes to express his thanks to you for purchasing this book. He hopes it helps in your clinical practice. This book is for guidance only, and the reader must take into consideration all aspects of the child's subjective history, followed by a thorough objective examination. Diagnosis should be confirmed using the appropriate scans where necessary to confirm diagnosis. If in any doubt, the reader should ask for a second opinion and should use further investigations where appropriate. Where possible, evidence-based research has been used to support the literature; however, because of the ever-changing world of research, the reader does need to consider this and further read the more up-to-date clinical research where necessary. Care has been taken to confirm accuracy of literature, but the author, editors, and publishers are not responsible for any human errors or omissions that may appear in this publication. All authors are experts in their fields, but their views remain personal and do not reflect on their current or past employers, or title or place of work.

Contributing Authors

Alexandra Chaplin, BSc (Hons), MSc
Senior Sports Rehabilitation Therapist
Specialist interest in children and adolescent sport
Anatomie Healthcare Clinic(s), London, United Kingdom

Richard Collinge MSc BSc MCSP SRP
Head of Performance, Cardiff City Football Club, United Kingdom
Senior Clinical Fellow, School of Emergency Medicine, Physiotherapy Department,
University of Hertfordshire, United Kingdom

Richard Goddard MSc, BSc, MCSP, SRP, AACP, ANUTR
MSc Human Nutrition and Public Health with Sports BSc Physiotherapy Register
of Exercise Professionals: Level 4 specialist exercise instructor
Arsenal Academy Football Club Physiotherapist, London, United Kingdom

Adam Kerr MSc, BSc (Hons), ASCC
MSc Sport Science (Strength and Conditioning)
BSc (Hons) Sport and Exercise Science
ASCC (Accredited Strength and Conditioning Coach
Arsenal Academy Football Club Sport Scientist, London, United Kingdom

Mr Robert S. Lee, BSc, MBBS, FRCS (Tr & Orth)
Consultant Orthopaedic and Spinal Surgeon
Royal National Orthopaedic Hospital, Brockley Hill, Stanmore, Middlesex, HA5
4LP, United Kingdom

Nelson Lopes, BSc (Hons), MCSP, SRP
Senior Physiotherapist
Specialist interest in children and adolescents
FirstPoint Health, Bushey, Herts, United Kingdom

Daniel Manzi BSc, MSc (PRM)
Sports Psychologist
Specialist interest in children and adolescent sport
London, United Kingdom

Stephanie Morgan, BSc (Hons)
Sports Rehabilitation Therapist
Specialist interest in children and adolescent sport
Anatomie Healthcare Clinic(s), London, United Kingdom

Georgia Parry, BSc (Hons)
Sports Therapist
Specialist interest in children and adolescent sport
Anatomie Healthcare Clinic(s), London, United Kingdom

Christian Schafer, BSc (Hons) Podiatry, MChS, LA (Cert) (local anaesthesia)
Musculoskeletal Podiatrist Lead, Alexandra Avenue Health and Social Care Clinic
Harrow Community Health Service
Ealing Hospital NHS Trust
Musculoskeletal Podiatrist, NHS Camden Physiotherapy Service, London, United Kingdom

Dr Richard Seah MBBS, MSc, MAcadMEd, MFMLM, MRCGP, FFSEM, DSEM, DCH
Consultant in Sport & Exercise Medicine
English Institute of Sport & Pure Sports Medicine, London, United Kingdom

Dr Jane Simmonds, PD, MS, PGDip Man Ther, PGCHE, BApp (Sc), BPE
Principal Lecturer, Programme Leader MSc Sport and Exercise Rehabilitation
University of Hertfordshire
Hatfield, Herts, United Kingdom

Faye Triggs, BSc (Hons)
Sports and Dance Therapist
Specialist interest in children and adolescent sport
Anatomie Healthcare Clinic(s), London, United Kingdom

Acknowledgements

I am grateful to Malcolm Hoppen and the staff of Anatomie Physiotherapy for the use of their sports medicine clinic(s); to Isobel Kilbey for her medical illustrations; to Andrew Caine, Georgia Parry, Dominic Sumpter, Triston Manzi, and Saskia Manzi for helping with the photographs; and also to all the contributing authors for their time, experience, and knowledge.

Preface

Solomon Abrahams

The number of children and young adolescents participating in sports is now increasing, even more so with the onset of early obesity (Carty, 1998). Similarly, sporting children are beginning sport at a much earlier age as they are encouraged to do so to become aspiring elite athletes (Raissaki, Apostolaki, & Karantanas, 2007).

Consequently, sports injuries in this young age group are also becoming more prevelant, not only due to the increasing incidence of youngsters participating in sport, but also because of the intensity, duration, and frequency of training which has also increased, especially at an elite level (Shanmugam & Maffuli, 2008).

In the United Kingdom (UK), 79% of children and young adolescents participate in some organised sport, sometimes at an elite level (Shanmugam & Maffuli, 2008. Similarly, in the United States (US), a total of 35 million children partake in organised sport (Soprano & Fuch, 2007), and some 2.7 million of them per annum have some type of sporting injury serious enough to visit the emergency room (Soprano & Fuch, 2007).

Some sports have a higher incidence of injuries such as rugby, football, wrestling, gymnastics, hockey, basketball, volleyball, baseball, American football, martial arts, and dancing (Micheli & Klein, 1991; Shanmugam & Maffuli, 2008).

In general, research suggests that the incidence of sports injuries also increases with the age of the child. The young adolescents, going through growth spurts, remain the most vulnerable (Shanmugum & Maffuli, 2008; Soprano & Fuch, 2007).

Thankfully, serious catastrophic injury remains rare in children and adolescents. However, sudden death, head trauma, and spinal cord injuries remain a potential risk in sport (Carty, 1998) and are discussed in this text.

The growing child is in constant evolution and continuously adapts from the moment they are born. With open growth plates, poor thermostatic control, explosive hormones, a thin body wall, fluctuating growing pains, tendons being pulled away from bones, an immature and rubbery skeleton vulnerable to fractures, precious developing trunk organs, and a fluctuating mental and emotional mind they remain a challenge to the sports medicine physician.

This text is designed to help provide sports medicine doctors, musculoskeletal clinicians, physiotherapists, sports therapists, osteopaths, rehabilitation therapists, and other respected colleagues with a simple guide to sports injuries in children and adolescents.

Injuries in children and adolescents tend to be unique due to the ever-changing physiology of the growing child and the psychology they normally present with. Understanding the anatomy, physiology, and pathophysiology of the child will hopefully give us every opportunity of identifying and managing their injuries better.

Simple orthopaedic testing, investigations and management of these injuries are discussed, with the help of evidence-based research. Prognosis and prevention of these injuries are paramount to ensure that the injuries do not cause any long-term disabilities.

References

Carty, H. (1998). Children's sports injuries. *European Journal of Radiology, 26*, 163–176.

Micheli, L., & Klein, J. (1991). Sports injuries in children and adolescents. *British Journal of Sports Medicine, 25*, 1.

Raissaki, M., Apostolaki, E., & Karantanas, H. (2007). Imaging of sports injuries in children. *European Journal of Radiology, 86*, 96.

Shanmugam, C., & Maffuli, N. (2008). Sports injuries in children. *British Medical Bulletin, 86*, 33–57.

Soprano, J., & Fuch, S. (2007). Common overuse injuries in the pediatric and adolescent athlete. *Clinical Pediatric Emergency Medicine, 21*, 5, 7–15.

Chapter 1

The Physiology of the Growing Child

Solomon Abrahams

Puberty and Sexual Maturation

Overview of the Growing Child Aged 6–12

Most children in this age group grow at a steady rate. Most of their bones, ligaments, muscles, cartilage, and nerves are fully formed and are predominantly functional, even though they continue to grow in strength and continually adapt to the environment (Patel, Greyanis, & Baker, 2009). The body at this age is continuously adapting.

Studies have shown (Stanitski, DeLee, & Drez, 1994) that most children in this age group should have a normal walking gait and a normal running gait despite having inferior coordination to adults. Studies have also shown that children in this age group who exercise and play some sport on a regular basis gain functional muscular strength, even though we suspect that this is due to neuromuscular adaptation rather than hypertrophy of muscle (Patel et al., 2009). Contrary to popular belief, regular training does not affect the height of the child and can result in an increase in aerobic capacity, even at this young age.

Children of this age group have enormous learning abilities. They seem to soak up knowledge and become very observant. They normally gain between 3 and 4 kg per annum and their height invariably increases at an average of 3 inches per annum. The child may have growth spurts also, even at this very young age, which can last from weeks to months (Boissonnault, 2012).

At the start of puberty, around the age of 10 in some, calorific intake increases and varies for both boys and girls. Typically, a boy's intake can be as much as 1800 calories per day, and up to 1600 calories for girls (Gidding, Dennison, & Birch, 2006).

Higher bone density and low percentage of body fat is seen more in males than females at this age. Lean body mass, which includes the essential lipid-rich stores seen in the bone marrow, brain, spinal cord, and internal organs, increases from 25 kg at 10 years to 42 kg in 16-year-olds for girls. Muscle mass in most boys increases from 12 kg at 9 years to 23 kg at 15 years. Girls also attain 2/3 of this lean body mass compared with boys during this age (MacGregor, 2001).

Vision is normally 20/20 at the age 7, and physical strength, coordination, sensitivity, and learning ability continuously increase (Neumann, 2002).

Boys and girls at this age are quite similar compared with boys and girls at the onset of puberty and during adolescence (Birrer, Greisemer, & Cataletto, 2002).

It is not until the age of 12, when physical strength diverges between boys and girls; it is mainly related to hormonal changes at this age. Also at this age, boys tend to become stronger than the girls, more so in endurance, speed, and agility. Girls begin to surpass boys at this age in flexibility and coordination. Gender differences certainly become more noticeable (Campbell, 2006).

Overview of the Growing Child 12–20 years

Between the age of 12 and 20 years, fundamental changes occur between boys and girls. Body size, body shape, physiology, social and psychological changes mainly occur. Except for the first year of life, this age group exhibits fast and exponential growth from childhood to adulthood. This can be uniform, but is more likely to be in the form of growth spurts. Most spurts vary from weeks to months. Aggressive spurts can cause aches and pains, specific pains at growth plates and significant emotional changes occur. This will be discussed later.

Studies have shown that adolescents at this age who exercise and play some sport on a regular basis gain functional muscular strength, causing significant hypertrophy of muscle (Patel et al., 2009).

Regular training at this age also can improve aerobic and anaerobic performance. Aerobic performance seems to be better in girls rather than in boys, but the adolescent male tends to be quicker and more aerobic (Birrer et al., 2002).

Sleep normally varies between 8 and 9.5 hours, but can be more during an active growth spurt (National Sleep Foundation, 2010).

Calorific intake also increases here compared with childhood years as discussed earlier. Cognitive development progresses to a more formal operational thinking, and decision making, morales, and academic learning become more obvious. Hormonal changes at this age also have a profound effect socially and emotionally. This can be a very turbulent time, as they try and identify themselves more.

During this age of fundamental change, girls – under the influence of oestrogen – acquire more body fat, particularly around the pelvis and shoulders, whereas boys – under the influence of testosterone – accumulate more muscle mass (MacGregor, 2001). The girls have higher amounts of essential body fat because of the tissue laid down in the breast and other sex-specific tissues. The absolute storage of fat in girls is actually equal to that in males, but because girls are normally lighter than boys, the relative storage is greater (MacGregor, 2001).

References

Birrer, R., Greisemer, B., & Cataletto, M. (2002). *Pediatric sports medicine for primary care* (2nd ed.). Philadelphia, PA: Lippincott Williams & Wilkins.

Boissonnault, W. (2012). *Primary care for the physical therapist* (2nd ed.). St. Louis, MO: Elsevier-Saunders.

Campbell, S. K. (2006). *Physical therapy for children* (3rd ed.). Philadelphia, PA: Saunders-Elsevier.

Gidding, S., Dennison, B., & Birch, L. (2006). Dietry recommendations for children and adolescents, a guide for practitioners. *American Academy of Pediatrics, 117,* 544–559.

MacGregor, J. (2001). *Anatomy and physiology of children* (2nd ed.). London: Routledge.

National Sleep Foundation (2010). Children and adolescent sleep patterns, National Sleep Foundation Website, WB&A.

Neumann, D. (2002). *Kinesiology of the musculoskeletal system: Foundations for physical rehabilitation pediatrics.* St. Louis, MO: Mosby.

Patel, D., Greyanis, D., & Baker, R. (2009). *Pediatric sports medicine* (3rd ed.). New York, NY: McGraw Hill Medical.

Stanitski, C., DeLee, J., & Drez, D. (1994). *Pediatric and adolescent sports medicine* (3rd ed.). Philadelphia, PA: W. B. Saunders.

Bone Growth in 6–18-Year-Olds

Anatomy and Physiology of Bone

Bone is a connective tissue made up of osteogenic cells (Bayliss, Mahoney, & Monk, 2012) and minerals such as calcium and phosphate (Bonjour, Gueguen, Palacios, Shearer, & Weaver, 2009).

There are different types of bones in the human skeletal system such as long bones, short bones, flat bones, irregular bones, and sesamoid bones (Khurana, 2009), with the structures of each varying depending on their function. The anatomy of bones includes the epiphysis, physis, diaphysis, metaphysis, periosteum, and bone marrow.

The epiphysis is the end of a tubular bone, and it contains spongy bone inside a thin layer of dense bone (Khurana, 2009). The physis is also known as the growth plate, and is composed of cartilage, bone, and fibrous components (Calmar & Vinci, 2002). It is only in children and adolescents, that the sizeand shape of bones are not fully established (Khurana, 2009). The diaphysis is the shaft of the bone (Khurana, 2009). The metaphysis is the funnel-shaped end of a long bone (Calmar & Vinci, 2002) occupying the area between the diaphysis and the physis or epiphysis (Khurana, 2009).

The periosteum is a thick fibrous membrane that covers the entire outer surface of all bones and is made up of two layers (Calmar & Vinci, 2002). The outer layer is a fibrous connective tissue containing fibroblasts, nerves, and blood vessels; the inner layer is an osteoprogenitor layer, which is capable of forming new bone (Khurana, 2009). Damage to this outer part of bone is normally very sore and sensitive in children.

Modelling of the Child's Bone

The production of bone, also known as bone modelling, is the process through which bone is formed by osteoblasts without prior bone resorption (Bilezikian, Raisz, & Martin, 2008). During growth, this process is vigorous and it produces a change in the bone shape and size. The change in shape may also be adapted according to physiological influences or mechanical forces placed on them (Clarke, 2008).

Wolff's law states that 'over time, the mechanical load applied to living bone influences the structure of bone tissue' (Ruff, Holt, & Trinkaus, 2006), which simply implies that a continual load across a bone would result in the bone becoming stronger and consequently more resistant to that load (Bayliss et al., 2012). This is essential in children and adolescents where their natural surroundings and the way they carry out activities can influence bone density and strength.

Weight-bearing activities in children promote healthy bone growth (injured and non-injured), but current research does suggest that these need to be weight-bearing or indeed functional (MacGregor, 2001).

Each bone constantly undergoes remodelling during life to help it adapt to changing biomechanical forces as well as remove old and micro-damaged bone and replace it with new mechanically stronger bone (Clarke, 2008).

Growth plate

The growth plate plays an important role in the growth of bones in children and adolescents. The growth plate is divided into three anatomic components: a cartilaginous component with specific histologic zones; a bony component, or metaphysis; and a fibrous component that surrounds the periphery of the plate (Calmar & Vinci, 2002). The histologic zones of the cartilage are divided into three parts, the reserve zone, the proliferative zone, and the hypertrophic zone (Calmar & Vinci, 2002; Karimian, Chagin, & Savendahl, 2011). New bone is formed longitudinally on the metaphyseal side of each growth plate (Calmar & Vinci, 2002), and this growth is driven by chondrocytes in the proliferating and hypertrophic zones of the growth plate (Rauch, 2012).

This type of growth is called endochondral ossification where cartilaginous tissue is synthesised into bone (Villemure & Stokes, 2009). Growth plates are present only during the growth period and vanish when sexual maturation is complete (Karimian et al., 2011), typically seen in late teens to early twenties. These plates are common fracture and injury sites and should always be examined in the presence of pain.

Growth plates during puberty are normally at their weakest and most vulnerable during growth periods. Some authors suggest that ligaments and tendons are stronger than the growth plates themselves during spurts of growth, hence the commonality of non-traumatic epiphyseal fractures (Shanmugam & Maffulli, 2008). During the early development of bone fusion in children and early adolescents, it has been shown that the ligaments and capsules can be up to 5 times stronger than the boney growth plate itself (Stanitski, 1994).

The growth plates remain the weakest link in the musculoskeletal system in children (Birrer, 2002).

Severe growth plate disturbances should be treated with urgency, as this can affect long-term disabilities (Caine, Difiori, & Maffulli, 2006), such as premature or early osteoarthritis in later age (Micheli & Klein, 1991).

Early Childhood 6–12 Years

The skeleton of a newborn contains 350 bones that gradually fuse together to form 206 bones in the adult skeleton (Salter, 1999).

Some authors suggest that the growth process of bones is influenced by hormones; however some suggest that the sequencing and timing of growth is influenced by genes. Furthermore, this can vary in different ethnic groups; for example, compared with other ethnic groups, Afro-black children grow faster in the first few years of life, and their bone density is higher at all ages, even though males and females show different tissue growth at puberty. Similarly, their lower limbs develop faster so they tend to be longer, and their functionality develops much quicker at this age (MacGregor, 2001).

Before the onset of growth spurts in adolescents, the skeleton in both sexes is much the same (Sharp, 2012).

In general, however, during the ages 6–12 years, the lower limbs are 15% of the total body weight compared with 30% seen in an adult and bone growth in females tends to be 2 years ahead of males, but carpal bones are not normally seen in either sex until the age 2 (MacGregor, 2001).

Spinal development starts early and the primary kyphotic curves are normally in place at birth. The lordotic curves develop in the first few years as the child becomes more upright and weight-bearing. Influences on posture here can make a difference to posture later on in life due to the elasticity and pliability of the spine. It is, therefore, essential that children adopt good posture from an early age, and not just through adolescence (Salter, 1999). Failure to do this can lead to postural and spinal abnormalities such as acquired scoliosis in later life.

Most of the spinal and discogenic joints go through a fusion process from the age of 7 and accelerate through adolescent age up to late teens/early twenties. The thorax and rib cage shape tend to be fully developed by the age 6, and hence the presence of a barrel-shaped chest is abnormal and can be associated with respiratory diseases such as childhood asthma (Goodman & Fuller, 2009).

During early childhood, typically between 6 and 12 years, the skeleton is fairly elastic and rubbery (Calmar & Vinci, 2002), where bone is significantly less dense, more porous, and is penetrated throughout by capillary channels. Therefore, in comparison to adult bone, paediatric bone has a lower modulus of elasticity, lower bending strength, and a lower mineral content (Calmar & Vinci, 2002). This makes them more vulnerable to fractures, particularly traumatic epiphyseal injuries. This is supported by studies by Mathew, Ramamohan, and Bennet (1998), who reviewed paediatric fractures in 88 children under the age of 14. They found that 91% of the children exhibited no bruising and concluded that external pressure was, therefore, minimal to cause the fracture in the first place, revealing bone fragility at this age.

In this age group, many factors can influence bone density. These include the amount of weight-bearing activities they do, the intensity of weight-bearing activities, various functional activities, early onset of hormones, and muscular development. It was found in a study of 9- and 10-year-olds, over a 10-month period, that lean body mass was significantly increased in shoulder and knee, and grip strength also increased after just three workout sessions per week and thirty minutes per session (Morris, Naughton, Gibbs, Carlson, & Waik, 1997).

In this age group, low-intensity exercises have also been shown to improve bone growth, whereas high-intensity exercises have been shown to inhibit bone growth (Shanmugam & Maffulli, 2008).

Incredibly, children's bones tend to heal more quickly than adult bones when damaged (Shanmugam & Maffulli, 2008). This can in the lower limb range between 4 and 6 weeks and between 2 and 3 weeks in the upper limb. This is simply because the bones are constantly adapting at this age, and moreover, the paediatric skeleton simply has a better blood supply compared with adults; thereby, healing time is reduced (Birrer, 2002).

As calcium is one of the key nutritional minerals essential for healthy bone growth in children, the recommended calcium intake over childhood rises with age. The requirement of calcium in children from ages 1 to 10 ranges from 800 to 1390 mg, whereas in children from ages 11 to 24 years, it ranges from 1200 to 1500 mg daily (Gallo, 1996).

Puberty

A large increase in bone mass occurs during childhood and accelerates greatly in puberty via endochondral bone formation (Gafni & Baron, 2007). Puberty has an essential role in the attainment of bone mass. Between the onset of puberty and young adulthood, skeletal mass approximately doubles (Saggese, Baroncelli, & Bertelloni, 2002).

Longitudinal studies of changes in bone mass during growth have confirmed that in girls, the greatest increases in bone mass occur between the ages of 12 and15 years, compared with 14–17 years in boys. Although the rate of change in bone mass slows dramatically between the ages of 16 and 18 years in females and between 17 and 20 years in males, uncertainty remains about the age at which accumulation of new bone stops and peak bone mass is attained (Davies, Evans, & Gregory, 2005).

As the skeleton matures through this period, bones are normally of the correct length and proportions and there is symmetry between the two sides of the body (Villemure & Stokes, 2009), but this can be affected by external factors such as severe trauma and posture.

Boys tend to have wider clavicles, wider shoulders, and straighter arms associated with muscle mass, explaining increased upper body strength. Girls tend to have wider pelvic bones at this age and retain more body fat (Sharp, 2012).

Some authors suggest that gender differences can also affect bone strength during this period, where ultimately, injuries in males can be double compared with injuries in females (Shanmugam & Maffulli, 2008). It still remains unclear from the available research whether this is related to the physiology of bone or the type of sporting demands of boys compared with girls.

Similarly, the spine and discogenic joints go through a fusion process from childhood, and this accelerates through adolescence up to the early twenties. However, given this natural development of accelerated growth during this unique period, adolescents become more susceptible to tumours. This can occur in long bones such as the femur or in spinal bones where continued unrelenting pain in this age group not consistent with mechanical signs and symptoms should be further investigated (Patel et al., 2009).

Other potential growth disturbances in this age group also include epiphyseal plate fractures and traction apohysitis injuries, which will be discussed later.

Eighteen-year-olds and peak bone mass

Late adolescence is critical for bone health development, which sets a basis for the rest of their adult life (Gordon, Bachrach, Carpenter, Karsenty, & Rauch, 2004). As discussed, in the first two decades of life, bone grows in both length and width, and bone mass grows steadily over childhood and more rapidly during adolescence, when peak bone mass is achieved (McDevitt & Ahmed, 2010).

Peak bone mass is defined as the maximum amount of bone mineral accumulated within the bone during childhood and adolescence (Davies et al., 2005). At peak bone mass, the amount of osteoclasts resorbing bone is exactly the same as osteoblasts forming bone (Davies et al., 2005).

Bone mass predominantly peaks at about the age of 18 years (Bonjour et al., 2009). Peak bone mass can be affected by several factors, which can stem from childhood. These can include the amount of stress on bones during their development, nutritional insufficiency, hormone onset, and, as some authors suggest, genetic factors, which happen to coincide with performance and intensity of exercise (MacGregor, 2001).

Hormones and bone growth

Childhood longitudinal bone growth is normally regulated by a number of key hormones including growth hormone, insulin-like growth factor-I (IGF-1), glucocorticoids, and thyroid hormone. During sexual maturation, sex steroids (androgens and estrogens), which are normally secreted by the body during adolescence, also contribute to this process (Karimian et al., 2011).

Growth hormone is important in the regulation of both bone formation and bone resorption (Giustina, Mazziotti, & Canalis, 2008). Other factors affecting body growth and peak mass are genetics, gender, race, dietary intake, endocrine factors, and other mechanical forces (Rizzoli et al., 2007; Villemure & Stokes, 2009; Zhu & Prince, 2012). This will be discussed in further detail later.

References

Bayliss, L., Mahoney, D. J., & Monk, P. (2012). Normal bone physiology, remodelling and its hormonal regulation. *Surgery (Oxford), 30*(2), 47–53.

Bilezikian, J. P., Raisz, L. G., & Martin, T. J. (2008). *Principles of bone biology* (Vol. 1, 3rd ed., p. 5). UK: Elsevier.

Birrer, R., Griesemer, B., & Cataletto, M. B. (2002). *Pediatric sports medicine in primary care* (2nd ed.). Philadelphia, PA: Lippincott Williams & Wilkins.

Bonjour, J-P., Gueguen, L., Palacios, C., Shearer, M. J., & Weaver, C. M. (2009). Minerals and vitamins in bone health: the potential value of dietary enhancement. *British Journal of Nutrition, 101*(11), 1581–1596.

Caine, D., Difiori, J., & Maffulli, N. (2006). Phyeal injuries in children and youth sport. *British Journal of Sports Medicine, 40,* 749.

Calmar, E. A., & Vinci, R. J. (2002). The anatomy and physiology of bone fracture and healing. *Clinical Pediatric Emergency Medicine, 3*(2), 85–93.

Clarke, B. (2008). Normal bone anatomy and physiology. *Clinical Journal of the American Society of Nephrology, 3*(3), S131–S139.

Davies, J. H., Evans, B. A. J., & Gregory, J. W. (2005). Bone mass acquisition in healthy children. *Archives of Disease in Childhood, 90*(4), 373–378.

Gafni, R. I., & Baron, J. (2007). Childhood bone mass acquisition and peak bone mass may not be important determinants of bone mass in late adulthood. *Pediatrics, 119*(2), pp. S131–S136.

Gallo, A. (1996). Building strong bones in childhood and adolescence. *Pediatric Nursing, 22,* 5.

Giustina, A., Mazziotti, G., & Canalis, E. (2008). Growth hormone, insulin-like growth factors, and the skeleton. *Endocrine Reviews, 29*(5), 535–559.

Goodman, C., & Fuller, K. (2009). *Pathology implications to the physical therapist* (3rd ed.). Philadelphia, PA: Saunders-Elsevier.

Gordon, C. M., Bachrach, L. K., Carpenter, T. O., Karsenty, G., & Rauch, F. (2004). Bone health in children and adolescents. *Current Problems in Pediatric and Adolescent Health Care, 34*(6), 226–242.

Karimian, E., Chagin, A. S., & Savendahl, L. (2011). Genetic regulation of the growth plate. *Frontiers in Endocrinology (Lausanne), 2*(113), 1–10.

Khurana, J. S. (2009). *Bone pathology* (2nd ed., pp. 2–3). Totowa, NJ: Humana Press.
MacGregor, J. (2001). *Anatomy and physiology of children* (2nd ed.). London: Routledge.

Mathew, M., Ramamohan, N., & Bennet, C. (1998). The importance of bruising, associated with fractures. *British Medical Journal, 317,* 1117–1118c.

McDevitt, H., & Ahmed, S. F. (2010). Establishing good bone health in children. *Paediatrics and Child Health,* 20(2), 83–87.

Micheli, L., & Klein, J. (1991). Sports injuries in children and adolescents, *British Journal of Sports Medicine, 25,* 1.

Morris, F., Naughton, G., Gibbs, J., Carlson, J., & Waik, J. (1997). Prospective ten-month exercise intervention in premenarcheal girls. *Journal of Bone and Mineral Research, 12,* 1453.

Patel, D., Greydanus, D., & Baker, R. (2009). *Pediatric sports medicine* (2nd ed.). New York, NY: McGraw Hill Medical.

Rauch, F. (2012). The dynamics of bone structure development during pubertal growth. *Journal of Musculoskelet Neuronal Interact, 12*(1), 1–6.

Rizzoli, R., Bonjour, J-P., & Chevalley, T. (2007). Dietary protein intakes and bone growth. *International Congress Series, 1297*(1), 50–59.

Ruff, C., Holt, B., & Trinkaus, E. (2006). Who's afraid of the big bad wolff? *'Wolff's Law' and Bone Functional Adaptation, 129*(4), 484–498.

Saggese, G., Baroncelli, G. I., & Bertelloni, S. (2002). Puberty and bone development. *Best Practice and Research Clinical Endocrinology and Metabolism, 16*(1), 53–64.

Salter (1999). *Textbook of musculoskeletal disorders* (3rd ed.). Baltimore, MD: Williams & Wilkins.

Shanmugam, C., & Maffulli, N. (2008). Sports injuries in children. *British Medical Bulletin, 86,* 33.

Sharp, C. (2012). Some features of the anatomy and exercise physiology of children, *Athletes Weekly, 2,* 1.

Stanitski, C., DeLee, J., & Drez, D. (1994). *Pediatric and adolescent sports medicine* (3rd ed.). London: WB Sounders Company.

Villemure, I., & Stokes, I. A. (2009). Growth plate mechanics and mechanobiology: A survey of present understanding. *Journal of Biomechanics, 42*(12), 1793–1803.

Zhu, K., & Prince, R. L. (2012). Calcium and bone. *Clinical Biochemistry, 45*(12), 936–942.

Muscle Growth in 5–18-Year-Olds

Introduction

During childhood and adolescence, the body is always growing and the changes that happen to the muscular system can affect the body greatly.

Early Childhood (6–12 years)

It all begins when the embryo develops in the womb, where muscle tissue is first developed. Mesoderm cells known as myoblasts develop muscle cells, and when several myoblasts fuse together, they form a muscle fibre. Cardiac and smooth muscle fibres can be formed from a single myoblast and display gap junctions due to this.

In the very early years, these cells become more specialised, and within the first year, muscle cells lose the ability to divide any further but are able to undergo hypertrophy and get bigger, especially in smooth muscle.

Muscular development in early childhood is mainly responsible for the increase in body weight during the early years. Typically, girls can gain 33.5 kg between the ages 7 and 18 years, which is essentially muscle mass and fat mass (Birrer, Greisemer, & Cataletto, 2002). Typically, boys can gain 43.8 kg between the ages 7 and 18 years, which composes of increased skeletal tissue and muscle mass, but, unlike in girls, fat tends to remain stable (Richard, Greisemer, & Cataletto, 2002).

As with bones, and compared with adults, children have an increased ability to repair and regenerate muscle cells more quickly when damaged. This is simply because the muscles are constantly adapting at this age, and moreover, the paediatric skeleton has a better blood supply compared with adults and consequently healing time is reduced (Birrer et al., 2002).

Interestingly, research suggests motor units are not able to be fully utilised until the age of 7. Before this age, this results in a decreased dimensionally normalised maximal torque. This simply means that any strength work before this age may not develop individual muscle strength to the same extent as that seen in an adolescent or in an adult (Xu, Nicholson, Wang, Alen, & Cheng, 2009).

It is not until later on in childhood that muscular development and strength accelerates, mainly under hormonal influences such as sex hormones like testosterone. However, it has been known for some time that very young children do possess muscle fibre numbers, types, and distribution ratios similar to those of adults (Stanitski, 1994).

This has been reinforced by Belanger and McComas (1989), who demonstrated that 6-year-old boys have histochemical and neurophysiology properties of fibre formation similar to 20-year-olds.

Muscle contraction can also be affected by age where normally children under the age of 10 have shorter contraction periods and half the relaxation times, which could explain why they are more susceptible to fatigue.

There is also evidence to suggest that twitch tensions increase steadily with age before a drastic increase when puberty is reached (Belanger & McComas, 1989).

However, some authors disagree, suggesting that very little evidence exists to show that distribution of fibre type and twitch tensions can change, even as a result of physical training in children or adolescents (Richard et al., 2002).

Even though gross muscle development is seen uniformly in children until pre-puberty, gains in strength have been reported to be significant in some studies, ranging from 30% to 50% according to the American Academy of Paediatrics.

Similarly, numerous studies have revealed significant functional improvements in vertical jump, sprint speed, long jump, agility time, isolated strength, and motor skills in this age group (Falk et al., 2009, Xu et al., 2009). This is further supported by other authors who suggest that in children, regular endurance training has the potential to modify the activities of oxidative enzymes whereas sprint training has the potential to modify glycolytic enzymes at a cellular level.

However, one area which does seem to be inferior is anaerobic power production in children compared with adults. The primary reason for this is a limitation in the activity of enzyme phosphofructokinase (PFK).

Apart from enzyme activity changes, gains can also be attributed to an increase in 'neuromuscular learning' and an increase in number of motor neurons firing per contraction, which explains why it can be achieved in low pre-androgen levels. Strength, therefore, in children can be attributed to neuromuscular learning or 'neural drive' with males normally showing advanced gender difference. The number of muscle fibres we are born with does not change – this remains genetic – but the size of the fibres can hypertrophy.

This is further supported by Falk et al. (2009), who highlight that high repetition training (low weights) can provide better opportunity for neuromuscluar learning through increase in adaptation of motor firing, discharge frequency, and motor unit recruitment as opposed to training with high weights and low repetitions in adults.

It was also found in a study of 9- and 10-year-olds, over a 10-month period, that lean body mass was significantly increased in shoulder and knee, and grip strength as well as bone mineral density increased after just 3 workout sessions per week at 30 minutes per session (Morris, Naughton, Gibbs, Carlson, & Waik, 1997). This has been attributed to the enzymal influences, neural drive, or both (MacGregor, 2001).

Generally, small repetitive loads actually strengthen the muscle cells, making them more resilient to further damage. However, repetitve heavy loads, where the cells do not have time to adapt, are more likely to fail (Birrer et al., 2002).

In pre-pubertal children, there was no sex difference in adjusted bone and muscle variables. There was a slight decrease in both muscle size and bone strength in girls as compared with boys, particularly in the 9–11 years age group (Högler et al., 2008). Similarly, a study involving children using submaximal contraction of various muscle groups (calf muscles and quads) found boys to be significantly stronger compared with their female counterparts (Belanger & McComas, 1989) in this age group.

However, not all authors agree. Leonard et al. (2010) found that there were no race or sex differences in the muscle strength identified in their study. This is further supported by (Shanmugam & Maffulli, 2008), who suggest that there is no difference in muscle mass between females and males pre-puberty.

Puberty and Adolescence

Muscle growth is more apparent during adolescence as the development of muscles is influenced by growth hormones, adrenal androgens, and also by testosterone in males. This is supported by the fact that full neuromuscular control of the muscle peaks during middle adolescence (Marieb & Hoehn, 2010).

Muscle mass increases steadily in males up to 10/11 years; then it spurts through teenage years and then dramatically increases thereafter until the age of 20. Type 2 fibres (fast twitch and sprint fibres) start to develop more functionally at 12–13 years of age (Patel et al., 2009).

Contraction time here is also significantly faster compared with pre-puberty (Belanger & McComas, 1989).

Also at this age, gender differences become more noticeable. It is here that adolescent males become physically stronger than females. This is further supported by Neu, Rauch, Rittweger, Manz, and Schoenau (2001), who found that isometric grip strength of the forearm in adolescents was specific to gender in puberty. They suggest that this is due to hormonal changes in the body. More specifically, girls at the age of 14 rarely develop their motor developmental skills and fine motor control any further whilst boys continue to develop throughout adolescence (Patel, Greydanus, & Baker, 2009).

However, this remains debateable. Some studies have suggested there is little difference in force generating capacity, fatigability, and twitch contraction speed between boys and girls during adolescence (Belanger & McComas, 1989).

Boys tend to have broader muscle mass in their arms and chest area giving them more upper body strength compared with girls (Sharp, 2012). Girls tend to retain more body fat around the pelvis and other areas of the body giving them increased body mass relative to surface area. These broader hips have been attributed to tightening the muscles that attach from the pelvis down to the knee, giving girls an increased likelihood of developing knee problems (Sharp, 2012).

Boys that tend to mature early are more likely to be taller and have greater muscle mass and strength. Their explosive power and grip strength as examples are more superior compared with late maturers (Patel et al., 2009).

Flexibility of the muscles tends to be poor in this age group. A number of studies indicate that children become less flexible as they age, reaching minimal levels between 10 and 12 years, then improving again during early adulthood (Stanitski, Delee, & Drez, 1994). Girls appear to be more flexible than boys, which tends to be sustained through adulthood. Flexibility in boys specifically decreases from mid-childhood to mid-adolescence (Patel et al., 2009).

Flexibility is particularly affected in hamstrings and lower leg muscles, which is consistent with lower limb growth during this period (Patel et al., 2009).

Some authors suggest that regular stretching can prevent the muscles from becoming too tight during these periods, and hence prevent them from becoming injured. However, recent published research indicates that stretching may not reduce the risk and incident of injury (Shrier, 2000).

It is also at this age, where the adolescent skeleton (bones) outgrows the muscles, which means that the muscular system struggles somewhat to keep its tension and length from the sudden growth spurt seen in the bones. This is seen more so in males than in females. This simply means that some adolescents have very tight muscles at this time, which can predispose them to injury. The muscles and tendons become so strong at this stage that they become stronger than the epiphyseal plate itself (Shanmugam & Maffulli, 2008), such as seen in Osgood–Schlatter disease (OSD).

In OSD, multiple small avulsion fractures occur within the apophysis during adolescence and is a self-limiting disorder. These occur due to the patella tendon and its traction on the tibial tuberosity. Usually it occurs during growth spurts and is commonly found in adolescents that actively take part in running or jumping activities (Gerbino, 2006; Gholve, Scher, Khakharia, Widmann, & Green, 2007).

Hormonal Effect

Growth hormone (GH) stimulates the majority of body cells (including muscle cells) to increase in size and divide (Marieb & Hoehn, 2010) and affects growth factors, particularly during puberty, although it is secreted all the way through life (BBC Health, 2012). GH has a large role to play in gaining lean body mass (LBM) (Hulthen et al., 2001).

GH promotes protein synthesis, but the effects are mediated by IGF-1 (Marieb & Hoehn, 2010). IGF-1 affects the muscle mass by gaining 20-fold during puberty (Serratrice, 2009). However, Mauras, Bishop, and Welch (2007) found that larger and stronger muscles in boys were because of additive effects of androgenic hormones and a greater sensitivity to GH and IGF-1.

Androgens are typically steroid hormones and are found predominantly in boys. They promote type 2A fibres of the muscle and prevent muscular atrophy during immobilisation. Androgen provides a proximate, not exclusive, stimulus in muscle growth and is increased during puberty (Hulthen et al., 2001) and has also been found to increase muscle weight independently from systematic or local IGF-1 production (Venken et al., 2007). However, GH receptor signalling and androgens both play a vital role in periosteal growth during puberty (Venken et al., 2007).

Testosterone, a type of androgen, is found in higher amounts in males than in girls. Influence of this hormone has a significant increase in muscle mass and bone growth and reduction in adipose fat (Rogol, Roemmich, & Clark, 2002; Schoenau, Neu, Mokov, Wassmer, & Manz, 2000). However, Gokhale and Kirschner (2003) found that LBM increases at a steady rate for both genders until 12–13 years of age. Afterwards, girls carry on with LBM increase until they are 15 years old and boys carry it on late into adolescence, almost twice as long as girls. Furthermore, Arsianian and Suprasongsin (1997) found that testosterone supplementation in late-pubertal boys increased the amount of fat-free muscle (FFM) and fat oxidation whilst decreasing the amount of fat muscle (FM) and leptin.

Conclusion

The human body grows all the way through childhood. However, during puberty, there is a substantial alteration in the structure and force produced by the muscles in the body. These changes can be due to androgens – the sex hormones oestrogen and testosterone specifically – and GH. IGF-1 works as the mediator of the GH and increases the size and rate of division of cells in the muscles.

In conclusion, a lot of factors affect the muscular system throughout childhood and puberty, but hormones have a massive part to play on the structure and composition of the body in males and females.

References

Arsianian, S., & Suprasongsin, C. (1997). Testosterone treatment in adolescents with delayed puberty: Changes in body composition, protein, fat, and glucose metabolism. *Journal of Clinical Endocrinology & Metabolism* [online]. Retrieved from http://jcem. endojournals.org/content/82/10/3213 [accessed on 13/11/12].

BBC Health (2012). *Human Growth Hormone* [online]. Retrieved from http://www.bbc.co.uk/ health/physical_health/conditions/human_growth_hormone.shtml [accessed on 13/11/12].

Belanger, A., & McComas, A. (1989). Contractile properties of human skeletal muscle in childhood. *European Journal of applied Physiology, 58,* 563–567.

Birrer, R., Greisemer, B., & Cataletto, M. (2002). *Pediatric sports medicine for primary care* (2nd ed.). Philadelphia, PA: Lippincott Williams & Wilkins.

Falk, B., Usselman, C., Dotan, R., Brunton, L., Klentrou, P., Shaw, J., & Gabriel, D. (2009). Child–adult differences in muscle strength and activation pattern during isometric elbow flexion and extension. *Applied Physiology, Nutrition and Metabolism* [online] *34*(4), 609–615.

Gerbino, P. G. (2006). Adolescent anterior knee pain. *Operative Techniques in Sports Medicine 14*(3), 203–211.

Gholve, P. A., Scher, D. M., Khakharia, S., Widmann, R. F., & Green, D. W. (2007). Osgood–Schlatter syndrome. *Current Opinion in Paediatrics* [online]. Retrieved from http://www.ncbi. nlm.nih.gov/pubmed/17224661 [accessed on 18/11/12].

Gokhale, R., & Kirschner, B. S. (2003). Assessment of growth and nutrition. *Best Practice & Research Clinical Gastroenterology* [online]. Retrieved from http://www.sciencedirect.com/ science/article/pii/S1521691802001439 [accessed on 13/11/12].

Högler, W., Blimkie, C. J. R., Cowell, C. T., Inglis, D., Rauch, F., Kemp, A. F., Wiebe, P., Duncan, C. S., Farpour-Lambert, N., & Woodhead, H. J. (2008). Sex-specific developmental changes in muscle size and bone geometry at the femoral shaft. *Bone* [online] *42*(5), 982–989. Retrieved from http:// www.sciencedirect.com/science/article/pii/S8756328208000148 [accessed on 18/11/12].

Hulthen, L., Bengtsson, B. A., Sunnerhagen, K. S., Hallberg, L., Grimby, G., & Johannsson, G. (2001). GH is needed for the maturation of muscle mass and strength in adolescents. *Journal of Clinical Endocrinology & Metabolism* [online] *86*(10), 4765–4770. Retrieved from http:// jcem.endojournals.org/content/86/10/4765.short [accessed on 13/11/12].

Leonard, M. B., Elmi, A., Moab, S. M., Shults, J., Burnham, J. M., Thayu, M., Kibe, L., Wetzsteon, J., & Zemel, B. S. (2010). Effects of sex, race, and puberty on cortical bone and the functional muscle bone unit in children, adolescents, and young adults. *Journal of Clinical Endocrinology & Metabolism* [online] *95*(4), 1681–1689. Retrieved from http://jcem.endojournals.org/ content/95/4/1681.short [accessed on 18/11/12].

MacGregor, J. (2001). *Anatomy and physiology of children* (2nd ed.). London: Routledge.

Marieb, E. N., & Hoehn, K. (2010). *Human anatomy & physiology* (8th ed.). San Francisco: Pearson International Edition.

Mauras, N., Bishop, K., & Welch, S. (2007). Growth hormone action in puberty: Effects by gender. *Growth Hormone & IGF Research* [online]. Retrieved from http://www.sciencedirect.com/science/article/pii/S1096637407000664 [accessed on 13/11/12].

Morris, F., Naughton, G., Gibbs, J., Carlson, J., & Waik, J. (1997). Prospective ten-month exercise intervention in premenarcheal girls. *Journal of Bone and Mineral Research, 12,* 1453.

Neu, C. M., Rauch, F., Rittweger, J., Manz, F., & Schoenau, E. (2001). Influence of puberty on muscle development at the forearm. *American Journal of Physiology, Endocrinology and Metabolism* [online] *283*(1), 103–107. Retrieved from http://ajpendo.physiology.org/content/283/1/E103.full#sec-8 [accessed on 18/11/12].

Patel, D., Greydanus, D., & Baker, R. (2009). *Pediatric sports medicine* (2nd ed.). New York, NY: McGraw Hill Medical.

Richard, B., Greisemer, B., & Cataletto, M. (2002). *Pediatric sports medicine for primary care* (2nd ed.). Philadelphia, PA: Lippincott Williams & Wilkins.

Rogol, A. D., Roemmich, J. N., & Clark, P. A. (2002). Growth at puberty. *Journal of Adolescent Health* [online]. Retrieved from http://www.sciencedirect.com/science/article/pii/S1054139X02004858 [accessed on 13/11/12].

Schoenau, E., Neu, C. M., Mokov, E., Wassmer, G., & Manz, F. (2000). Influence of puberty on muscle area and corticol bone area of the forearm in boys and girls. *Journal of Clinical Endocrinology & Metabolism* [online]. Retrieved from http://jcem.endojournals.org/content/85/3/1095.full [accessed on 13/11/12].

Serratrice, G. (2009). Building muscle. *Joint Bone Spine,* 76(4):324-6.

Shanmugam, C., & Maffulli, N. (2008). Sports injuries in children. *British Medical Bulletin, 86,* 33.

Sharp, C. (2012). Some features of the anatomy and exercise physiology of children. *Athletes Weekly, 2,* 1.

Shrier, I. (2000). Stretching before exercise; an evidence-based approach. *British Journal of Sports Medicine, 34,* 324–325.

Stanitski, C., Delee, J., & Drez, D. (1994). *Pediatric and Adolescent Sports Medicine* (3rd ed.). New York: W. B. Saunders.

Venken, K., Moverare-Skrtic, S., Kopchick, J. J., Coschigano, K. T., Ohlsson, C., Boonen, S., Bouillon, R., & Vanderschueren, D. (2007). Impact of androgens, growth hormone, and IGF-1 on bone and muscle in male mice during puberty. *Journal of Bone and Mineral Research* [online]. Retrieved from http://onlinelibrary.wiley.com/doi/10.1359/jbmr.060911/abstract [accessed on 13/11/12].

Xu, L., Nicholson, P., Wang, Q., Alen, M., & Cheng, S. (2009). Bone and muscle development during puberty in girls: A seven-year longitudinal study. *Journal of Bone and Mineral Research* [online] *24*(10), 1693–1698. Retrieved from http://onlinelibrary.wiley.com/doi/10.1359/jbmr.090405/full [accessed on 18/11/12].

Ligaments and Cartilage Growth in 5–18-Year-Olds

In children and adolescents, connective tissue is one of the main types of tissue in the body. It is an abundant tissue coming in various forms (Saladin, 2012). Connective tissues often have a high density of collagen fibres which bind together, giving them high tensile strength which is necessary for connective tissues that support and protect the body/joints from external forces/stressors (Lodish, Berk, Zipursky, et al., 2000).

This is an essential structure for ligaments and cartilage in the growing child.

Early Childhood 6–12 years

Ligaments are a form of dense connective tissue, comprising of closely packed collagen fibres that span to help protect and stabilise a joint (Frank, 2004). The collagen fibres within the ligaments form in the direction of the applied mechanical load (Altman et al., 2002), which further provides high levels of resistance to forces acting upon the ligaments.

From early childhood, as age increases, the stresses applied also increase via changes in body mass/size and often increased levels of activity. These stresses actually help to consolidate the collagen bundles within the ligaments and help configure their alignment structure, which prepares them for future external forces. These ligaments are constantly adapting and remodelling from an early age depending on the activity and changes within the child. Because most children in this age group grow uniformly, injuries to ligaments and joints tend to be less.

In children, cartilage is another form of connective tissue found in abundance. It is a tough but flexible tissue which provides rigidity to supported structures, especially within the joints.

Cartilage is necessary for bone growth because the ends of bones are used in joint movement. Bone growth cannot occur directly at the ends of bones. In children, premature ossification cannot occur due to the constant proliferation of chondrocytes/cartilage within the epiphyseal plates (Vortkamp, Kaechoong, et al., 1996).

Epiphyseal plates only exist in children and adolescents, where bone maturation is not complete. Ossification of cartilage within the epiphyseal plates as well as production of new cartilage causes bone to grow. This causes elongation of bones and may well lead to some instability during childhood and early adolescence due to constant remodelling (Malanga & Ramirez-Del toro, 2008). This essentially is what causes aches and pains (known as growing pains) at some growth plates. This also remains a vulnerable area where fractures can occur in children.

Cartilage development in children is laid down by osteoblasts which, in this age group, has been seen to be stimulated by weight-bearing activities and functional activities, within moderation (MacGregor, 2001).

From 10 to 15 years, growth is more rapid due to increased levels of growth hormones accelerating physical development. Ligament and cartilage density increases as more collagen fibres are produced to deal with the increased demand placed on the musculoskeletal system by the body, due to more dramatic and accelerated increases in stature, weight, and body composition.

Adolescent

In adolescents, growth accelerates more in the limbs than in the trunk. Specifically, the bones grow quicker than the muscles and tendons even though they do adapt after a short period. At this time, this can give rise to high levels of overuse and traction type injuries of the tendons as they become tighter, especially at insertion sites on to the bone (particularly around the pelvis and knee); this is why we tend to see more growth-related injuries here.

Closing of epiphyseal plates prevents further production of cartilage to be ossified thereafter, preventing increase in bone length. Closure of epiphyseal plates occurs in the late or end stage of adolescence and is an indicator of adulthood. Growth from childhood is rapid, but as time goes on, month-to-month gains become less consistent.

As individuals enter adolescence, there is an increase in sex hormones (e.g. testosterone/oestrogen), where these sex hormones accelerate bone deposition and skeletal growth. This acceleration, however, results in closure of the epiphyseal cartilganious plates. Closure of the epiphyseal plates limits further bone growth and hence the physical characteristics that are related to it e.g. height. Oestrogen causes a more rapid acceleration than testosterone, explaining the short periods of growth for females (Martini, 2004). Towards late adolescence, the epiphyseal plates become completely closed (Thibodeau & Pattons, 1993) and cartilage formation is now complete in the adolescent, early adult.

Conclusion

The ligaments and cartilage follow the same stimulus as bones and muscles. The more functional the child, the stronger the ligaments and cartilage become for that specific function, making them highly adaptive.

References

Altman, G. H., Horan, R. L., Martin, I., Farhadi, J., & Stark, P.R. (2002) Cell differentiation by mechanical stress. FASEB J 16:270–272. 26.

Davidson, J., Klagsbrun, M., Hill, K., Buckley, A., Sullivan, R., Brewer, P., & Woodward, S. (1985). Accelerated wound repair, cell proliferation, and collagen accumulation are produced by a cartilage-derived growth factor. *Journal of Cell Biology, 100*(4), 1219–1227.

Frank, C. (2004). Ligament structure, physiology and function. *Journal of Musculoskeletal and Neuronal Interactions, 4*(2), 199–201.

Lodish, H., Berk, A., Zipursky, S. L., et al. (2000). *Collagen: The fibrous proteins of the matrix.* Retrieved from http://www.ncbi.nlm.nih.gov/books/NBK21582/ [accessed on 10/11/2012].

MacGregor, J. (2001). *Anatomy and physiology in children* (2nd ed.). London: Routledge.

Malanga, G., & Ramirez-Del toro (2008). Common Injuries of the foot and ankle in the child and adolescent athlete. *Physical Medicine and Rehabilitation clinics of North America, 19*(2), 347–371.

Saladin, K. (2012). *Connective tissue.* Retrieved from http://www.biologyreference.com/Ce-Co/Connective-Tissue.html#b. [accessed on 10/11/2012].

Thibodeau, G., & Pattons, K. (1993). *Anatomy and physiology* (2nd ed., p. 831). St Louis: Mosby.

Vortkamp, A., Kaechoong, L., et al. (1996). Regulation of rate of cartilage differentiation by Indian hedgehog and PTH-related protein. *American Association for Advancement of Science, 273*(3), 613–622.

The Nervous System in Children and Adolescents

At birth, the brain weight is 25% of that of an adult brain, and within 6 months, the brain weight is doubled. The brain reaches 90% of its adult size by 6 years of age.

The central nervous system starts its amazing journey from birth.

The Baby's Nervous System

Babies are born with nervous systems that mature fully over the first few years of their life. From as early as 4 weeks old, the first brain cells, called 'neurons', start developing at a rate of 250,000 per minute. These neurons form links with other neurons and builds up connections between cells, forging intricate links and putting everything in its place (Healy, 1994; Shore, 1997).

Myelination of the peripheral nervous system is also present in birth mostly, giving the newborns every advantage to learn about their surroundings. All cranial nerves are also myelinated (apart from the optic nerve) and are present at birth. However, a child's control of movement is somewhat faulted at an early age until total myelination of all peripheral nerves takes place, which normally isn't until later childhood (MacGregor, 2001).

Once the foetus leaves the womb, development continues through the central nervous system and the visual cortex – here the rate of development is dependent on the amount of stimulation the infant is able to withstand. When a child is born with a visual abnormality, it is vital to correct this in the best way possible so as not to allow the brain to forget how to use the eye, as the baby brain sculpts itself. Crying is a baby's way of communicating with its environment, and it may also represent the baby's inability to cope with all the stimuli in its environment. In maturing a baby's nervous system, a mother's maternal bonding is vital, so is the need for social, physical, and emotional contact (Healy, 1994; Jensen, 1998; Shore, 1997).

The Child's Nervous System

At this stage, as the central nervous system (CNS) matures, complex behavioural and cognitive abilities become possible. Scientists have demonstrated that up to age 1, babies respond to language with the whole of their brain, and then gradually, once a language has been acquired, language centre switches to the left hemisphere. A growth spurt occurs in the brain during middle childhood, and at the age 8 or 9, a child's brain is almost the size of an adult brain.

The frontal lobe and corpus callosum are two structures that grow significantly during childhood. Any damage or injury to these parts of the brain will result in erratic emotional outburst, poor judgement, and the inability to plan. However, as the size of the frontal lobe increases, children are better able to engage in more difficult cognitive tasks (Giedd et al., 1991; Shore, 1997; Siegel, 1999).

Before age of 6, the growth of a child's head results in development of nerve tracts and creation of nerve fibres within the brain. After age 6, head size continues to increase but development of nerve tracts and fibres begins to slow until they are fully developed. The age of full development of the nervous system has previously been stated as 3 years for the CNS and 10 years for the complete nervous system. However, further research has suggested that due to the impact of puberty, a fully developed and mature nervous system is not achieved until late teens (Giedd et al., 1991)

Motor skills such as walking are continously developing in children, and by age 7, they normally attain 60% of the fundamental motor skills required for daily life (MacGregor, 2001).

Similarly, other studies have supported this work, suggesting that developing children can increase their coorindation skills with the help of repetitive actions in pre-school children. It still, however, remains unclear how this is achieved, but motor patterning in the brain could be one of the reasons rather than fine motor control from the peripheral nerves (Stanitski, Delee, & Drez, 1994).

However, some studies also suggest that some 6-year-old children still do not have the motor patterns to voluntarily contract certain muscle groups efficiently, thereby affecting their gait (Belanger & McComas, 1989). However, they further admit their population size was small and more research is required in this area.

Boys tend to attain throwing and kicking motor skills earlier than girls, but girls seem to attain hopping and skipping earlier (Malina & Bouchard, 1991). Ball-handling skills such as dribbling, catching, and aiming seem to be superior in boys with incremental improvements being seen throughout childhood up to adolescence, when they plateau (Stanitski et al., 1994). Girls have better balance at this age compared with boys, and their fine motor skills tend to be more superior (Patel, Greydanus, & Baker, 2009).

Until a child is fully developed, their behaviour is predominantly reflective due to the immaturity of the system. At this age, a child's neuromotor development is plastic, which can be influenced by many factors including functionality and sport. Intensity of sport and its duration can also have an effect on nerve plasticity (MacGregor, 2001).

The Adolescent Nervous System

By puberty, between the ages of 12 and 16 years, the brain would be 100% of the adult brain weight. The development of the central and peripheral nervous system is well established before adolescence.

The adolescent years extend well beyond the teenage years. During adolescence, the nervous system is changing at a striking rate, acquiring hormones, and the centre for reasoning and impulse control continues to develop. During the late teen years and even into the early twenties, the brain continues to grow; research has shown that there is a second wave of overproduction of grey matter at this stage. After which, there is a pruning phase where neuron connections that are used regularly are kept, and those that are not used are withered away. This pruning process is thought to make the nervous system more efficient by strengthening the existing neuron connections (Begley, 2000; Dahl & Spear, 1999; Giedd et al., 1999).

The prefrontal cortex is in its final stage of development during adolescence. This area of the nervous system is responsible for executive functions such as reasoning, advance thoughts, and impulse control. As the front region of the brain is not fully developed, adolescents must rely, to a great extent, on other parts of the brain responsible for emotions when making decisions. Additionally, a change in the brain's neurotransmitters also takes place in this stage of development. And as such, the behaviour of adolescents remain very unstable and involves greater risks, and they mostly partake in activities that give higher stimulation in order to receive similar excitement as in their younger years (Dahl & Spear, 2004; National Institute of Mental Health, 2001; Siegel, 1999; White, 2001).

Functionally, females perform balance tasks better compared with boys at this age, but motor development involving fine motor skills rarely progresses beyond the age of 14 in girls whereas this continues in males (Patel et al., 2009). However, there is a brief period, typically between the ages of 12 and 14 years where males in particular go through a period of un-coordination (Sullivan & Anderson, 2000). It typically lasts for 6 months or so and is often a temporary disturbance during an aggressive growth spurt which affects their balance centres (Patel et al., 2009).

As adolescents mature, they continue to experience an improvement in their balance and reaction time with practice. The refinement of these skills is influenced by many factors including somatotype, gender, motivation, age, and, more importantly, intensity and duration of training. The adolescent nervous system is highly plastic and adaptive at this age, and will normally mould to the functionality of the sport or function well (Patel et al., 2009).

References

Begley, S. (2000). Getting inside a teen brain. *Newsweek, 135*(9), 58–59.

Belanger, A., & McComas, A. (1989). Contractile properties of human skeletal muscle in childhood, *European Journal of Applied Physiology, 58,* 563.

Dahl, R., & Spear, L. (2004). Adolescent brain development: Vulnerabilities and opportunities, *Annals of the New York Academy of Sciences,* A collection of more than 60 research papers and essays.

Giedd, J., Blumenthal, J., Jeffries, N., Castellanos, F., Liu, H., Zijdenbos, A., Paus, T., Evans, A., & Rapoport, J. (1999). Brain development during childhood and adolescence: A longitudinal MRI study. *Nature Neuroscience, 2*(10), 861–863.

Healy, J. (1994). *Your child's growing mind: A practical guide to brain development and learning from birth to adolescence.* New York: Doubleday.

Jensen, E. (1998). *Teaching with the brain in mind.* Alexandria, VA: Association for Supervision and Curriculum Development.

MacGregor, J. (2001). *Anatomy and physiology of children* (2nd ed.). London: Routledge.

Malina, R., & Bouchard, C. (1991). *Growth, maturation and physical activity.* Champaign, IL: Human Kinetic.

National Institute of Mental Health (2001). *Teenage brain: A work in progress.* National Institute of Mental Health Publication. Retrieved from www.nimh.nih.gov/publicat/teenbrain.cfm.

Patel, D., Greydanus, D., & Baker, R. (2009). *Pediatric sports medicine* (2nd ed.). New York, NY: McGraw Hill Medical.

Shore, R. (1997). *Rethinking the brain: New Insights into early development.* New York, NY: Families and Work Institute.

Siegel, D. J. (1999). The developing mind. New York, NY: Guilford Press.

Stanitski, C., Delee, J., & Drez, D. (1994). *Pediatric and adolescent sports medicine* (3rd ed.). New York, NY: W. B. Saunders.

Sullivan, A., & Anderson, S. (2000). Health care of young athletes. *American Academy of Paediatrics* (3rd ed.). *American Academy of Orthopedic Surgeons,* 243-258.

White, A. (2001). *Alcohol and adolescent brain development.* Retrieved from http://www.duke.edu/~amwhite/alc_adol_pf.html.

Hormonal Changes in the Musculoskeletal System

The most important hormones in the process of growth during childhood and adolescence are the growth hormone and sex hormones. Other hormones that are involved include insulin and thyroid hormones (Chan & Mantzoros, 2005; Stanfield, 2011).

Growth Hormone and Insulin-like Growth Factor

Bone growth begins at infancy and persists right the way through to late adolescence under the influence of growth hormone (GH) and insulin-like growth factor (IGF) (Saggese, Baroncelli, & Bertelloni, 2002).

Growth hormone is important in the regulation of both bone formation and bone resorption (Giustina, Mazziotti, & Canalis, 2008). GH is also responsible for increases in bone mineral content and muscle mass (Roemmich, Clark, & Walter, 2000).

IGF is a protein that stimulates the effects of GH within bones and muscles (Gunnell, Miller, Rogers, & Holly, 2005).

Throughout the first phase of puberty, in both boys and girls, the amount of GH and IGF secretion (Mauras, Bishop, & Welch, 2007) doubles in quantity (Saenger, 2003). This then peaks in the second phase as described later (Rogol, 2002).

Boys are more sensitive to GH and IGF than girls, leading to greater bone length and mass in boys (Mauras et al., 2007). This is influenced by the increasing levels of testosterone and IGF (Lang, 2011).

Sex Hormones – Testosterone and Oestrogen

During puberty, sex hormones stimulate growth spurts in conjunction with GH and IGF (Harel et al., 2007; Saggese et al., 2002).

Remer et al. (2003) describe them as 'the engine' that stimulates bone growth during the transition from childhood to adulthood. The sex hormones, along with IGF, deposit and regulate the distribution of body fat during puberty. Testosterone is the male sex hormone and oestrogen the female sex hormone (Marieb, 2009), and both play a very important role in development.

The larger and stronger skeletal muscle mass in males is partly influenced by the added effects of testosterone (Mauras et al., 2007; Rogol, 2002). The growth in muscle and bone is parallel in nature (Lang, 2011), and without the increase in testosterone during puberty, boys would be unable to achieve substantial muscle mass (Smolak, Murnen, & Thompson, 2005).

Oestrogen, the female sex hormone, increases bone growth and remodelling in girls (Schoenau, Neu, Rauch, & Manz, 2002) in conjunction with GH and IGF (Van Coeverden et al 2002). There is an increase in bone length, mass, and strength as opposed to muscle mass (Rittweger et al., 2000). This is because females have an increased secretion of oestrogen and a decreased secretion of testosterone (Lang, 2011). Pajamaki et al. (2008) also found that oestrogen increases bone rigidity. Oestrogen also pays an important role in males as well as females during development. Mackie et al. (2008) explain that the fusion of epiphyseal plates (growth plates) in boys and girls is significantly influenced by the secretion of oestrogen.

Childhood

Linear bone growth begins at infancy (Saggese et al., 2002) and continues during childhood until the epiphyseal plates fuse (Robson, Siebler, Shalet, & Williams, 2002) in the late teens or early twenties. This process is a result of endochondral ossification and is regulated by different genetic and hormonal factors (Eerden, Karperien, & Wit, 2003). The regulators of bone growth and development in children are GH, IGF-I, glucocorticoids, and thyroid hormone (Eerden et al., 2003; Robson et al., 2002) and each play an important role in longitudinal skeletal growth (Giustina et al., 2008).

Puberty

Marieb (2009) explains that puberty begins between the ages of 10 and 15 years, and during this time, there are a number of growth spurts. The pubertal growth spurt begins at 13 for boys and 11 for girls (Stanfield, 2011) and can be split into three phases: the first phase, where there is minimal growth; the second phase, where there is peak growth; and the third phase, where growth slows down again.

Throughout the first phase of puberty, in both boys and girls, the amount of GH and IGF secretion (Mauras et al., 2007) almost doubles (Saenger, 2003). This then peaks in the second phase (Rogol, 2002).

It has long been established that sex hormones are important for longitudinal growth, especially during puberty (Eerden et al., 2003).

Sex hormones stimulate growth spurts and epiphyseal fusion (Robson et al., 2002) in conjunction with GH and IGF (Harel et al., 2007).

Remer et al. (2003) describe them as the powerhouse that stimulates bone growth during the transition from childhood to adulthood. Boys are more sensitive to GH and IGF than girls, leading to greater bone length and mass (Mauras et al., 2007). This is influenced by the increasing levels of testosterone and IGF (Lang, 2011). The growth in muscle and bone is parallel in nature (Lang, 2011) and without the increased testosterone during puberty, boys are unable to achieve substantial muscle mass (Smolak et al., 2005). Boys peak at difference ages/times and hence this is normally when testosterone levels begin to increase. Noticeably, not only does the boy grow suddenly, but other changes occur, including a deepening of the voice.

Adolesence

During adolescence, the critical role of GH and IGF-I is to maintain and achieve peak bone mass (Eerden et al., 2003; Giardina, 2011). During adolescence, these hormones are secreted in large amounts and in spurts, hence there are growth spurts.

References

Chan, J. L., & Mantzoros, C. (2005). Role of leptin in energy-deprivation states: Normal human physiology and clinical implications for hypothalamic amenorrhoea and anorexia nervosa. *Lancet, 366*(9479), 74–85.

Eerden, B., Karperien, M., & Wit, J. (2003). Systemic and local regulation of the growth plate. *Endocrine Reviews, 24*(6), 782–801.

Giardina, P. (2011). Pain in thalassemia – An emerging complication. *Thalassemia Reports, 1*(2), 83–85.

Giustina, A., Mazziotti, G., & Canalis, E. (2008). Growth hormone, insulin-like growth factors, and the skeleton. *Endocrine Reviews, 29*(5), 535–559.

Gunnell, D., Miller, L., Rogers, I., & Holly, J. (2005). Association of insulin-like growth factor I and insulin-like growth factor-binding protein-3 with intelligence quotient among 8- to 9-year-old children in the Avon Longitudinal Study of Parents and Children. *Pediatrics, 116*(5), 681–686.

Harel, Z., Gold, M., Cromer, B., Bruner, A., Stager, M., Bachrach, L., Wolter, K., Reid, C., Hertweck, P., Nelson, A., Nelson, D., Coupey, S., Johnson, C., Burkman, R., & Bone, H. (2007). Bone mineral density in postmenarchal adolescent girls in the United States: Associated biopsychosocial variables and bone turnover markers. *Journal of Adolescent Health, 40*(1), 44–53.

Lang, T. (2011). The bone–muscle relationship in men and women. *Journal of Osteoporosis, 2011*(1), 1–11.

Mackie, E., Ahmed, Y., Tatarczuch, L., Chen, K., & Mirams, M. (2008). Endochondral ossification: How cartilage is converted into bone in the developing skeleton. *International Journal of Biochemistry & Cell Biology, 40*(1), 46–62.

Marieb, E. (2009). Essentials of human anatomy and physiology (9th ed.). San Francisco: Pearson.Mauras, N., Bishop, K., & Welch, S. (2007). Growth hormone action in puberty: Effects by gender. *Growth Hormone & IGF Research, 17*(1), 463–471.

Pajamäki, I., Sievänen, H., Kannus, P., Jokihaara, J., Vuohelainen, T., & Järvinen, T. (2008). Skeletal effects of estrogen and mechanical loading are structurally distinct. *Bone, 43*(4), 748–757.

Remer, T., Boye, K., Hartmann, M., Neu, C., Schoenau, E., Manz, F., & Wudy, S. (2003). Adrenarche and bone modeling and remodeling at the proximal radius: Weak androgens make stronger cortical bone in healthy children. *Journal of Bone and Mineral Research, 18*(8), 1539–1546.

Rittweger, J., Beller, G., Ehrig, J., Jung, C., Koch, U., Ramolla, J., Schmidt, F., Newitt, D., Majumdar, S., Schiessl, H., & Felsenberg, D. (2000). Bone-muscle strength indices for the human lower leg. *Bone, 27*(2), 319–326.

Robson, H., Siebler, T., Shalet, S., & Williams, G. (2002). Interactions between GH, IGF-I, glucocorticoids, and thyroid hormones during skeletal growth. *Pediatric Research, 52*(2), 137–147.

Roemmich, J., Clark, P., & Walter, K. (2000). Physical activity energy expenditure, body composition, and abdominal fat distribution during puberty. *American Journal of Physiology-Endocrinology and Metabolism, 1*(1), 1426–1436.

Rogol, A. (2002). Androgens and puberty. *Molecular and Cellular Endocrinology, 198*(1), 25–29.

Saenger, P. (2003). Dose effects of growth hormone during puberty. *Hormone Research, 60*(1), 52–57.

Saggese, G., Baroncelli, G., & Bertelloni, S. (2002). Puberty and bone development. *Best Practice & Research Clinical Endocrinology & Metabolism, 16*(1), 53–64.

Schoenau, E., Neu, C. M., Rauch, F., & Manz, F. (2002). Gender-specific pubertal changes in volumetric cortical bone mineral density at the proximal radius. *Bone, 31*(1), 110–113.

Smolak, L., Murnen, S., & Thompson, K. (2005). Sociocultural influences and muscle building in adolescent boys. *Psychology of Men & Masculinity, 6*(4), 227–239.

Stanfield, C. (2011). *Blackboard for principles of human physiology* (4th ed.). Alabama: Pearson.Van Coeverden, S., Netelenbos, J., de Ridder, C. M., Roos, J., Popp-Snijders, C., Delemarre-van de Waal, H. (2002). Bone metabolism markers and bone mass in healthy pubertal boys and girls. *Clinical Endocrinology, 57*(1), 107–116.

Puberty and Sexual Maturation

Dr Solomon Abrahams

Everyone has heard the phrase 'you should act more mature', whether it was directed at them or they were the ones saying it. However, maturity is much more complex and is not entirely dependent on one's action. There are three components to maturation; these include physical, mental, and cognitive maturity phases. The physical and mental components of maturity can easily be identified, especially as they are evident from the bodily changes of both males and females during puberty (Healthy Futures, 2013). The cognitive component is much more complex and deals more with aspects of mature judgement, abstract thinking, and rational decision making. Cognitive maturity is developed from both puberty and life experiences and choices, while physical maturity and mental maturity are mostly developed just from puberty onwards (Healthy Futures, 2013).

Puberty is defined as the period of human development during which physical growth and sexual maturation occur (Stöppler, 2013). Puberty involves biological, or physical, transformation as well as emotional development in both males and females.

Females typically start the maturation process before males. One of the first signs of puberty in girls is the beginning of breast development. This is followed by growth of pubic and armpit hair as well as menstruation (Stöppler, 2013).

For males, the process begins with the enlargement of the reproductive organs followed by the growth of pubic and armpit hair as well as an increase in muscle size and deepening of vocals (Stöppler, 2013). These sequences in puberty for both males and females is referred to as the Sexual Maturity Rating (SMR) which allows doctors to classify their patients in different stages (Stöppler, 2013).

Aside from sexual maturation, there are many other physical changes that occur during puberty. Males and females both experience a growth spurt where they grow rapidly in height. Close to 20% of an adult's height comes from the growth spurt during puberty (Stöppler, 2013).

With this sudden growth in height comes a growth in bones and bone density as well as changes in body weight. These weight changes are typically caused from mostly muscular growth in males and an increase in body fat in females. Inside the body, there is significant growth in the heart and the lungs, which leads to an increase in endurance and strength (Stöppler, 2013). Another physical change in both males and females is the medical condition of inflammation of the sebaceous glands and hair follicles, most commonly known as acne – discussed later.

Physical changes that both male and female adolescents go through during puberty give rise to mental and emotional changes. Many adolescents feel self-conscious about their changing body, which can lead to them feeling embarrassed, being under pressure to look different, and being treated differently by their peers (Better Health Channel, 2012). The sudden release of hormones that bring about these physical changes can cause young people to have mood swings, but they are usually only temporary (Better Health Channel, 2012). Another change that is often experienced is in their energy levels. Adolescents can experience large rushes in energy followed by quick crashes. These energy changes are complemented by changes in sleep patterns. The body's sleep–wake cycle is influenced by hormones that control a 'circadian rhythm' (Oswalt, 2010). When these hormone levels change, it creates a shift in this rhythm and causes teens to often at times feel more awake at night, which can lead them to sleep in late on the weekends (Oswalt, 2010). These mental and emotional changes should not be confused with cognitive changes in adolescents, which are changes in how one thinks and reasons.

Cognitive maturity is less understood because it branches from recent breakthroughs in neuroscience, which is much harder to study and draw conclusive evidence from compared with physical and mental changes that have tangible evidence to back them up.

In adolescents, cognitive thinking changes from basic abilities to think in concrete ways that are learnt between the ages of 6 and 12 years to more complex, abstract thinking (Lucile, 2013). Adolescents develop the ability to think systematically about logical relationships, consider different viewpoints, and think about the process of thinking (Healthy Futures, 2013). Everyone develops their own view of the world through complex cognitive maturity, but it takes time for adolescents to apply these views and ways of thinking to their personal decisions.

Cognitive maturity can be broken into three different development stages. The first stage is during early adolescence when 'the use of complex thinking is focused on personal decision making in school and home environments' (Lucile, 2013). This can include questioning authority standards and verbalising own thoughts and views on various topics.

The second stage of cognitive maturity is the middle adolescence stage when the use of complex thinking is focused on philosophical and futuristic concerns (Lucile, 2013). This includes analysing and questioning things more, creating a code of ethics, and developing a self-identity. The third and final stage of cognitive maturity is the late adolescence stage when complex thinking is focused on 'less self-centred concepts as well as personal decision making' (Lucile, 2013). This includes developing idealistic views on topics, making career decisions, and thinking about emerging into having a role in an adult society. Cognitive maturation is the way that people truly separate themselves from their peers apart from physical appearance (Healthy Futures, 2013). It is who we are, how we think and react to dilemmas, and how we view the world around us. People have different philosophies on life and politics, express their concerns and views in different ways, connect with other people, and form relationships mainly based on their cognitive thinking. Cognitive maturity is the lifeblood that makes us all unique.

Every adolescent will experience puberty and all the many changes that come with it. Some people will develop faster than others, attain more or less athleticism than others, get more or less acne than others, and develop different ways of viewing the world around us. All these differences are derived from puberty and maturation and are what make us all unique individuals (Better Health Channel, 2012).

References

Better Health Channel (2012). *Puberty*. Retrieved from *http://www.betterhealth.vic.gov.au/bhcv2/bhcarticles.nsf/pages/Puberty* [accessed on 5/2/2013].

Healthy Futures (2013). *Maturation of the teen brain*. Retrieved from *http://ontheirlevel.org/whats-happening/maturation-of-the-teen-brain/* [accessed on 5/2/2013].

Lucile Packard Children's Hospital (2013). *Cognitive development*. Retrieved from *http://www.lpch.org/DiseaseHealthInfo/HealthLibrary/adolescent/cogdev.html* [accessed on 5/2/2013].

Oswalt, A. (2010). *Mental/emotional/social changes through puberty*. Retrieved from *http://www.mentalhelp.net/poc/view_doc.php?type=doc&id=38408&cn=1276* [accessed on 5/22013].

Stöppler, M. C. (2013). *Puberty*. Retrieved from *http://www.medicinenet.com/puberty/article.htm* [accessed on 5/2/2013].

Other Parts of the Developing Child An Overview

The Child's Heart and Circulation

Over childhood, cardiac muscles increase seven times in size with the cardiac blood vessels increasing proportionately. (MacGregor, 2001). Research in this area still remains limited due to ethical considerations.

Cardiac output of children and adolescents are lower than that of adults at any given level of oxygen uptake (MacGregor, 2001). Cardiac output, and hence pulse, begins to lower as the child becomes older. Typically, a 5-year-old's pulse is around 95 beats per minute, whereas a 10-year-old's is 75 beats per minute and a 15-year-old's is typically 70 beats per minute at rest. Obviously, this is dependent on many factors (Hazinski, 1992).

From the age of 6 years, children's maximal heart rate is higher than adults', upto 200 beats per minute. Girls have a similar sub-max heart rate, but normally it is higher compared with boys of the same age group (Armstrong & Welsman, 1997). This potentially is due to sex-related differences in autonomic cardiac regulation, which might also explain why boys have faster recovery of heart rate following exercise.

Heart rate during sleep differs from heart rate while being awake. Children below 10 years have a daytime heart rate between 70 and 110 beats per minute as opposed to a sleep heart rate of between 60 and 100 beats per minute. Normally, from 10 years of age, through adolescence and early adulthood, this changes. Daytime rates range from 55 to 90 beats per minute during normal activities, whereas sleeping heart rates range from 50 to 90 beats per minute (Wong, 1995).

The Heart

As the child grows bigger, the heart also grows and produces a larger stroke volume. Boys who have more lean tissue which has a higher metabolic rate require larger hearts to service this and, consequently, have a pulse rate that is similar to pulse rate at a young age, slowing in the pubertal spurt when testosterone is released (MacGregor, 2001).

In an overweight child, the pulse is higher as the heart has to work harder to feed oxygen around the child's body. If the child is underweight, the pulse may also be faster due to the constant release of small quantities of adrenaline, a response from the sympathetic nervous system. MacGregor (2001) also suggests that this can be because of high amounts of thyroxine but does not explain why.

Interestingly, Rowland, Geoff, and Popowski (1998) report children do not develop left ventricular hypertrophy as seen in some adult long distance runners, and they only improve their maximum oxygen uptake by 5–10% when training.

Blood Pressure

Resting blood pressure rises throughout childhood as the heart becomes stronger and bigger (MacGregor, 2001). Typically, the blood pressure in a 10-year-old is about 100/62 when alert, whereas the blood pressure of an adolescent, from 15 years old, is about 115/65 and it is 121/70 in an adult of 20 years (Wong, 1995).

The Child's Blood

Red blood cells are made in the bone marrow, which occupies most of the spongy spaces and medullary cavities of the child's skeleton. However, by puberty the red marrow is replaced by yellow marrow containing fat, and red cell production only remains in the adolescent upper shaft of the femur and humerus, vertebrae, sternum, ribs, and scapula (MacGregor, 2001).

Essentially, the child's diet is essential for normal red cell production. This includes a balanced diet including amino acids, vitamin B12, iron, vitamin B6, and folic acid.

Interestingly, haemoglobin, the essential protein within blood cells which carries the oxygen around the body, increases dramatically in boys when they go through their growth spurts and there is the onset of testosterone hormone. However, girls show an increase with the onset of menarche only; therefore, this could explain why boys show superiority in endurance sports at this age (MacGregor, 2001).

The Respiratory System

From age 5 to puberty, the weight of the lungs increases threefold. Total volume of the lungs increases with age and this is seen equally in boys and girls. Respiratory frequency is slightly higher in boys possibly because of the lean muscle tissue they possess (MacGregor, 2001).

Maturation of lung tissue is complete by age 8, and from 8 years to puberty, increased air space occurs through enlargement of alveoli and airways. Lung capacity correlates with age, but also with changing body height (Rowland et al., 1998).

Respiratory rate generally slows down as the child ages, due to accommodation of lung volume. The average respiratory rate of a 6-year-old is 20–26 per minute, 18–24 in a 10-year-old and 12–20 in a mature adolescent. Anything above 30 suggests hyperventilation or respiratory distress (MacGregor, 2001).

Armstrong and Welsman (1997) found boys' maximum oxygen uptake increases by 150% from 8 to 18 years, whereas girls only demonstrate an increase of 80% during puberty. They continue to suggest that an accumulation of body fat in girls during puberty restricts their maximal oxygen uptake, whereas consistency in increasing muscle mass and height in boys explains this increase in oxygen uptake.

Water Balance and Dehydration

Water balance in children is quickly affected by environmental temperature and humidity, more so than in adults.

Dehydration in children can sometimes be hard to identify. Severe dehydration would normally lead to a dry mouth, with the mucous membrane of the mouth between the lip and gums being very dry, a smaller tongue, lack of salivation, irritability and tiredness (MacGregor, 2001). Dehydration in children is common after respiratory tract infections, sore throats, and fever.

Water and salt is important for normal osmoregularity in children, but too much salt (e.g. seen in some foods) will cause fluids to be withdrawn from interstitial tissues of the body into the blood and essentially cause cellular dehydration (MacGregor, 2001).

Kidneys

The child's kidneys are fully developed and functional by the age of 2 years. Normally, children dehydrate more quickly than adults due to their surface area compared with adults (MacGregor, 2001).

Urine in children should be 'straw-coloured' or a light yellow. It is common for children to develop urine infections in early childhood, but this becomes less of an issue as they get older. Strong-smelling urine, red or dark yellow/orange-coloured urine could be an indication of infection or dehydration. Urine output varies with age, but generally, 5–8-year-olds normally expel between 600 and 1200 ml of urine, 8–14-year-olds normally expel 1000–1500 ml of urine, and 14-year-old-plus normally expel over 1500 ml of urine (MacGregor, 2001).

Heat Regulation in Children

Children produce more heat per kilogram of weight compared with adults, making them inefficient at temperature regulation (Sharp, 2012). In general, pre-pubertal boys and girls sweat/perspire the same, although less in absolute terms. They possess more sweat glands compared with adults, but they produce far less sweat (Stanitski, Delee, & Drez, 1994). Children also have higher skin temperatures normally, which hinders the flow of heat from the body core to the peripherals making their hands and feet more colder compared with those of the average adult (Sharp, 2012). Similarly, children do not acclimatise well to heat or cold compared with adults, and may require more time (Stanitski et al., 1994).

The Stomach

The stomach in children is normally located high in the abdomen and is orientated horizontally rather than vertically up to the age of 10 years. Because of its position, children's appetites may not be significant as the capacity remains small. Typically, a child up to 10 years will have a minimum stomach capacity of only 750 ml. However, after this age, it increases dramatically, and nearly doubles up to the age of 16 years – normally around 1500 ml – and then can double again, depending on the person's appetite to 3000 ml (MacGregor, 2001).

Expected Weight Gains

Children up to 10 years of age normally make modest weight gains, approximately 2–3 kg per annum, with height increasing by 5 cm per annum.

In females, from 10 to 14 years, 7–25 kg is expected per annum. 95% of the height is achieved at the onset of menarche.

In males, from 10 to 14 years, 7–30 kg is expected per annum, with 95% of the height being achieved by age 15. (Campbell & Glasper, 1995).

The Child's Eye

Normally, children by the age of 4 have 20/20 vision. The lens in children continues to grow throughout life, and at 14 years, it is adult size. Sadly, at 60 years, it is only 1/3 smaller than a young 20-year-old's (MacGregor, 2001).

Child's Sleep

As children mature, the quality and quantity of sleep changes. Family influences, social expectations and cultural variations can affect a child's sleep. The duration of a child's sleep decreases as the child ages.

However, some authors suggest that this is not entirely true, as adolescents require more sleep during periods of growth spurts (Campbell & Glasper, 1995). They also stipulate that a child's sleep patterns are further disrupted by other external factors such as emotional factors, environmental issues, overcrowding, poverty, mental health, and physical health. Some authors actually suggest that sleep disturbance in children is common through to adolescence, affecting 25% of all children (Mindell, Moline, Zendell, Brown, & Fry, 1994).

It has also been documented that children and adolescents who do have sleep disturbances do replenish their sleep in the morning and late evening. In particular, this is seen in adolescents more so due to the enormous growth spurts they exhibit and academic demands (Yarcheski & Mahon, 1994).

Cognitive Function 6–10-Year-Olds

Children at this age understand simple present and past questions, but are unable to relate this to future events. They also engage in magical thinking, believing they have unique powers so nobody can do them harm (Patel, Greydanus, & Baker, 2009). They are exceptionally naive at this age, are still learning about their surroundings, and can be very gullible. If they watch wrestling on television, for example, they believe they can throw people around similarly (Patel et al., 2009).

The attention span begins to develop at this age, and they can follow simple instructions. Their memory improves, but problem-solving remains difficult for some. They understand rules and judgement and begin to separate those that are intelligent and those who are not (Patel et al., 2009).

From a sports-specific point of view, they are now able to distinguish between good players and below-average players and understand the competitive nature of sport.

Cognitive Function 10–15-Year-Olds

At the beginning of puberty, abstract thinking, analytic abilities, problem-solving, and transitional skills begin to come together. Selective attention and memory begin to improve, and they begin to remember complex strategies, such as understanding certain tactics within a game (Patel et al., 2009).

Language differences become more understandable. They become more concerned about their body image, which can be very important in terms of their communication with members of the opposite sex. They become more aware of themselves as a person and the people and family that surround them. Reasoning and explanations become more difficult, which may make them disagree and argue more. Magical thinking is now in the past, and they begin to realise that the external world can be challenging (Patel et al., 2009).

From a sports-specific point of view, they now begin to demonstrate different attitudes, making some conversations rather difficult.

Cognitive Function 15-Year-Plus

Late adolescents become more self-aware and have realistic goals. Because their complex motor abilities are now fully enhanced, they become more competitive and strive to become the best they can. At this age, they become more aware of future aspirations as they now begin to understand the realistic chances of how good or not good they are with particular sports (Patel et al., 2009).

Growing Pains

Growing pains still remain a mystery, and clinical research remains inconclusive (Birrer, Griesemer, & Cataletto, 2002). The incidence of growing pains ranges from 5% to 42% and normally affects 3–5-year-olds and 8–12-year-olds. It also tends to affects girls more than boys.

Pains tend to be deep-seated, cramping sensations which can affect day or night, sometimes even waking the child. The pains are normally intermittent, normally affecting legs more than arms. They can last 3 months and can be intermittent during this period (Birrer et al., 2002).

Differential diagnosis should eliminate infection, malignancy, arthritis, and hypermobility syndrome.

The Healing Process in Children

The healing process in most children tends to be quicker than in adults because of their adaptability at this age. This all begins with the inflammation cycle, just like in adults, which occurs over the first 5–7 days.

Following any soft tissue injury, the child will have hemorrhage as a result of tissue damage, which begins to infiltrate cells. This activates cellular chemicals, mainly degradative enzymes and vasoactivators such as histamine, prostaglandins, and kinins which begin the vasodilation and increase permeability of the cells. This also triggers oedema and pain, which sadly produce discomfort for the child. The degradative enzymes begin to mop up the debris and damaged cells.

Within this period, it is important that the basic principles that apply to adults are applied to children. Rest, ice, compression, and elevation are required to reduce any further bleeding of tissue and limit pain. If necessary, painkillers such as Calpol analgesic or limited amounts of paracetamol should be used rather than non-steroidal anti-inflammatory drugs, which interfere with the normal inflammatory response.

The next stage of inflammation in children is profileration of collagen where fibroblasts form a cellular matrix which is mesh like. This normally begins anywhere from 5 to 7 days. Collagen here is laid down in a haphazard matrix, but stretching and functional exercises realign the collagen in the direction of force, thereby improving the collagens tensile strength. Scar tissue formation is also reduced with stretching of tissues (Birrer et al., 2002).

References

Armstrong, N., & Welsman, J. (1997). Children in sport and exercise. *British Journal of Physical Education, 30*(2), 33.

Birrer, R., Griesemer, B., & Cataletto, M. (2002). *Pediatric sports medicine for primary care* (2nd ed.). Philadelphia, PA: Lippincott Williams & Wilkins.

Campbell, S., & Glasper, E. (1995). *Children's nursing* (1st ed.). London: Mosby.

Hazinski, M. (1992). *Nursing care of the critically ill child.* St. Louis, MO: Mosby.

MacGregor, J. (2001). *Anatomy and physiology of children* (2nd ed.). London: Routledge.

Mindell, J., Moline, M., Zendell, S., Brown, L., & Fry, J. (1994). Pediatricians and sleep disorders, *Pediatrics, 94*(2), 194–200.

Patel, D., Greydanus, D., & Baker, R. (2009). *Pediatric sports medicine* (3rd ed.). New York, NY: McGraw Hill Medical.

Rowland, T., Geoff, D., & Popowski, R. (1998). Cardiac responses to exercise in child long distance runners, *International Journal of Sports, 19*, 385.

Sharp, C. (2012). Some features of the anatomy and exercise physiology of children, *Athletes Weekly, 2*, 1.

Stanitski, C., Delee, J., & Drez, D. (1994). *Pediatric and adolescent sports medicine* (3rd ed.). Philadelphia, PA: W. B. Saunders.

Wong, D. (1995). *Clinical manual of pediatric nursing* (4th ed.). St Louis, MO: Mosby.

Yarcheski, A., & Mahon, N. (1994). A study of sleep during adolescence, *Journal of Pediatric Nursing, 9*(6), 357.

CHAPTER 2

Premedical Assessment in Children and Adolescent Sport

Solomon Abrahams

Before a young athlete joins your club, a thorough examination (with the parents or guardian present) should be conducted to help exclude any potential risk factors that may affect them.

There is no reliable standard assessment to date, and furthermore, little evidence suggests that gaining blood results, scans, and investigations can prevent illness or injury if its onset is late or even exercise-induced. For example, exercise-induced asthma is undiagnosed in up to 14% of young athletes, as it may not be picked up on a standard examination (Birrer, Griesemer, & Cataleto, 2002). Clinicians need to bear this in mind when conducting the examination and revealing the results to parents, coaches, and management. All examinations should be done in a medical type room (see Fig. 2.1) with the parents or a chaperone present.

Past Medical History

A thorough medical history is important in determining future risk of illnesses and injuries in the young athlete. Also, any potential patterns to the injuries should be assessed. This may give an indication of any potential pathology that may have been undiagnosed previously and help prevent any future events, for example hypermobility syndrome.

Continuous days taken off school, days in hospital, and days off sport due to an injury or illness should all be collated. Any past surgery should be documented, and visits (consistent) to their local general practitioner (GP) or family physician should be recorded.

Any previous investigations into any heart problems should be highlighted and any investigations to any previous joint or neurological pathology should be reviewed.

Cardiac History

Cardiac history should be recorded, including that of any family members with cardiac problems, specifically those with problems with exercising. Sudden death in children and adolescents is very rare, but more than 95% of all sudden death occurs before 30 years of age, with the incidence being 5 times more likely in males (Birrer et al., 2002). Any chest pains, shortness of breath, easy fatigue, palpitations, and persistent dizziness linked with exercise should be further investigated.

Pulmonary History

Pulmonary history should be recorded, in particular any history of asthma, bronchitis or any other breathing difficulties in the family as well as of the child. Any breathing difficulties that worsen with weather conditions, including cold or extreme weather, should also be noted.

Neurological History

Any neurological disorders or conditions should be recorded. This includes any previous head injuries, persistent headaches, dizziness, numbness, or increasing fatigue. Any night sweats or persistent fevers should be recorded.

Orthopaedic History

Any previous orthopaedic problems should be reviewed, including surgical and non-surgical. Previous fractures, ligament damage, or any persistent musculoskeletal pathology should be further documented.

Visual, Auditory, and Dermatological History

Any visual problems as well as auditory problems should be recorded.

Any previous history of dermatological pathology must be recorded, whether this be eczema, head lice, or infections.

Immunisation and Nutritional Status

Immunisation history and nutritional status should be recorded, and any supporting evidence must be submitted.

Lower Abdominal History

Any history of irritable bowel or persistent abdominal pathology is to be recorded. Similarly, any previous surgery to the abdominal area, such as to the appendix, should be recorded. Any hospitalisation for any abdominal complaint should be further investigated.

More sensitive issues including sexual history (and whether protection was used) in males and females, frequency of partners, and any drug or solvent abuse should be documented. In females, onset of menstrual cycle and regularity of the cycle must be recorded. Any history of lower abdominal cramps or pains may indicate endometriosis, fallopian cysts, ectopic pregnancy, or pregnancy. In males, questions about sexual activity, any spots on the penis, or any pains on urination should be sensitively asked.

Drug and Allergy History

Any current medication and any current allergies should be recorded. Names and details of the physicians should also be recorded in the event that you need to contact them regarding any medications that may or may not interact with their sport, or any medication you wish to give them.

Allergies should also be recorded in the event the child has a reaction to anything on and off the field of play.

Family History

Asking parents about their illnesses and injuries (as a child or adult) may also give an indication of future illnesses or injuries the child may present with in the future. For example, some illnesses have a genetic component, such as asthma or vision problems in the family. If anyone in the family smokes, this may have a bearing on the child. Any family history of cardiomyopathy (hypertrophy), congenital heart disease, arrhythmia, or sudden death should be particularly highlighted. The family should be asked about any history of multi-joint pains or hypermobility, and any history of rheumatoid arthritis and other such pathologies should be reviewed.

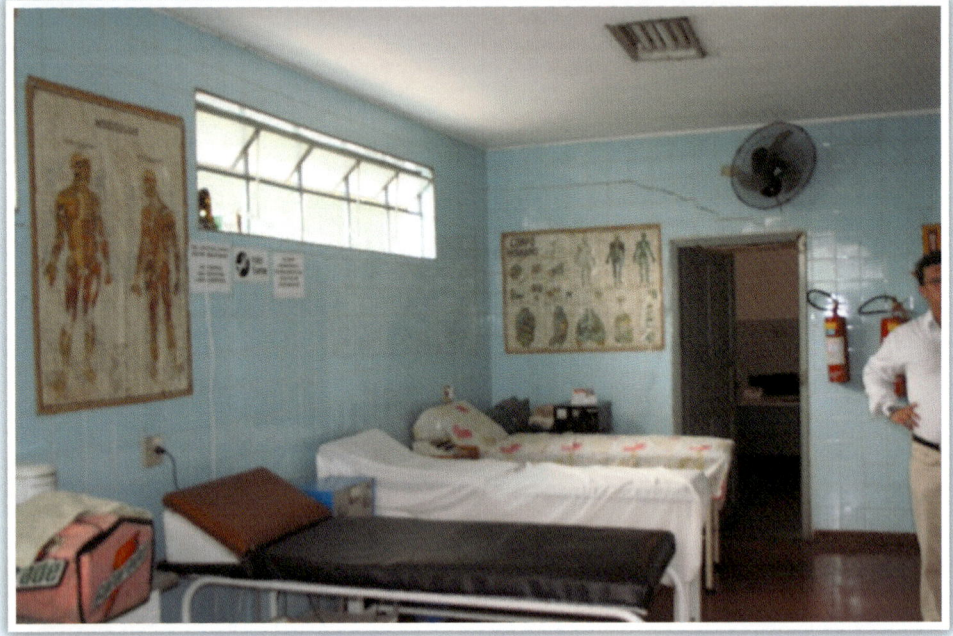

Fig. 2.1 Typical medical room in small professional clubs

Physical Examination

In the presence of the parents or a chaperone, the following physical examination can be further conducted, but should not be exclusive.

General appearance should be observed. Pale-looking skin could be an indication of anaemia or tiredness or an underlying infection. Long arms, for example, could be an indication of Marfan's syndrome, which may have cardiac implications. General posture should be visualised for kyphosis or Scheuermann's disease.

Height and weight should be assessed for obesity or underweight, which may indicate an eating disorder or a digestive disorder. This should be benchmarked against other children at the club to give a more functional evaluation rather than making comparisons with non-sporting children.

Vitals

Blood pressure, heart rate, and respiratory rate should be examined in standing and sitting positions. Arguably, these should also be assessed following exercise or function. Additionally, having this recording can act as a benchmark so future recordings can be easily compared.

Any abnormalities from the norm (see previous chapter on physiology) should be documented and further investigated.

Cardiac and Pulmonary Examination

Cardiac and pulmonary auscultation should be recorded. All central and peripheral pulses should be taken (bilaterally). Any arrhythmias should be documented but not necessarily be regarded as significant. If in doubt, exercise echocardiogram (or ECG stress tests) can be further used and the examination repeated. Murmurs in the paediatric population are common, but any systolic murmur rated 3/6 or greater or any diastolic murmur or a mumur which grows louder on a Valsalva manoeuvre may require further investigation (Birrer et al., 2002).

The sound of any fluid or any wheeze or reduced or hyper-resonant sounds on inspiration and expiration should be further investigated, and if necessary, a computed tomography (CT) or magnetic resonance imaging (MRI) scan should be taken. Depth of breath at all fields of the lungs is to be clearly examined. See Fig. 2.2.

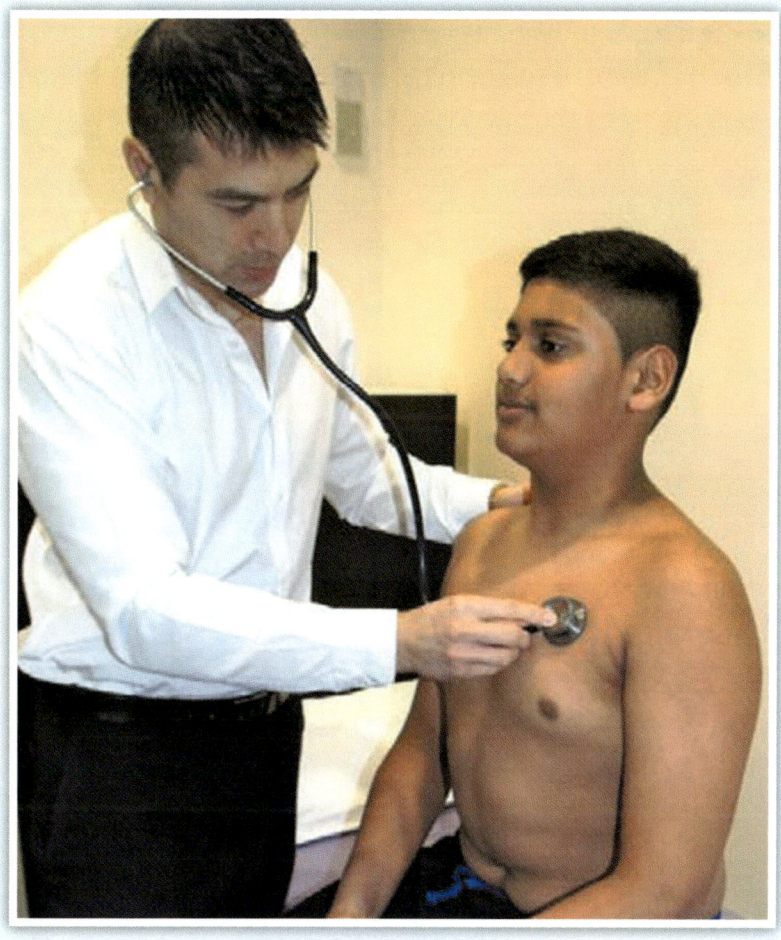

Fig. 2.2 Auscultation of the chest

Lower Abdominal Examination

Abdominal examination should involve auscultation for bowel sounds and percussion sounds and palpation of all quadrants for tenderness, masses, enlargement, rigidity, tension, and apprehension. The spleen, liver, kidneys, appendix, and abdomen should be specifically palpated and reviewed. (See Fig. 2.3.)

In girls (with female chaperone), palpation of uterus externally, fallopian tubes, and breasts (if appropriate) should be carried out. Any evidence of pain, tenderness, apprehension, lumps and bumps, or enlargement should be further investigated with diagnostic ultrasound, if appropriate.

In boys (with male chaperone), shaft or penis should be palpated for tenderness, spots, rash, and irritation. Testicles should be palpated for position (with and without cough). The inguinal area should be palpated and examined for hernia and glands.

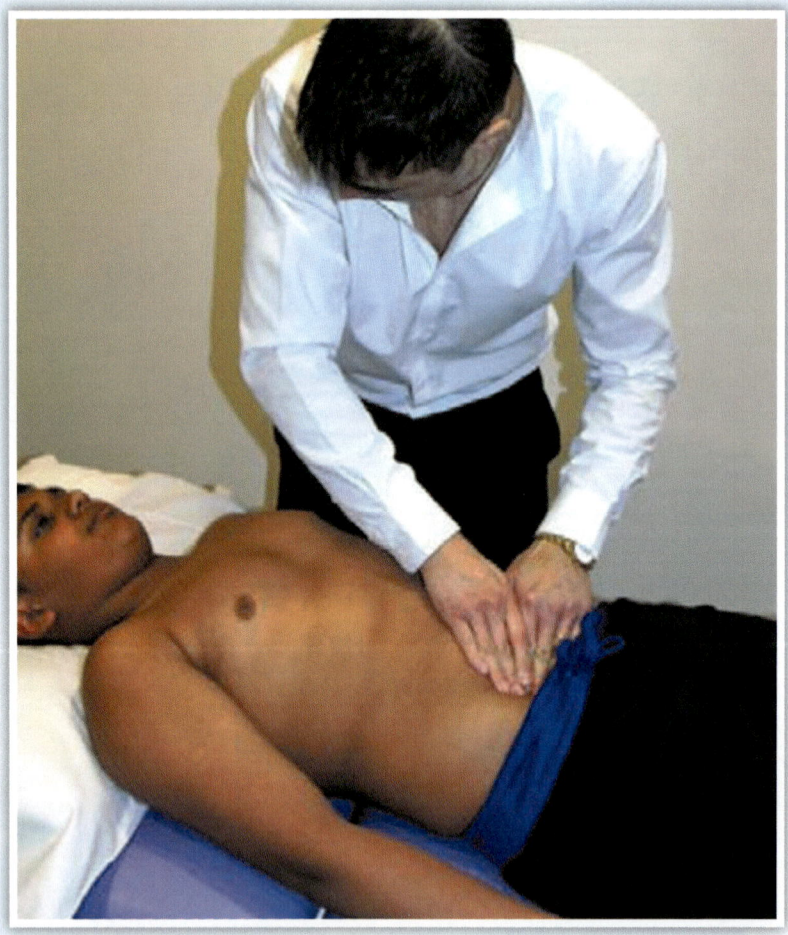

Fig. 2.3 Abdominal palpation

Neurological Examination

Neurological examination should never be underestimated. The cranial nerves should be screened, and the cerebellar and cognitive functions (again for benchmark) should be assessed. Myotomes, dermatomes, and reflexes of the body should be recorded. Functional tests appropriate for sport may also be employed to be more sports-specific.

Others (Eye, Ear, Nose, and Throat)

Other areas of interest for examination include eye, ear, nose, and throat.

Examination of eye should include checks for infection, pupil size (and reaction to light) for baseline unless underlying pathology is found, movements of the eye, and focus of peripheral and central vision.

Throat examination should consist of visualisation of the glands, gums, and tongue. Possibilities of infections, ulcers, and bleeding should be re-examined and excluded.

Ear examination should involve simple tests for hearing and the internal and external drum should be checked for damage.

Nose examination should reveal any previous fracture/deviated septum (for benchmark), nasal polyps, and unilateral nasal inspiration.

Musculoskeletal Examination

All joints should be examined with special attention and any relevant or significant information revealed in the subjective examination should be tested. For example, if there is a history of ankle sprains, the examiner should focus on specific tests for ankle instability. Some of the information are provided in this section; however, specific information on testing (if appropriate) can be found in main text under pathology.

General standing posture and asymmetries should be noted.

The spine should be observed from the back to identify scoliosis or any pelvic asymmetries. Hip creases, knee creases, and shoulder height should be looked at.

Bony and muscular asymmetries should be documented. If necessary, sitting and running posture should also be evaluated for any functional indiscrepencies.

Spinal Examination

The active range of motion of the spine (lumbar, thoracic, and cervical) should be examined. Passive overpressure should be applied to assess end feel for excessive or restricted movements (see Fig. 2.2). Again, this can be diagnostic and useful for benchmarking purposes. In a neurological examination, straight leg raise, slump test, and tests of dermatomes and myotomes of upper and lower limbs are done along with checking of reflexes. (See Fig 2.4.)

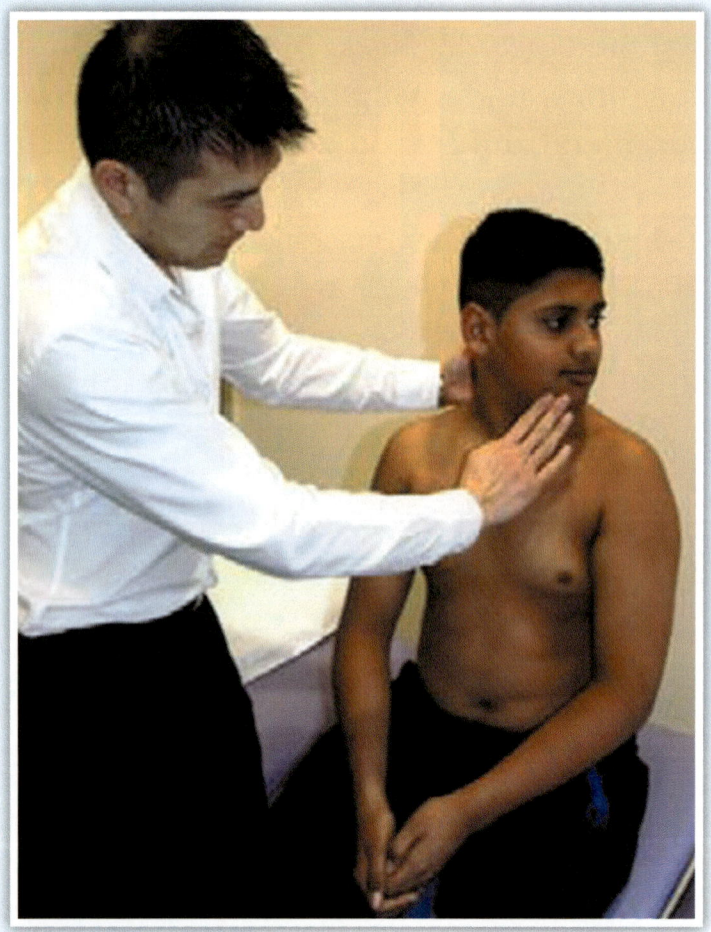

Fig. 2.4 Examination of the cervical spine

Palpation of the spinous process, transverse process should be performed and muscle tone assessed. Individual spinal tests can be done on a case-by-case basis, depending on the results of the subjective examination.

Some of these tests are discussed in the text under the different pathologies.

Specific traction apophyseal regions (see traction apophysitis) and any specific regional osteochondritis juvenilis (see osteochondritis juvenilis) should be palpated and assessed.

Shoulder Examination

This should involve active range in flexion, abduction, elevation, rotation (medial and lateral), adduction, and combined movements (see Fig. 2.5). End feel movements (with passive overpressures) should be looked at for instability or stiffness. Resisted movements should be conducted for strength testing as well as for pathology. The acromioclavicular (AC) joint, sternoclavicular joint, glenohumeral joint (tuberosities), subacromial joint (lateral edge of acromio-humeral joint), and the specific ligaments should be palpated and tested for pain, sensitivity, apprehension, and stiffness.

Specific tests for individual pathologies may be found under the sections dealing with different pathologies. Specific traction apophyseal regions (see traction apophysitis) and any specific regional osteochondritis juvenilis (see osteochondritis juvenilis) should be palpated and assessed. All readings should be recorded for benchmarking, comparing left to right.

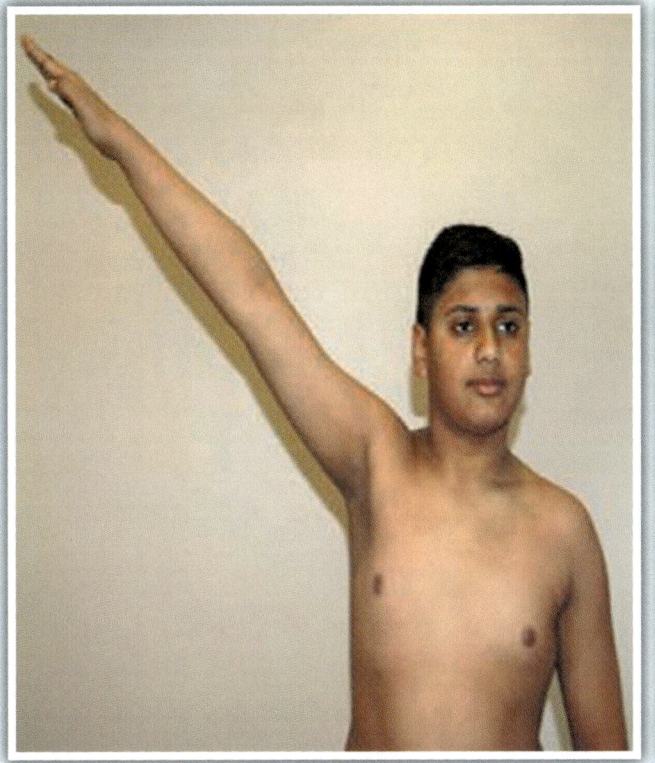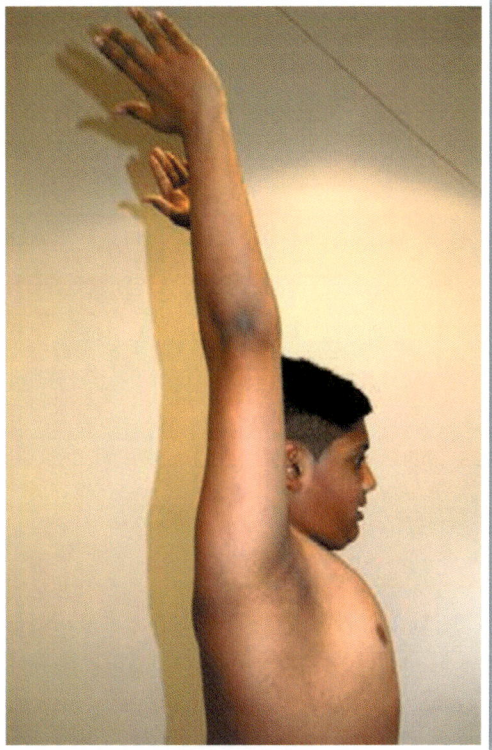

Fig. 2.5 Examination of shoulder

Elbow Examination

This should involve active and passive (with overpressures) flexion, extension, supination, and pronation. Resisted movement tests should be conducted for evaluating the patient's strength as well as for pathology. The lateral epicondyle, medial epicondyle, radial head, radiohumeral joint, and the shaft of radius and ulnar and distal humerus should be palpated and assessed. Specific ligaments should be tested for pain, sensitivity, apprehension, and stiffness.

Specific tests for individual pathologies may be found under the sections dealing with the different pathologies. Specific traction apophyseal regions (see traction apophysitis) and any specific regional osteochondritis juvenilis (see osteochondritis juvenilis) should be palpated and assessed. All readings should be recorded for benchmarking.

Wrist and Hand Examination

This should involve looking at active and passive (with overpressure) movements to include extension, flexion, and ulnar and radial deviation. End feel movements (with passive overpressures) should be looked at for instability or stiffness. Resisted movements should be conducted for strength testing as well as for pathology. Palpation of distal radius and ulnar, scaphoid, lunate, hamate, and all carpal and metacarpal bones should be done. All joints should be looked at for pain, sensitivity, apprehension, and stiffness in specific ligaments.

Specific tests for individual pathologies may be found under the sections dealing with the different pathologies. Specific traction apophyseal regions (see traction apophysitis) and any specific regional osteochondritis juvenilis (see osteochondritis juvenilis) should be palpated and assessed. All readings should be recorded for benchmarking.

Hip Joint Examination

This should involve testing for active range of motion in hip flexion, adduction, abduction, extension, medial and lateral rotation, and circumduction. End feel movements (with passive overpressures) should be looked at for instability or stiffness. Resisted movements should be conducted for strength testing as well as for pathology. Palpation of the hip joint itself, trochanteric area, traction aphophyseal areas (see pathology sections), and individual muscles should be done.

Specific tests for individual pathologies may be found under the sections dealing with the different pathologies. Specific traction apophyseal regions (see traction apophysitis) and any specific regional osteochondritis juvenilis (see osteochondritis juvenilis) should be palpated and assessed. All readings should be recorded for benchmarking.

Knee Examination

This should involve active and passive range of motion in flexion and extension and medial and lateral rotation of the knee joint. The superior tibiofibular joint should also be examined for pain or hypermobility. Also, check range of motion of patella, medial and lateral glide, and inferior and superior glide. Where necessary, passive overpessures should be applied for instability or stiffness issues. Resisted movements should be conducted for strength testing as well as for pathology. The knee joint, femoral condyles, medial and lateral ligaments, distal femur, patella, and joint lines should be palpated and assessed.

Specific tests for individual pathologies may be found under the sections dealing with the different pathologies. Specific traction apophyseal regions (see traction apophysitis) and any specific regional osteochondritis juvenilis (see osteochondritis juvenilis) should be palpated and assessed. All readings should be recorded for benchmarking.

Ankle examination

This should involve active and passive range of motion in plantarflexion, dorsiflexion, inversion, and eversion of the ankle. Where necessary, passive overpessures should be applied for instability or stiffness issues. Resisted movements should be conducted for strength testing as well as for pathology. The ankle joint lines, malleoli, subtalar joint, Achilles insertion, ligaments, and tendons should be palpated and reviewed.

Specific tests for individual pathologies may be found under the sections dealing with the different pathologies. Specific traction apophyseal regions (see traction apophysitis) and any specific regional osteochondritis juvenilis (see osteochondritis juvenilis) should be palpated and assessed. All readings should be recorded for benchmarking.

All joints should be compared bilaterally and should be the same (albeit some strength abnormalities are normally seen on the dominant side of body).

Conclusion

The physical assessment of any child is for guidance only and does not guarantee that the child will never have problems in the future. Obviously, however, if any faults are revealed, and subsequently confirmed and managed appropriately, then this may play a preventative role and highlight potential issues that may require continual assessment.

Key Points

- There is no reliable assessment tool for children's premedical assessment.

- There is no reliable evidence that premedical assessments prevent serious illness/injury.

- Family history is very important to exclude congenital conditions such as heart problems.

References

Birrer. R., Griesemer, B., & Cataleto, M. (2002). *Pediatric sports medicine for primary care* (2nd ed.). Philadelphia, PA: Lippincott Williams & Wilkins.

CHAPTER 3

Traction Apopysitis in Children and Adolescent Sport

Solomon Abrahams

Definition

Apophysitis occurs at the apophyseal joints; these are the points at which the muscle insertions attach on to an apophysis. An apophysis is a prominent bony outgrowth upon the surface of a bone which the bone does not/has not moved upon e.g. a tuberosity (Kent, 2005). Some authors suggest that traction apophysitis is actually many micro avulsions of the tendon insertion rather than just one traction injury (Soprano & Fuchs, 2007).

Apophysitis happens mostly in adolescents, before the apophyseal joints have ossified and are therefore weaker than the myotendinous unit (Schultz, Houglum, & Perrin, 2010). Apophysitis itself normally remains asymptomatic, but triggers such as excessive activity can exacerbate pain. Research suggests that inflammation itself is minimal, even though this can remain very painful (Birrer, Greisemer, & Cataletto, 2002).

Common areas for this pathology include the tibial tuberosity insertion (Osgood Schlatters) (see Fig. 3.1), patellar tendon (Sinding-Larsen-Johansson) patellar tendon (see Fig. 3.3), Achilles tendon insertion (Severs), hamstring insertion (ischial), anterior inferior iliac spine insertion (rectus), anterior superior iliac spine (sartorius) (see Fig. 3.4), lesser trochanter (iliopsoas), greater trochanter (gluteus maximus), iliac crest (abdominal obliques) (see Fig. 3.2), medial epicondyle (little league pitchers), olecranon (triceps), and various parts of the thorax and lower spine. Once traction or a pull tears the muscle from the bones, an area of ossification is always left behind, which can be seen either later on in life, such as that seen in Osgoods Schlatters (Patel, Greydanus, & Baker, 2009; Shanmugam & Maffuli, 2008).

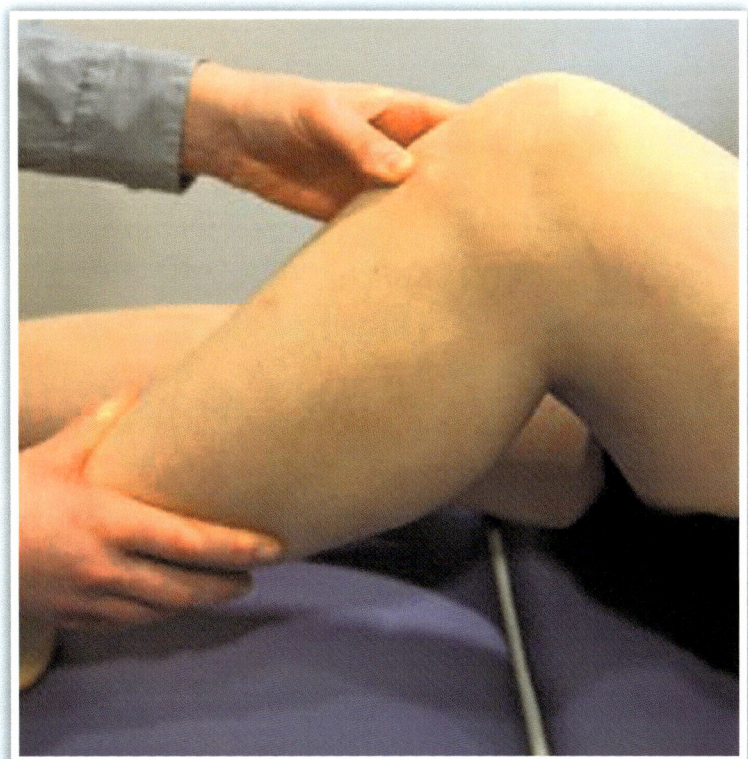

Fig. 3.1 Palpation of the tibial tuberosity to identify Osgood–Schlatter disease

The sports that are mainly involved, but in no way exclusive, are running and kicking sports, such as football, hurdling, gymnastics, and skiing (Carty, 1997).

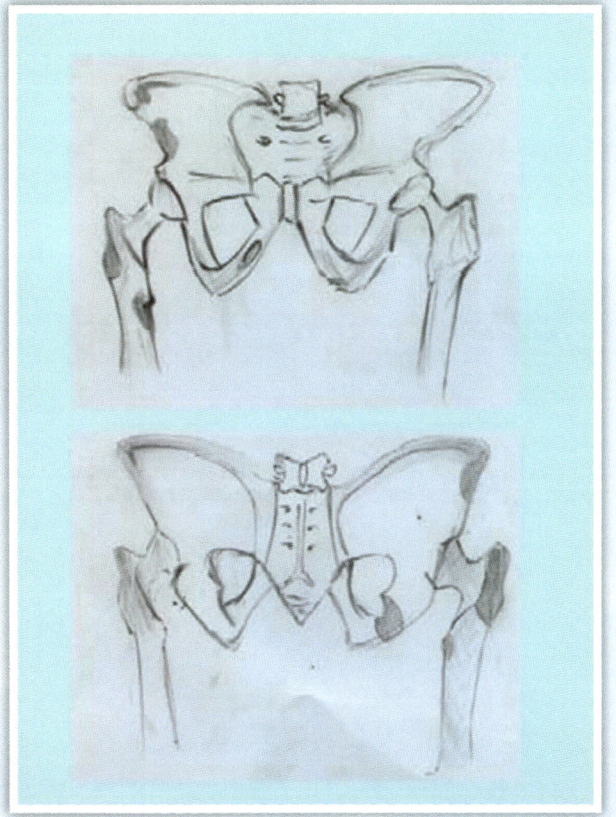

Fig. 3.2 Anterior and posterior pelvis where traction apophysitis can originate from

Cause

Apophysitis is caused by repetitive strain, in the direction of separation (tractioning), upon the apophysis at the area of tendon insertion. If the apophysis is weaker than the connecting muscle pull, then irritation, inflammation, and partial avulsion can occur. Typically, it is caused by repetitive submaximal loading (Wilson & Rodenberg, 2011). For example, the patellar tendon can avulse from its insertion, the tibial tuberosity, from constant kicking movements. Changes in training such as duration, intensity, and frequency can be potential triggers. Change in footwear, camber, type of training can all affect this injury.

Prevalence

Apophysitis occurs mostly in the skeletally immature (Wilson & Rodenberg, 2011), hence most apophyseal injuries occur between the ages of 14 and 20 years. Some authors suggest that it can affect adults until the age of 25 (Patel et al., 2009).

With regard to the ischial apophysis, it is more likely here that avulsion will occur, mainly as the hamstring muscles that attach to it are so strong (Yamamoto et al., 2004). Conversely, apophysitis of the hip flexor insertion on the lesser trochanter is less likely than other forms of apophysitis around the hip and pelvis (Patel et al., 2009).

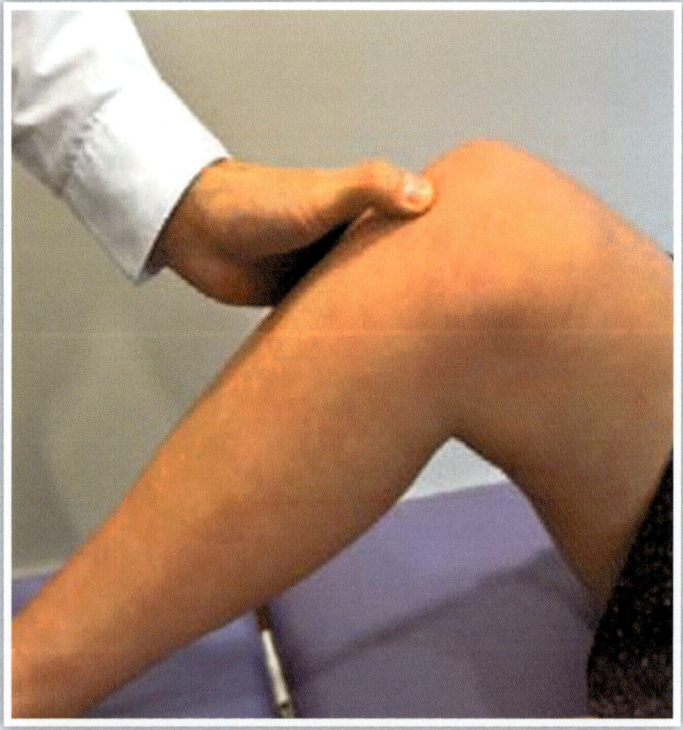

Fig. 3.3 Palpation of the inferior patella where the patellar tendon can avulse from the patella, namely jumpers knee

Signs and Symptoms

A child suffering with apophysitis will present with onset of pain following exercise and will not normally recall a specific reason for the onset.

The signs and symptoms are similar to that of muscle strain. The patient will have point tenderness at the myotendinous insertion; also, enlarged bony prominence and crepitus may be observed (Schultz et al., 2010).

There is a lack of bruising compared with when avulsion occurs; this helps with differentiation between the two pathologies. Pain increases with activity and decreases with rest, and is reproduced by passive stretching of the affected muscle (Wilson & Rodenberg, 2011).

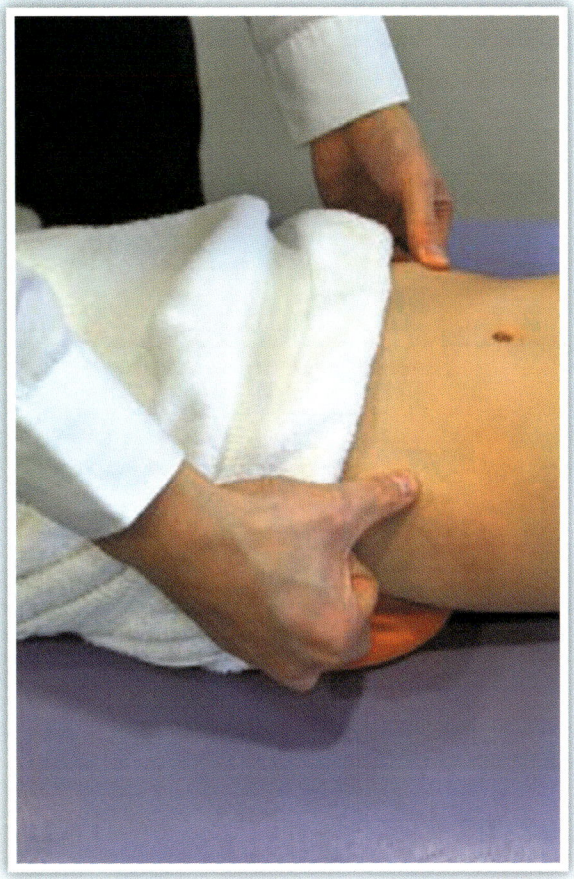

Fig. 3.4 Palpation of bilateral ASIS, traction apophysitis of sartorius tendon

Tests

The main techniques used to diagnose apophysitis are X-rays, CT scans, and MRIs. Diagnostic ultrasound may also be used for diagnosis provided that the technician is skilled enough. Along with these imaging methods, range of motion and manual muscle testing will reproduce pain allowing a therapist to pinpoint the site of injury. (See Fig. 3.5 and Fig. 3.6.)

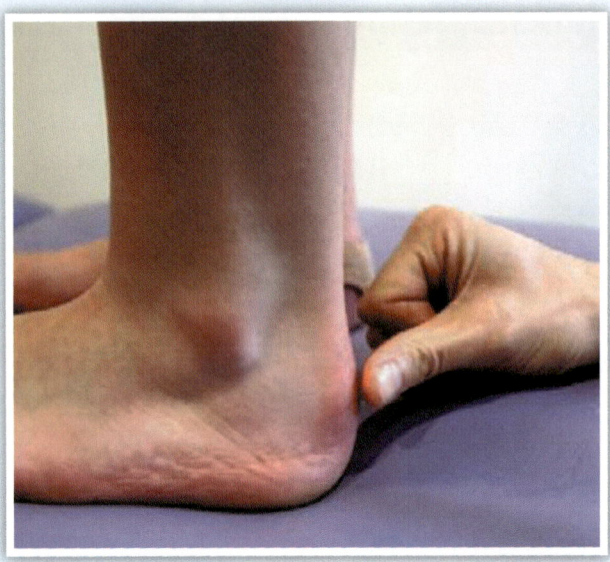

Fig. 3.5 Point tenderness of Sever's disease (Achilltes tendon inserton)

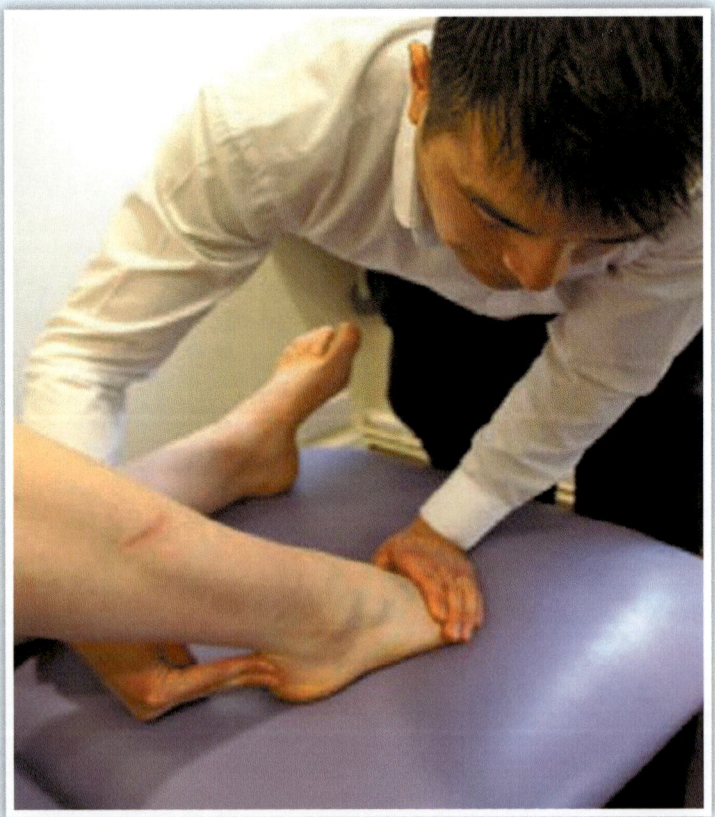

Fig. 3.6 Quick test for Sever's disease with a patient in long sitting

Treatment and Management

Apophysitis is an overuse injury, and the treatment method of it is mostly conservative. In extreme cases, anti-inflammatory drugs may be prescribed to reduce inflammation and allow for pain-free movement, but this should be used sparingly and in severe cases only (Soprano & Fuchs, 2007). Ice and compression can also be used in acute cases.

The basis of overuse injuries are often removed once internal and external factors are corrected. External factors are caused by environmental conditions, for example weather and training/playing surface. Internal factors are physiologically based, for example mal-alignment or muscle strength imbalances (Bahr & Maehlum, 2004).

Activity and training volume should be decreased, because of the cause of the injury being overuse. Work should then be done to decrease predisposing factors such as muscle tightness/strength imbalances and poor loading patterns. Stretching should be done, but only once the pain has fully settled (see Fig. 3.3). Stretching should also be recommended (see Fig. 3.7) on discharge consistently to help prevent reoccurrence. Once these points have been addressed, the child should begin stability and flexibility exercises to improve proprioception and maintain muscle balance.

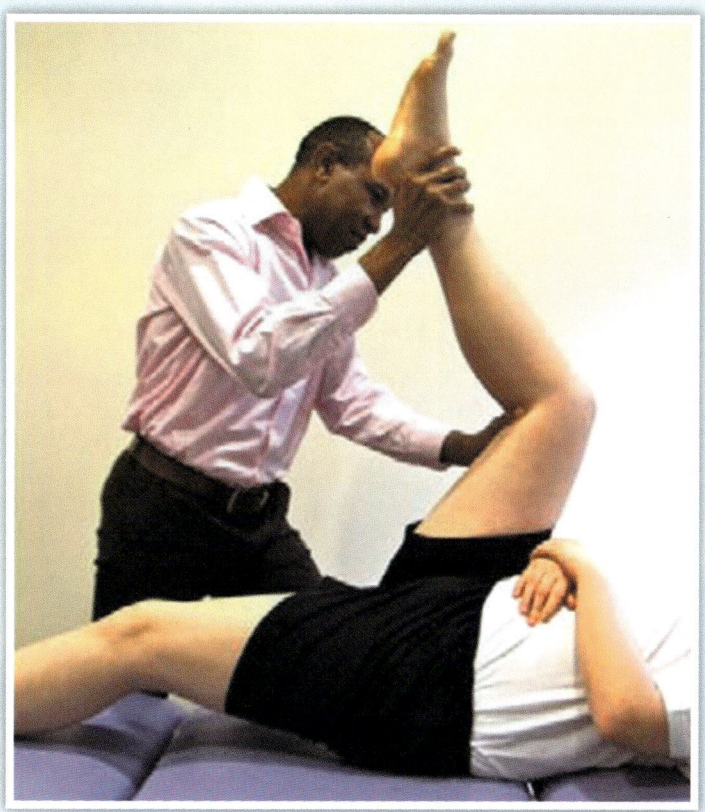

Fig. 3.7 Stetch the upper hamstring only once the pain has fully settled

As the child progresses, loading can be gradually increased to build upon the secondary ossification sites, and finally towards the end stage of rehabilitation, gentle and progressive plyometrics may be introduced to prepare the child for a return to sporting activity (if applicable).

Some authors suggest that if apophysitis doesn't respond to rest or conservative treatment within a few weeks, then alternative diagnosis should be considered. Ogden, Ganey, and Hill (2004) found that some young patients who presented with 'Severs' did not respond to normal conservative treatment. Following MRI scans, they suggest stress fractures to be the pathology which gave the children persistent heel pain. This then required further immobilisation. However, they are not suggesting that an apophysitis is due to stress fractures; more research in this area is currently underway (Soprano & Fuchs, 2007).

Key Points

- Apophysis is weaker than the ligaments of the joint by up to 5 times.
- Avulsion fractures are common from hamstring.
- Most avulsions come from the origin.
- Most are asymptomatic until they are triggered.

References

Adirim, T., & Cheng, T. (2003). Overview of injuries in the young athlete. *Sports Medicine, 33*(1), 75–81.

Bahr, R., & Maehlum, S. (2004). *Clinical guide to sports injuries* (p. 29). Oslo: Gazzette Book.

Birrer, R., Greisemer, B., & Cataletto, M. (2002). *Pediatric sports medicine for primary care* (2nd ed.). Philadelphia, PA: Lippincott Williams & Wilkins.

Carty, H. (1997). Children's sports injuries. *European Journal of Radiology, 26,* 163.

Kent, M. (2005). *Oxford dictionary of sports science and medicine* (3rd ed., p. 48). Oxford: Oxford University Press.

Ogden, J., Ganey, T., & Hill, J. (2004). Severs injury: A stress fracture of the calcaneus metaphysis. *Journal of Orthopaedic Paediatrics,* 24, 5, 55-68.

Patel, D., Greydanus, D., & Baker, R. (2009). *Pediatric practice sports medicine* (2nd ed.). New York, NY: McGraw Hill Medical.

Schultz, S., Houglum, P., & Perrin, D. (2010). *Examination of musculoskeletal injuries* (3rd ed., pp. 453–498). Leeds: Human Kinetics.

Shanmugam, C., & Maffuli, N. (2008) Sports Injuries in Children, British Medical Bulletin, 86; 33-57.

Soprano. J., & Fuchs, J. (2007). Common overuse injuries in the pediatric and adolescent athlete. *Clinical Pediatric Emergency Medicine, 8*(1), 7–14.

Wilson, J., & Rodenberg, R. (2011). Apophysitis of the lower extremities. *Contemporary Pediatrics, 12*(1), 342-390.

Yamamoto, T., et al. (2004). Apophysitis of the ischial tuberosity mimicking a neoplasm on magnetic resonance imaging. *Skeletal Radiology, 33*(12), 737–740.

CHAPTER 4

Osteochondritis Juvenillis in Children and Adolescent Sport

Faye Triggs and Solomon Abrahams

Definition

Osteochondritis is a localised pathological disorder (Edge & Porter, 2011) of subchondral bone and its covering articular cartilage (Ganley, Gaugler, Kocher, Flynn, & Jones, 2006). It is regarded as the separation of a fragment of articular surface (Pudas, Koskinen, Hiltunen, & Mattila, 2012), the bone and the cartilage, either as a lesion, partial break or full break, due to it becoming necrotic tissue (Hefti, 2007). The necrotic tissue may detach from the rest of the bone to become a loose body (Freemont, 2010) and remain within the joint (Hefti, 2007), causing a mechanical disruption. It is most common in the knee joint, but it is also present in the elbow, hand, spine, knee, ankle, and hip (Kulkarni, 2008).

Savoie (2008) has described osteochondritis as an inflammatory condition, but Pudas et al. (2012) disagree, suggesting that no inflammatory cells are present in the disorder.

Osteochondritis is usually seen in an adolescent age range (Bruce, 2012), typically after the age of 10 years (Hefti, 2007). Although the juvenile form can happen in children from the age of 5 up to 15 years (Ganley et al., 2006), this is where the epiphyseal growth plate is open (Edge & Porter, 2011) and the skeleton is deemed immature (Freemont, 2010).

Osteochondritis juvenilis is most commonly seen in physically active children and adolescents (Kramer & Kocher, 2008) and remains the most common cause of a loose body in the sporting adolescent (Edge & Porter, 2011).

Types of Osteochondritis Diseases

Kienbock's disease affects the lunate in the wrist (Desy, Bernstein, Harvey, & Hazel, 2011). The disease causes avascular necrosis which is then followed by the fragmentation of the lunate bone (Kawoosa, Dhar, Mir, & Butt, 2007) and can lead to pain and loss of function in the wrist. Kienbock's disease usually affects the dominant wrist (Yazaki, Nakamura, Nakao, Iwata, Tatebe, & Hattori, 2005).

Freiberg's disease affects the metatarsal heads in the foot (Hefti, 2007). It tends to occur in the second metatarsal (Atanda, Shah, & O'Brien, 2011) but can affect any of the others. It is the only osteochondritis that is found more in females than in males (Capar, Kutluay, & Mujde, 2007).

Kohler's disease is an osteochondritis that affects the navicular bone in the foot (Freemont, 2010). It frequently affects 4–9-year-olds (Tarrago et al., 2011).

Legg–Calvé–Perthes affects the femoral head and is an avascular necrosis of the head of the femur which causes flattening of the superior surface.

Scheuermann's disease is a common cause of thoracic back pain (Atanda et al., 2011) in children and adolescents and has been defined as a rigid kyphosis or humpback deformity (Weiss, Turnbull, & Bohr, 2009). It is a disorder affecting the ring apophysis of the vertebral body next to the vertebral disc (Freemont, 2010). Scheuermann's disease has been estimated to affect 1–8% of the population (Damborg, Engell, Nielsen, Kyvik, Andersen, et al., 2011).

Specific areas of osteochondritis will be discussed in more detail under the relevant anatomical regions of the body.

Causes

There have been many causes linked to osteochondritis; athletic activity (Bruce, 2012), microtrauma produced by repetitive forces (Mihara, Tsutsui, Nishinaka, & Yamaguchi, 2009), overuse (Fleisher & Ludwig, 2010), genetics (Hefti, 2007), disruption of the vascular supply (El Hajj, Sebaaly, Kharrat, & Ghanem, 2012) which can cause ischemic necrosis (Kulkarni, 2008), and abnormal ossification (Fleisher & Ludwig, 2010). The most common cause in general literature does point to some kind of avascular necrosis. Stanitski, Delee, and Drez (1994) suggest the vascular supply to the physis is crucial, and any impediment of this will close the plates prematurely, leading to a complete avascular necrosis.

Previous injury has also been reported in 40% of patients (Kulkarni, 2008). Freiberg disease can also be caused by improper shoewear (Atanda et al., 2011), and Kienbock's disease can be caused by faulty biomechanics at the radiocarpal joint (Desy et al., 2011).

Prevalence

Osteochondritis occurs in approximately 250 people per million of the population, and around 75% of the affected are from the juvenile population (Freemont, 2010). It occurs in 5–15-year-olds with open growth plates (Ganley et al., 2006). It is less prevalent in children under 10 (Edge & Porter, 2011).

Kramer and Kocher (2008) stated that juvenile osteochondritis occurred in 15–29 cases per 100,000 physically active children. Boughanem, Riaz, Patel, and Sarwark (2011) quoted a study by Lindén that identified the prevalence to be 18 in 100,000 in females and 29 in 100,000 in males. Although, Edge said that the prevalence of osteochondritis of the knee is estimated as 3 to 6 cases per 10,000 adult population (Edge & Porter, 2011). Osteochondritis juvenilis affects both males and females in a 2–3:1 ratio (Edge & Porter, 2011).

Osteochondritis can affect any synovial joint; the knee is the most commonly involved joint in about 70% of cases, followed by the capitellum of the humerus at the elbow in around 6% of cases, and the superior articular surface of the talus in 4% of cases (Freemont, 2010).

Pathophysiology

There is a tendency for the convex surfaces of joints to be affected by this disease, particularly load-bearing joints like the knee (Bruce, 2012), or joints that frequently have a strong weight through it.

Although the articular surface of a joint can be affected by osteochondritis (Bruce, 2012), this involves a process of events that includes the softening of the articular cartilage with an intact articular surface (Boughanem et al., 2011) which then leads to the early articular cartilage separation (Edge &

Porter, 2011), and if forceful activity is continued, partial detachment of the articular lesion may occur (Ganley et al., 2006), followed by complete separation with loose body formation (Fleisher & Ludwig, 2010).

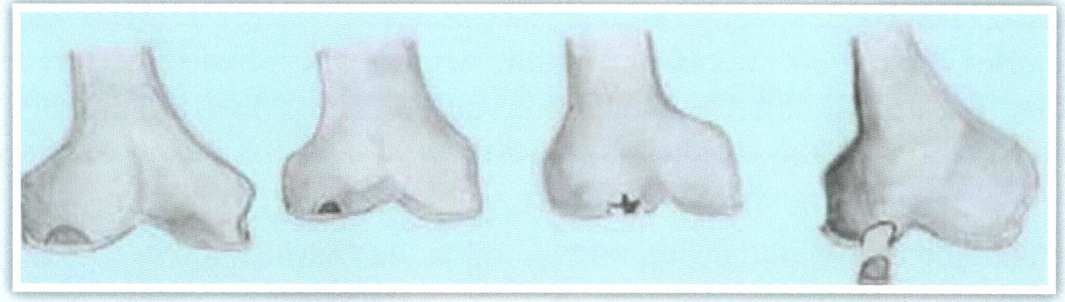

Fig. 4.1 Diagram of osteochondral fragment becomes loose during avascular nercrosis

The partially separated fragment becomes avascular and may form a loose body within the joint, causing pain and maybe inflammation (Edge & Porter, 2011) (see Fig. 4.1). The failure of revascularisation then leads to subchondral bone and articular cartilage degeneration (Boughanem et al., 2011). Since the arteries supplying blood to the subchondral bone are end arteries, the necrotic bone is effectively an infarct in the distribution of one or a small number of end arteries (Freemont, 2010). If left untreated, osteochondritis can lead to the development of degenerative arthritis secondary to joint incongruency and abnormal wear patterns (Edge & Porter, 2011).

The classification of osteochondritis can be based on age, location of lesion, and radiographic and MRI findings (Boughanem et al., 2011).

Grade 1 is a lesion with a continuous but softened area covered by intact cartilage.

Grade 2 is a lesion with partial discontinuity of articular surface.

Grade 3 is a complete discontinuity of articular surface but fragment is not yet dislocated.

Grade 4 is an empty defect with loose fragment in joint or loose within bed (Bruce, 2012).

Signs and Symptoms

Symptoms develop gradually over several months (Fleisher & Ludwig, 2010); there may be mild aching after activity, and the signs will worsen slowly over time (Savoie,

2008). The joint will become tender (Ganley et al., 2006), the pain may radiate (DiGiovanna, Schiowitz, & Dowling, 2005), range of motion may be limited (El Hajj et al., 2012), and the joint may swell (Fleisher & Ludwig, 2010).

As time goes on, the symptoms will usually worsen with physical activity and will improve with rest, although this recovery may take longer as the condition progresses (Bruce, 2012). When there is a presence of a loose or free fragment, the joint may catch, grind (Freemont, 2010), or lock (Edge & Porter, 2011), or it may give the patient a feeling of the joint giving way when loaded (Savoie, 2008).

With Kienbock's disease, there may be pain, stiffness (Desy et al., 2011), and loss of function in the dorsal medial aspect of the wrist (Kawoosa et al., 2007). Kohler's disease will present pain in the midfoot and the medial foot, and the patient may also limp (Atanda et al., 2011). Freiberg's condition could show pain in the forefoot (Atanda et al., 2011) and restricted movement, specifically extension, due to synovitis (Capar et al., 2007). Patients with Scheuermann's disease will show a painful trunk deformity of an excessive thoracic kyphosis (Summers, Singh, & Manns, 2008), where there might be compensation in the lumbar and cervical spine (Weiss et al., 2009).

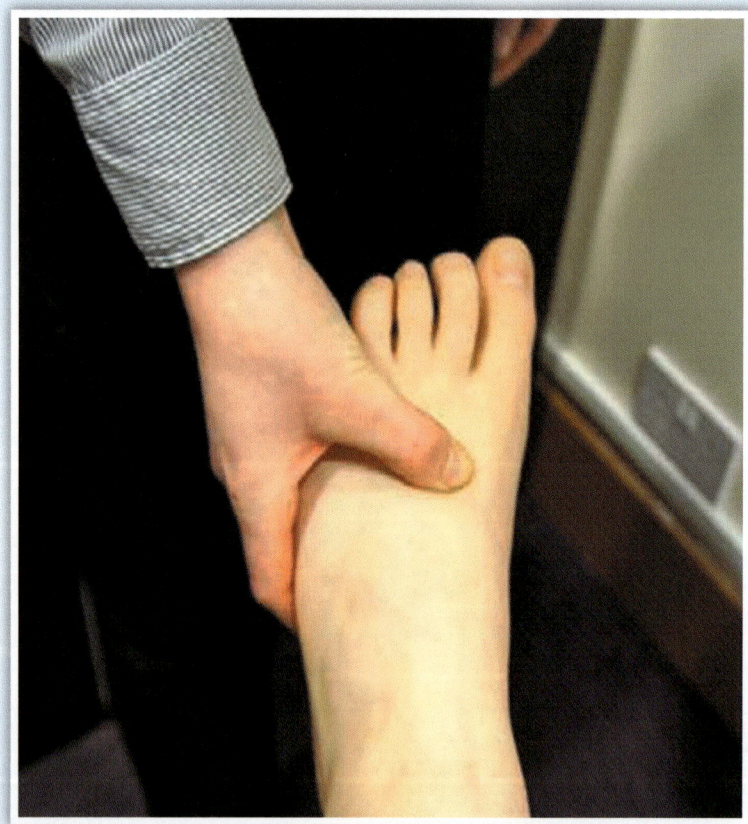

Fig. 4.2 Palpation of second metatarsal (Freibergs)

Diagnosis

Diagnosis is mainly made by X-rays (Hefti, 2007) and MRI (Kramer & Kocher, 2008) scans after a physical exam. Other diagnostic imaging options are radiographs, MR arthrography, and technetium bone scans (Ganley et al., 2006). During the physical exam, the clinicians should listen to the patient for the signs and symptoms mentioned above; they should then feel for pain and tenderness along the joint line (Kramer & Kocher, 2008) and swelling, and if the condition is in the advanced stage, the clinician may be able to palpate the loose body within the joint. Normally, the area is sore on direct palpation. (See Fig .4.2.)

The physical examination of Scheuermann's disease shows a humpback deformity that does not correct with back extension (Atanda et al., 2011).

Treatment

The type of treatment used depends on the patient's age and the size, joint alignment, the nature of the lesion, stability, and size of the osteochondral fragment (Freemont, 2010).

A grade 1 lesion is stable, and the treatment used is non-operative. Grade 2, 3, and 4 are classed as unstable, where operative treatment options may be arguably included (Bruce, 2012).

Non-operative

Temporary relief can be achieved from non-steroidal anti-inflammatory medication (Savoie, 2008) and icing the affected joint (Morrey & Sanchez-Sotelo, 2009). The patient would be advised to rest, reduce physical activity (Hefti, 2007), and even restrict weight bearing (Boughanem et al., 2011). Bracing (Kramer & Kocher, 2008) and immobilisation (Freemont, 2010), where the patient uses crutches to walk for up to 8 to 10 weeks (Kulkarni, 2008), would help limit activity (Morrey & Sanchez-Sotelo, 2009) and promote healing in the lower limb.

Rest and limited weight bearing prevent repetitive forces (Kramer & Kocher, 2008) on the articular cartilage and bone and stop it from softening. This works better for juveniles as the disturbed bone will revascularise (Freemont, 2010) and prevent further damage. Prolonged immobilisation is not recommended as it will lead to muscle atrophy (Freemont, 2010).

Physiotherapy is used to recover range of motion (Edge & Porter, 2011), and additional active and passive movements such as flexion and extension exercises can be used (Freemont, 2010) and eventually resisted exercises where strength around the joint can be improved (Edge & Porter, 2011). The motion of the joint aids in articular cartilage nutrition (Kramer & Kocher, 2008).

The duration of non-operative treatment can range from 3 months (Boughanem et al., 2011) to 18 months (Kramer & Kocher, 2008), but it has been said that the juvenile can take 10–18 months to heal (Brown & Neumann, 2004).

Osteochondritis juvenilis is generally managed with non-operative treatment as studies have shown that 50% of juvenile cases show spontaneous healing (Ganley et al., 2006), especially with joint immobilisation (Edge & Porter, 2011) combined with daily range of motion exercises (Freemont, 2010).

Initial management of Scheuermann's disease includes physiotherapy for postural improvement, with emphasis on hamstring, pectorals stretching, and trunk extensor strengthening as well as improving function (Polousky, 2011). Bracing of the spine in patients may also be required (Weiss et al., 2009).

Freiberg disease can be treated using orthotics (Capar et al., 2007) and metatarsal pads (Atanda et al., 2011).

Operative

Operative treatments are used for patients with detached lesions (Ganley et al., 2006), those approaching epiphyseal closure (Boughanem et al., 2011), and those who have not responded to non-operative treatment (Kramer & Kocher, 2008). The type of surgery depends on the type and grade of lesion (Boughanem et al., 2011). The goal of the procedure is to secure or remove loose fragments and support and restore bone and articular cartilage healing (Ganley et al., 2006).

Type of operations include drilling to expose bone marrow (Freemont, 2010), bone grafting (Boughanem et al., 2011), removal of fragment (Bruce, 2012), and reconstruction and internal fixation of the articular surface (Bruce, 2012). Operations are usually successful in 85% of cases over the short term (Freemont, 2010).

Rehabilitation

After operative treatment, the joint is placed into a brace and made non-weight-bearing; physiotherapy is started 2 weeks after surgery, and the range of motion is limited for the first 6 weeks. This is also when the brace comes off and full range of the joint is allowed. At 12 weeks, the patient is allowed to gradually return to sport. Radiographs are obtained to document healing (Kramer & Kocher, 2008).

Conclusion

Osteochrondritis can remain asymptomatic for some time but should never be underestimated due to the prognosis.

Suspicion should always be there if any pain develops at these particular areas in a child or teen until proven otherwise.

Key Points

- Osteochondritis can affect 5–15-year-olds.

- It is common in knees of youth as loose bodies.

- Freibergs is the only osteochondritis more common in females.

- Most osteochondritis remain asymptomatic until triggered.

- It can affect elbows and the humerus.

References

Atanda, A., Shah, S. A., & O'Brien, K. (2011). Osteochondritis: Common causes of pain in growing bones. *American Family Physician, 83*(3), 285–291.

Boughanem, J., Riaz, R., Patel, R. M., & Sarwark, J. F. (2011). Functional and radiographic outcomes of juvenile osteochondritis dissecans of the knee treated with extra-articular retrograde drilling. *American Journal of Sports Medicine, 39*(10), 2212–2217.

Brown, D. E., & Neumann, R. D. (2004). *Orthopedic secrets* (3rd ed., p. 349). Philadelphia, PA: Hanley & Belfus.

Bruce, C. E. (2012). *Operative elbow surgery* (pp. 223–230). Oxford: Elsevier.

Capar, B., Kutluay, E., & Mujde, S. (2007). Dorsal closing-wedge osteotomy in the treatment of Freiberg's disease. *Acta Orthopadeica et Traumatologica Turcica, 41*(2), 136–139.

Damborg, F., Engell, V., Nielsen, J., Kyvik, K. O., Andersen, M. O., & Thomsen, K. (2011). Genetic epidemiology of Scheuermann's disease: Heritability and prevalence over a 50-year period. *Acta Orthopaedica, 82*(5), 602–605.

Desy, N. M., Bernstein, M, Harvey, E. J., & Hazel, E. (2011). Kienbock's disease and juvenile idiopathic arthritis. *McGill Journal of Medicine, 13*(2), 8–13.

DiGiovanna, E. L., Schiowitz, S., & Dowling, D. J. (2005). *An osteopathic approach to diagnosis and treatment* (3rd ed., p. 538). Philadelphia, PA: Lippincott Williams & Wilkins.

Edge, A., & Porter, K. (2011). Osteochondritis dissecans: A review. *Trauma, 13*(1), 23–33.

El Hajj, F., Sebaaly, A., Kharrat, K., & Ghanem, I. (2012). Osteochondritis of the distal tibial epiphysis. *Case Reports in Medicine, 2012*(1), 1–7.

Fleisher, G. R., & Ludwig, S. (2010). *Textbook of pediatric emergency medicine* (6th ed., pp. 1581–1583). Philadelphia, PA: Lippincott Williams & Wilkins.

Freemont, T. (2010). Osteochondritis. *Orthopaedics and Trauma, 24*(6), 410–415.

Ganley, T. J., Gaugler, R. L., Kocher, M. S., Flynn, J. M., & Jones, K. J. (2006).

Osteochondritis dissecans of the knee. *Operative Techniques in Sports Medicine, 14*(3), 147–158.

Hefti, F. (2007). *Pediatric orthopedics in practice* (pp. 294–297). Berlin: Springer.

Kawoosa, A. A., Dhar, S. A., Mir, M. R., and Butt, M. F. (2007). Distraction osteogenesis for ulnar lengthening in Kienbock's disease. *International Orthopaedics, 31*(3), 339–344.

Kramer, D. E., & Kocher, M. S. (2008). Juvenile osteochondritis dissecans of the knee. *Operative Techniques in Sports Medicine, 16*(2), 70–76.

Kulkarni, G. S. (2008). *Textbook of orthopaedics & trauma* (Vol. 4, 2nd ed., pp. 2994–2997). New Delhi: Jaypee Brothers Medical Publishers.

Mihara, K., Tsutsui, H., Nishinaka, N., & Yamaguchi, K. (2009). Nonoperative treatment for osteochondritis dissecans of the capitellum. *American Journal of Sports Medicine, 37*(2), 298–304.

Morrey, B. F., & Sanchez-Sotelo, J. (2009). *The elbow and its disorders* (4th ed., pp. 288–295). St. Louis, MO: Saunders Elsevier.

Polousky, J. D. (2011). Juvenile osteochondritis dissecans. *Sports Medicine & Arthroscopy Review, 19*(1), 56–63.

Pudas, T., Koskinen, S. K., Hiltunen, A., & Mattila, K. T. (2012). Osteochondritis dissecans of the humeral capitellum in identical twins. *Acta Radiologica Short Reports, 1*(7), 1–3.

Savoie, F. H. (2008). Osteochondritis dissecans of the elbow. *Operative Techniques in Sports Medicine, 16*(4), 187–193.

Stanitski, C., Delee, J., & Drez, D. (1994). *Pediatric and adolescent sports medicine* (3rd ed.). Philadelphia, PA: W. B. Saunders.

Summers, B. N., Singh, J. P., and Manns, R. A. (2008). The radiological reporting of lumbar Scheuermann's disease: An unnecessary source of confusion amongst clinicians and patients. *British Journal of Radiology, 81*(965), 383–385.

Tarrago, A., Yebra, J., Steiner, M., Bonsfills, N., Albillos, J. C., Sanchez, A., Cid, L., & Canete, A. (2011). Kohler's disease secondary to tarsal pyogenic arthritis. *International Journal of Clinical Medicine, 2*(5), 633–635.

Weiss, H-R., Turnbull, D., & Bohr, S. (2009). Brace treatment for patients with Scheuermann's disease – A review of the literature and first experiences with a new brace design. *Scoliosis, 4*(22), 1–17.

Yazaki, N., Nakamura, R., Nakao, E., Iwata, Y., Tatebe, M., & Hattori, T. (2005). Bilateral Kienböck's disease. *Journal of Hand Surgery, 30*(2), 133–136.

CHAPTER 5

Spinal Pathologies in Children and Adolescent Sport

Solomon Abrahams

Neck injuries

Introduction

Injuries to the neck are always of concern when it comes to children. A child's lack of fine motor control and weak neck muscles relative to the superior weight of the head makes the neck a rather vulnerable area in the developing child.

Because the child is constantly developing until the age of 18 years, the neck (cervical spine) also undergoes fundamental changes which can depict the type of injuries commonly seen.

Spinal injuries in children are surprisingly high – as many as 75% of all sports injuries seen within the Accident and Emergency Department. These may be soft-tissue-related or a serious, spinal pathology (Birrer, Greisemer, & Cataletto, 2002).

In general, children under the age of 8 years rarely sustain neck injuries or neck problems (Stanitski, DeLee, & Drez, 1994).

Anatomy and Physiology

The cervical spine in children is different from that in adults due to the nature of its immature bone development, immature muscle development, and its increased range of motion. In very early childhood, normally below the age of 1 year, most of the bones are non-ossified. However, from 3 to 8 years, progressive ossification of the bones occurs posteriorly and then moves anteriorly (Carty, 1997).

By the age of 6 years, the internal diameter of the spinal canal, which encases the spinal cord, is fully developed. The angulation of the facet joints in the upper cervical spine undergo vast changes compared with the lower cervical spine. This can sometimes, in children, lead to occasional pseudosubluxation and potentially pseudolocking of the upper cervical spine. Segments commonly problematic include C2, C3, and C4 in this age group (Birrer et al., 2002). This is common and should not be treated as pathologic; rather the ever-changing and evolving spine seen in children.

Cervical flexion in children originates from the upper cervical spine before the age of 8, when there is greatest range of motion and when the ligaments are highly extensible. As the child grows older, range of motion in flexion is distributed lower, to the lower cervical spine.

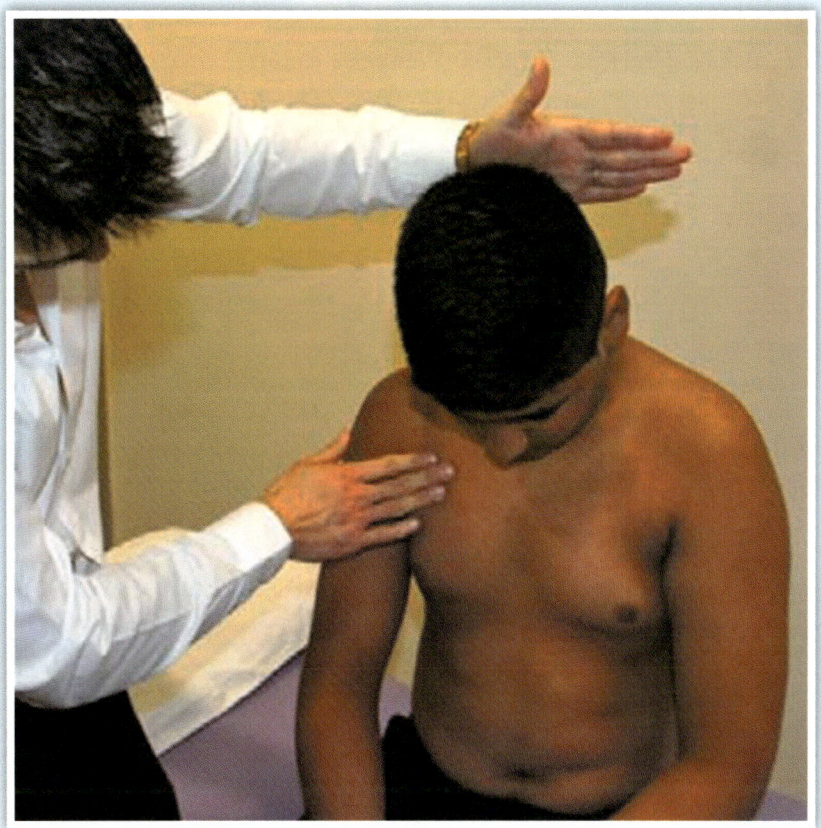

Fig. 5.1 Cervical flexion in a child

Even though the ligaments are highly extensible at this age, where the joints can stretch an extra 5 cm without injury, the spinal cord at this age remains fragile and rather inflexible, only allowing 0.64 cm of movement; hence, it is more likely to be injured during hyperflexion/hyperextension movements (Birrer et al., 2002).

When the neck is in 30 degrees of flexion (see Fig. 5.1), it becomes a straight segmented column. Axial pressures at this angle places full force down the spine, rather than the normal extension position it holds in standing (Stanitski et al., 1994).

The vertebral discs in children up to 12 years are enormously water-filled and hydrated compared with adults and even late teens. Because of the high water and collagen content, and hence in some part the spine's hyperflexibility, the forces transmitted up and down the spine at this early age are normally unremarkable. However, as the child enters teens, the water content and collagen slowly begin to decrease, which may explain why some endplate fractures and increase in Schmorl's nodes can be seen in this age group. It may also explain why more osseous injuries are also seen in the older teens (Wilberger, 1998).

As the child progresses to 12 years, the cervical spine exhibits movements similar to that of an adult; hence, more flexion occurs at lower cervical spine levels, C5 and C6.

As with adults, injuries at levels above C4, should be treated seriously and as an emergency if necessary due to the nerve supply involved in respiration. Below this level, spinal cord involvement affects the upper limbs as seen in adults. Lesions of individual nerves can give unilateral symptoms, bilateral symptoms, sensory loss, motor loss, and pain.

The nerves from C5 to T1 combine to form the brachial plexus in children, and whilst injuries to these nerves are rare, they are always of concern due to potential long-term disability. As in adults, children's nerves are thought to repair very slowly, at a rate of 1 mm per day (Birrer et al., 2002).

Sensory nerve distribution in children is similar to adults. C5 (predominantly the auxillary nerve) supplies the lateral aspect of the upper arm. C6 supplies sensation to the lower arm and some parts of the hand as it innervates the thumb, index finger, and radial portion of the middle finger. C7 supplies part of the middle finger, via the radial nerve. C8 supplies the ringer finger and parts of the little finger, and finally, T1 supplies most of the medial arm via the branch of the medial brachial cutaneous nerve (Moore, 1992).

The motor nerves are similar again to that seen in adults. C5 normally supplies the deltoid muscle and some of the biceps. C6 motor nerve supplies the bicep muscle and some of the wrist extensors. C7 motor nerve can be tested with triceps, wrist flexors, and finger extension. C8 can be tested resisting the small interossei muscles and finger flexors, whilst T1 tests finger abduction (Moore, 1992).

Hyperflexion is the most common mechanism of injury seen in children's sports. This can result in wedge fractures of the vertebral body, avulsion fractures of the body, and spondylolysis (fracture of the pars inticularis) and spondylolisthesis (slippage of vertebral body). The most common site it affects is C5 and C6, especially in the older child. Damage can also be seen at the posterior soft-tissue structures such as the posterior longitudinal ligament and interspinous ligaments and facet joint ligaments (Birrer et al., 2002). Diving, rugby, wrestling, gymnastics, martial arts, and football are common sports where an injury like this can occur.

Hyperextension injuries normally result in damage to the anterior portion of the child's cervical spine. Damage to the anterior longitudinal ligament as well as to all the connective tissue surrounding the spine is common. The anterior muscles of the neck are normally weaker in the child compared with the posterior neck muscles, and apart from the facet joints blocking further hyperextension, nothing else of significance blocks excessive movement. This normally results in more serious injury compared with hyperflexion, and fractures (until proven otherwise) as well as nerve damage should always be suspected (Birrer et al., 2002).

Contusions

Contusions of the child's neck remain rare, but they are more common in certain sports such as rugby, cricket, and martial arts. They are normally direct blows from an object such as a ball, an arm, or a flying object.

Contusions anteriorly can affect the larynx, cricoid, thyroid and upper airway causing distress, panic, and pain. This injury causes haemorrhage and oedema, which can cause a choking-like symptom which can be very scary to the child and his/her parents (Patel, Greydanus, & Baker, 2009).

Airway obstruction should always be treated as an emergency, and ensuring a clear airway should always be the priority. Ice should always be applied, as with any soft-tissue contusion, to reduce further bleeding and improve prognosis.

Any contusion to the anterior neck should be treated as a head injury, due to potential damage of the veterbral artery, discussed later (Birrer et al., 2002).

Contusions posteriorly can also be quite alarming. Cord concussion can occur, causing temporary paralysis (motor and sensory), but normally full recovery does occur within a few days. Any child with this should be sent to hospital immediately to also exclude other potential damage including fractures of the spinous process (which would be particularly painful on palpation).

Contusions rarely cause spinal cord damage unless followed by hyperflexion or hyperextension. Children's spines are normally very pliable and flexible, unlike the spinal cord.

Strain and Sprains

Strains and sprains of the neck are common in children's sports. A larger and heavier head in proportion to body size, weak neck muscles, and poor technique are some examples of vulnerability.

Any form of hyperflexion or hyperextension injury can cause soft-tissue injury, as discussed in the introduction earlier. Damage to the child's ligaments, joints, and muscles can occur, and if the injury is violent, nerve damage and spinal cord damage can also be present. However, spinal cord damage remains rare in children due to flexibility and elasticity of the spinal segments.

There will always be a mechanism of injury in these children, and injuries like these normally take 6 weeks to repair. Strains and sprains are graded according to their severity (Patel et al., 2009).

Grade 1 Strain

The most common strain of the child's neck remains a grade 1 strain – less than 30% disruption of the soft tissues. This normally causes pain but movement is within 75% of normal, with no neurological signs/symptoms, and function is not normally affected to any great restriction (Stanitski et al., 1994).

These injuries should be treated initially with ice (followed by heat after 24 hours), analgesics where necessary, and advice to try and keep the neck moving within pain-free range. As with any injury to the neck, the parents should be present when giving advice, warning them to visit their general practitioner or family physician if symptoms worsen or last more than a week.

Grade 2 Strain

Grade 2 strains (30–70%) tend to be less common but more serious. Pain in the neck, moderate restriction in movement, and more neck spasm is common. Children (and of course depending on the age of the child) tend to be more anxious and scared during episodes like these, so there is also likely to be more apprehension.

Sometimes, the child may exhibit neurological symptoms which can be unilateral or bilateral due to the tethering of soft tissues in proximity to the nerves or resultant oedema of the damage area. Headaches, shoulder pain, and vertigo may accompany the other symptoms, but temporarily only (Birrer et al., 2002). A full neurological examination should be untaken, and any extreme pain or localised tenderness should be further explored for fracture.

These injuries normally cause distress to the child and the parents, and as such, the usage of a soft collar for 48 hours is sometimes warranted and justified. Further reassessment should be considered after a few days to allow initial pain, distress, and spasm to calm down and allow a more thorough assessment. Remembering that the child's spine is hypermobile, instability tests should be considered (discussed later) or any indication of instability (discussed later) should be re-examined and scanned if necessary (Stanitski et al., 1994).

Ice (and eventual heat) and rest for the first few days should be advised, followed by encouragement of movement within pain-free range. Once pain has settled, rehabilitation of the muscles should be encouraged to prevent the atrophy of muscles caused by pain inhibition and immobility.

Return to sport should be encouraged once full range of motion has been re-established and the child is happy to return, in consultation with the parent and coaching staff.

Grade 3 Strain

Grade 3 strains (70% + damage to soft-tissue structures) are the most serious and should be treated like a head injury in the initial stages. For example, if there are any worsening signs including extreme tiredness or more serious symptoms, the patient should be sent for further examination.

Severe pain, severe restriction in movement of the neck, severe spasm of muscle with neurological symptoms are more common. Spinal shock can also be common, indicating damage to the spinal cord rather than complete resection. X-rays/MRI scans should always be considered here due to hyperflexibility of the child's spine, and hence its vulnerability, to exclude fracture, instability, or cord damage.

Initially, these injuries should be collared due to the distress that the child may be in and to comfort the parents. Pain control (analgesics), if necessary, should be considered, along with ice (heat after 24 hours) and encouragement of movement. Emphasis should be placed on the fact that the child should not get too reliant on the collar or immobility of the spine. Children with grade 3+ strains should not return to sport for a minimum of 8–10 weeks following the onset of injury, or unless a scan reveals full recovery. Studies have shown that many of these children are at higher risk for a more extensive injury if they return within an 8–10-week period (Osenbach, 1992).

Infantile Torticollis

Infantile Torticollis or wry neck is spasm of the sternocleidomastoid muscle on one side, causing a tilting and rotation of the neck. This pathology is generally uncommon in the child. The exact cause remains unknown, but sleeping in a bad position can sometimes exacerbate the pathology.

Signs and Symptoms: Pain and stiffness with physical deformity of the neck. Normally tilts to one side. Pain on movement of the neck. Rarely refers (Crawford & Hamblen, 1990).

Test: Clinically, with active and passive range of motion which will be limited in rotation and side flexion.

However X-rays of the neck may exclude other pathology.

Management: Early physiotherapy to gently stretch the neck and heat normally help. If symptoms persist and do not settle within 3 to 4 days, the child should see their general practitioner or family physician.

Fractures and Dislocatons

Fractures and dislocations of the cervical spine in children rarely cause severe neurological pathology due to the increased space in the spinal canal in children, which accommodates displacement and the flexibility of the spine itself.

However, fractures of physis and growth plates should never be underestimated in certain age groups. Whereas the majority of fractures in adults occur in the lower cervical spine, 70% of fractures seen in children and teens normally affect the upper cervical spine, mainly due to the size of the large skull in proportion to the spine (Stanitski et al., 1994).

Fractures of C1 (Jefferson Fracture)

Fractures of C1 in children tend to be rare, but severe axial compression, such as a fall directly on top of the head or a force loaded on to the head can cause a Jefferson fracture. This can happen in gymnastics, rugby, horse riding, and diving.

A Jefferson fracture can simply be a fracture in four places, two anterior and two posterior fractures of the condyles of the atlas C1 bone (Patel et al., 2009). These fractures are very difficult to pick up, but constant neck and occipital pain with limitation in rotation of the neck are good indications. The child may report dizziness and feeling unstable. X-ray and/or CT scan can confirm diagnosis.

Any suspicion of this pathology requires immediate bracing and referral to orthopaedic consult.

Fractures of C2 (Odontoid)

Odontoid fractures in children normally come from a hyperextension of the neck, where the ring of C1 compresses the odontoid process. This is normally a physis fracture of the synchrondrosis (Loder, 1996).

Pain will be quite localised with some residual headache or referred upper-neck-occipital pain. As with any bony fracture, localised tenderness over C2 maybe evident, and not necessarily will there be any indication of instability as one might suspect. Protraction of the chin and deep flexion of the neck can be painful. Open mouth X-ray confirms diagnosis. Any child with this suspected fracture should be immediately immobilised in a hard collar and scanned.

Fractures of Bilateral Pars C2 (Hangman's Fracture)

This is simply a fracture of bilateral pars of C2. Mechanism of injury and symptoms are similar to that of odontoid fractures.

C3 and C4 Fractures

Fractures of C3 and C4 are generally rare in children and are mainly attributed to their positioning within the cervical spine and pathomechanics.

C5 and C6 Fractures

C5 and C6 fractures in children normally result in neurological injury due to the dimensions of the child's spinal cord (Birrer et al., 2002).

C5 is the most commonly fractured vertebrae, and in 10% of all fractures of this bone, a secondary fracture can occur and should not be excluded. These fractures normally require immobilisation and a neurological consult should be considered (Birrer et al., 2002).

C7 Fractures (Clay-Shoveler's Fracture)

C7 fractures are again rare, but clay-shoveler's fracture is an avulsion fracture of the spinous process. Hyperextension of the neck with force is the normal mechanism of injury and normally the aggravator during examination. Neurological pathology is rare and patient normally recovers well with conservative management.

Wedge-Compression Fractures

Wedge-compression fractures of the cervical spine are normally caused by hyperflexion of axial loading. It is a rare pathology not normally seen in the child but is normally a stable fracture and only requires conservative management in most cases. Most of the wedging is anteriorly rather than posteriorly, which can be easily picked up by a competent surgeon on X-ray.

Upper Cervical Spine Dislocations

Upper spine dislocations normally involve the atlantooccipital joint or atlantaxial joint. These are normally very rare and simply involve slippage of the joint in an anterior, posterior, or longitudinal direction.

Anterior dislocations involve forward movement of the cranium on the atlas, and the most common in children is a longitudinal distraction of the cranium on the atlas. Lastly, a posterior dislocation involves posterior displacement of the cranium on the atlas (Birrer et al., 2002).

These pathologies are normally traumatic and violent and normally result in serious prognosis or fatality due to the severity and region of injury.

Lower Cervical Spine Dislocations

(1) Unilateral facet dislocation
Unilateral facet dislocation is normally caused by axial loading combined with rotation and flexion. A fall within a rugby scrum or a diving injury can be an example. Normally, the shift causes compression within the vertebrae foramen and can be associated with fractures of the facet itself. Neurological deficit can be a sign, and the child's neck cannot normally move due to intense spasm of muscle (Birrer et al., 2002). In fact, any child who is unable to move their neck following trauma should be X-rayed to exclude fracture.

(2) Bilateral facet dislocations
Bilateral facet dislocations tend to be more unstable with damage to the spinal cord more likely as the slippage tends to be more intense. These require surgery to stabilise the spine to prevent further damage to the spinal cord. Symptoms and mechanism are similar to unilateral facet dislocation (Birrer et al., 2002).

Neurological Injuries in the Cervical Spine

There are three distinct classifications of nerve injuries (excluding spinal cord) in children.

First-degree nerve damage or neuropraxia is reversible, and even though it affects the motor nerves, functionality is normally restored within 2–3 weeks of initial trauma.

Second-degree injury is axonotmesis and involves severe disruption of the axon of the nerve and surrounding myelin (Birrer et al., 2002). Sensory and motor nerves are normally affected, and within 72 hours of trauma, the most distal motor nerve normally loses its function.

Third-degree nerve damage is the most severe, and because of disruption to the endoneurium, functional regeneration of the nerve is not likely. Damage to the epineurium and perineurium can, with sufficient time and rehabilitation can be helped, but damage to the endoneurium normally is irreversible (Patel et al., 2009).

The rate of nerve repair in children is not too dissimilar to that of adults, albeit it is at a slightly higher speed at 1 mm per day. Nerve conduction tests should always be considered with any potential nerve damage to ascertain the severity of nerve damage and likely prognosis (Birrer et al., 2002).

Spinal Shock

Spinal shock is a 'concussion' of the spinal cord following trauma. Normally, symptoms can last up to 48 hours, and eventually, movement and/ or sensory deficit is restored.

Prognosis of spinal shock in the initial stages is difficult to determine until a full MRI/CT scan has been done to see the extent of the damage. Motor and sensory weakness is common with absent reflexes. The shock could be due to the swelling within the spinal canal following the initial trauma; hence it is prudent to wait 48 hours to determine full prognosis.

Spinal Cord Damage

Spinal cord damage can be very distressing to all concerned. Normally, there is motor and sensory loss in the affected dermatomes and myotomes. Partial transection normally has a fairly good prognosis in children due to the speed of repair in children and their adaptability. However, complete transection is normally not a good prognosis and can result in quadriplegia (Birrer et al., 2002).

The exact anatomical location of the damage to the spinal cord sometimes depicts likely seriousness of pathology. Damage to the anterior spinal cord from compression, which normally involves hyperflexion-type injuries, tends to involve the motor nerves, and hence it causes motor weakness more so than sensory deficit. This tends to be more common in children (Birrer et al., 2002).

Central lesions of the cord normally involve paralysis of upper and lower limbs with motor and sensory deficit. This is normally caused by hyperextension-type injuries.

Stanitski et al. (1994) reports that in a long-term clinical study involving children and teens involved in neck trauma without radiographic abnormality, results in 52% experienced the onset of spinal cord problems (serious and not serious) on average 14 days after injury.

Brachial Plexus Injuires

Brachial plexus injuries in children's sport is common and usually results in pain or tingling down the arm, normally from trauma to the neck or shoulder. The symptoms can last for minutes or days, depending on the severity of the trauma.

Two potential mechanisms can cause the irritation – tractioning or an overstetch of the brachial plexus, or a nerve root compression with subsequent impingment within the neural foramen. Younger players are more likely to sustain the traction-type injury.

Symptoms include sensory loss in a dermatomal pattern and motor loss in a myotomal pattern. C5 and C6 are most commonly affected in children, resulting in numbness or tingling of parts of their arm.

If symptoms persist for more than a few days, an MRI scan should be considered to determine extent and seriousness of injury.

Brachial plexus lesions are normally unilateral rather than bilateral, and bilateral symptoms should be further investigated.

Vascular Injuries

Injuries to the carotid and veterbrae arteries are rare in children due to the flexibility of all soft-tissue structures and the spine. Injuries to these vessels can cause an occlusion and clotting, which can result in an embolus and ultimately a stroke.

Any fracture dislocation of the neck in children should be checked for injury to the arteries as these potential events (such as emboli causing stroke) can take a weeks to manifest (Birrer et al., 2002). This can be achieved with an MRI scan or Doppler ultrasound scan.

Disc Injuries

Disc injuries in children such as a herniation within the cervical spine remains rare.

Congenital and Structural Abnormalities of the Cervical Spine

Klippel–Feil syndrome is a congenital abnormality of bones in and around the neck area. The most common finding is a reduced range of motion at the neck joints in lateral flexion and rotation. Cervical radiculopathy is also a common finding, and congenial cervical fusion may also be present.

Other features may also include a congenital scoliosis, congenital elevation of the scapula (Sprengel's deformity), hearing impairment, renal impairment, and congenital heart disease.

Conclusion

Any child who is unable to move their neck following trauma should be X-rayed to exclude fracture. Similarly, any child who sustains any neck injury should receive a follow-up just to ensure that no pathology has materialised in the interim. This should be performed 5 to 10 days after the initial injury (Stanitski et al., 1994).

Key Points

- Pseudolocking of C2, C3, and C4 is common in children.

- Cervical spine ligament can stretch up to 5 cm, but the spinal cord can stretch only up to 0.64 cm.

- Hyperflexion injuries are the most common in children.

- Spinal concussion can last up to 48 hours.

- Children with head or neck trauma should always be reassessed after 5 days following initial trauma.

Mid-Back and Lower Back Injuries

Solomon Abrahams

Back injuries in children from sport can account for between 10% and 15% of all sports injuries, but they can be as high as 30% in some sports such as rowing, weightlifting, and some of the power sports (Patel et al., 2009).

Children rarely complain of back pain unless it is persistent or interferes with their sport (Stanitski et al., 1994). Similarly, children and teens who consistently keep complaining of repeated back pains are more likely to have a bony injury such as spondylolysis rather than a repeated strain (Stanitski et al., 1994).

In adults, the vertebrae consists of 33 bones: 7 cervical, 12 thoracic, 5 lumbar, and 5 sacral bones. The sacral bones are normally fused, with the coccyx being the tail-end bone. (See Fig. 5.1a.)

However, in children, this is not entirely the case. Certainly, all the main bones are present, but the five sacral bones remain cartilaginous until the end of infancy and don't fuse until this time. The vertebral arches also remain cartilaginous until the age of 6 to 7 years, and even though the main vertebra is bone, most are still ossifying and adapting in bone density (Moore, 1992).

Most ossification takes place by the age of 14 (Patel et al., 2009), but ossification of the arches of the vertebrae is not completed and they do not fuse until early to mid-twenties; therefore, it is very easy to make mistakes in identifying fractures of the spine on X-ray by an inexperienced doctor confusing them for the epiphysis plate (Birrer et al., 2002).

The spinal column in children can be stretched by up to 5 cm because of its elasticity at this age and high water content. Unfortunately, the spinal cord can only be stretched by up to 1 cm before damage occurs. This is why X-rays sometimes do not show pathology as the spine will look normal, but spinal cord damage could be present; this is also known as spinal cord injury without radiological abnormaility or spinal cord injury without radiological abnormalities (SCIWORA) (Patel et al., 2009).

All the main bones, muscles, ligaments, and intervertebral discs are within their anatomical regions by infancy, all fully functional, but all still adapting to the traumas and daily activities the child puts them through. The intervertebral discs of a child are more resilient than the adult disc due to their elasticity and higher water content (Moore, 1992).

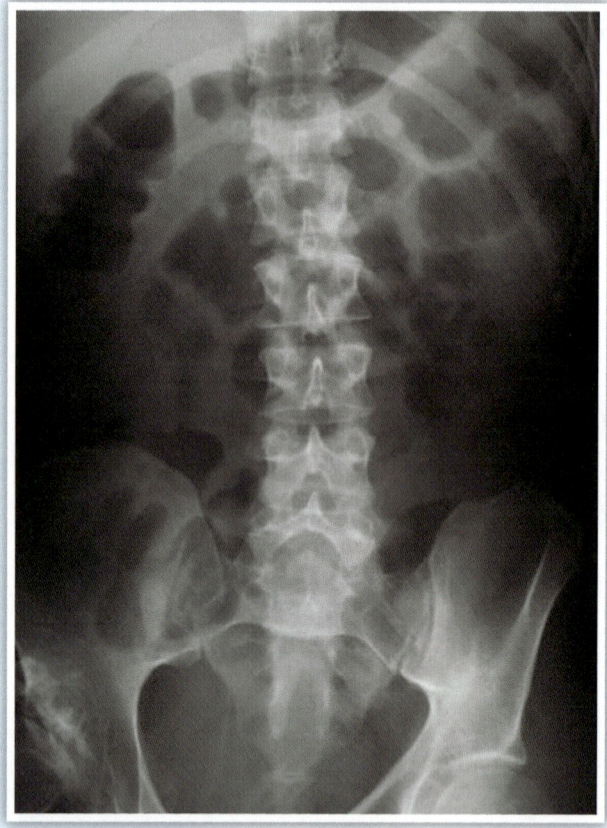

Fig. 5.1a X- ray of the lumbar/thoracic spine

Subjective Examination

Asking a young child questions to ascertain the pathology can be somewhat tricky at times. The type of questions you ask and the way you ask the questions and relate to the children are just as important as the questions themselves. Making sure that the child understands the questioning is vital to help not only your examination but also to help build up a rapport with the child.

Questions should be simple and straightforward. Anatomical terms should be avoided, and basic terminology appropriate for the child's age should be used.

Try relating to the child – asking questions like who their favourite footballer is or what they got on their last birthday can often help to build up a positive rapport with the child – rather than making the conversation purely medical-based. Similarly, as parents will normally be in the room with you, they will feel at ease with the clinician if you form a good rapport with the child early.

Where possible, the child should be asked the questions rather than the parents, to help build up trust and rapport. However, there will be times where you may have to get some feedback from the parents, especially in the case of young children.

Asking the age is an important factor as spondylolysis and cartilaginous end plate abnormalities and infections are the most common cause of persistent back pain in 10–15-year-olds, whilst discogenic pathology and mechanical back pain is more common in the older adolescents (Stanitski et al., 1994).

Subjective questions such as where the site of pain is, how long have they had the pain for, and how did it start, should be asked. Aggravating factors and easing factors, sleep patterns, and 24-hour pattern should be discussed. For example, continuous pain at night in children could involve neoplasm, whereas fever at night may involve an infection. Diffused generalised pain may involve an inflammatory disorder, or pain in the lumbar spine that worsens with extension and rotation may reveal a spondylolysis, especially if the children are involved in a sport which involves hyperextension such as gymnastics. Lower back pain following an acute upper respiratory chest infection may reveal a potential infection within the discs.

Obviously, bladder, bowel, gait disturbances, bilateral weakness could indicate serious spinal pathology and should be further investigated. Fevers, chills, lethargy, bruising, lack of concentration, and weight loss could indicate infection or malignancy.

Family history and social history should be taken from the parents to give further evidence of any potential hereditary problems, and understanding any issues at home or school could give further evidence of more non-medical-related issues. For example, spondylolysis and scoliosis have strong family links (Stanitski et al., 1994).

Objective examination should consist of gait analysis, sit-to-stand activities, and functional activities, where possible before they are formally introduced to you. When examining the child's spine, it is important that the whole spine, from the cervical spine to the lumbar spine, be examined. Postural abnormalities and excessive kyphosis and scoliosis in sitting and standing positions should be examined.

Examination of the extremities for hamstring and tightness of the calf and sciatic nerve should be observed and recorded, especially in adolescents who may be going through active growth spurts at the time.

All ranges of motion, including flexion, extension, lateral flexion, and rotation, and even combined movements should be reviewed. For example, observation of a rib hump during flexion in children may indicate Scheuermann's disease (discussed later), or excessive movement may indicate hypermobility syndrome. Pain in extension combined with rotation may indicate spondylolysis, especially in a sport which involves hyperextension such as gymnastics, swimming, or diving.

Bone tenderness should also be noted, and any referred pains should be investigated.

Neurological examination should always be performed including myotomes (see Fig. 5.2), dermatomes, reflexes, and straight leg raise test (or any other nerve tests you feel appropriate), remembering that a child's response will be similar to that of an adult.

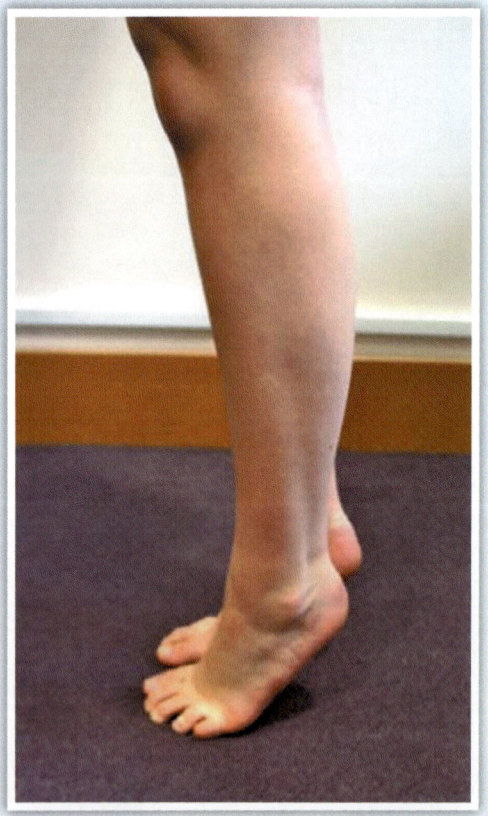

Fig. 5.2 Standing on tiptoes tests S1/S2 myotome

Differential Diagnosis of Lower Back Pain

Sources of back pain in children can be various. These include mechanical, developmental, traumatic, inflammatory, neoplastic, visceral, psychogenic, and metabolic. Not all pains may come from a mechanical origin, which is why subjective questioning is important. (See Table 5.1.)

For example, children with continuous night-time pain relieved only with non-steroidal anti-inflammatory drugs should be further investigated for osteoid osteoma or osteoblastoma.

Pain associated with chills, fever, or weight loss may indicate malignancy or infection. Back pain following a serious bout of upper respiratory infection or ear infection could indicate discitis.

Joint aches and pains in the morning, relieved with movement in the day with or without other associated issues (such as eye problems) may indicate arthropathies such as juvenile ankylosing spondylitis, juvenile chronic arthritis, or juvenile rheumatoid arthritis.

Examples include:

Developmental, Scheuermann's disease, Postural abnormality, Spondylolysis, Spondylolisthesis, Lumbar epiphysitis

Mechanical/Traumatic, Disc bulge/herniation, Ligamentous and muscular strain, sprains, contusions, Facet joint syndrome, Spondylolysis or spondylolisthesis, Slipped vertebrae apophysis, Postural pains, Overuse injuries

Inflammatory, Juvenile rheumatoid arthritis, Ankylosing spondylolysis, Enteropathic arthritis, Juvenile chronic arthritis

Infection, Discitis, vertebrae osteomyelitis, Tuberculosis spondylitis, sacroiliac joint infection

Neoplastic, Benign osteoid osteoma, osteoblastoma, Histiocytosis, Leukaemia, Lymphoma, Osteosarcoma, Wilm tumour, Ewing tumour, Spinal cord tumour, Neuroblastoma, Astrocytoma

Visceral, Appendicitis, Pneumonia, Renal calculi, Pleuritis, Pancreatitis, Renal stones, Pelvic inflammatory disease, Retroperitoneal mass, Ectopic pregnancy, Endometriosis, Collitis, Urinary tract infection

Table 5.1 Examples of different pathologies causing spinal pain (Patel et al., 2009)

Red Flags in Children

Red flags in children and teens vary, but referral to a specialist should be considered if a child under 10 years has consistent back pain; wakes up at night with back pain; has pain for more than 2 months; has severe progressive pain, constant pain, pain at rest; or shows severe neurological signs and associated systemic symptoms or signs (Patel et al., 2009).

Common Pathologies of the Middle and Lower Spine

Solomon Abrahams

Scheuermann's Disease

Scheuermann's disease is characterised with a very stiff and kyphotic thoracic spine, sometimes, accompanied by pain, though not always (Stanitski et al., 1994). It is a structural and developmental pathology which is thought to be caused by an avascular necrosis (part of the osteochondritis juvenilis family of pathologies, discussed earlier) which causes wedging of the vertebrae of more than 5 degrees.

It can affect the end plates, which are thought to be aggravated during certain growth spurts in adolescents rather than small children (Birrer et al., 2002). Scheuermann's disease and the wedging seen on X-rays is uncommon below the age of 10 years (Patel et al., 2009).

The exact cause of Scheuermann's disease remains controversial (Shanmugam & Maffulli, 2008). Some specialists postulate an avascular necrosis of the spine during growth spurts, but some postulate hormonal abnormalities, collagen defects, vitamin deficiency, and genetic predisposition (Patel et al., 2009).

There are two types of Scheuermann's disease, atypical and typical.

Atypical Scheuermann's disease affects the thoracolumbar and lumbar spine. Typical Scheuermann's disease affects the thoracic spine only, in partilcular regions in and around T7 to T9 vertebrae. It is more common in males, and onset normally begins at 10 years but does not normally become noticeable or symptomatic until teens.

The child or teen normally presents with mid-thoracic and/or lumbar spine pain with a very round back (kyphosis). Sometimes, spondylolysis and/or spondylolisthesis may accompany the pathology, possibly due to the hyperlordotic lumbar spine, which is compensatory to the kyphosis.

Pain normally comes on with activity, especially extension sports. Tight hamstring and tight hip flexors can also be present. Once the growth spurt begins to end, the pain does normally begin to settle.

Some authors suggest that a family history of Scheuermann's disease or at least a severe kyphosis maybe present (Patel et al., 2009).

Clinical Examination

An excessive kyphosis of the mid/ lower back is normally indicative of a postural kyphosis or Scheuermann's disease. Some children or teens present with pain in the back; most however, do not. Parents are often the first ones to notice the hump or poor posture and are unaware of the condition (Patel et al., 2009). If pain is present, it is normally exacerbated with sitting or standing for long periods.

During lumbar spine flexion, an egg-shaped spine at the thoracic spine is more indicative of postural kyphosis, which may be ever present in young teens who are tall and going through very fast growth spurts. An egg-shaped back at the lower end of the thoracic spine is more indicative of Scheuermann's disease (Birrer et al., 2002). Thoracic spinal curvature is considered normal between 20 degrees and 40 degrees, and a kyphosis beyond 45 degrees is considered abnormal (Patel et al., 2009).

Pain on lumbar extension may also be sore, due to compensatory pains, or a spondylolisthesis/spondylolysis at the lumbar spine.

Neurologcial examination is normally unremarkable, but tightness in hamstring and sciatic nerve could be present.

Test

A simple lateral X-ray should reveal Scheuermann's disease easily. Failing this, MRI and bone scans can also confirm diagnosis. X-rays should show irregular end plates and vertebrae wedging of 5 degrees or more. Disc narrowing maybe present along Schmorl's nodes.

Treatment and Management

Management is normally conservative. Monitoring and reassurance are important to ensure the condition doesn't worsen. Postural correction and awareness in sitting and standing position is essential. Core stability and abdominal control is important. Stretching of the leg muscles and nerves of the lower limbs and self-taught exercises will also help ease the condition and will empower the child.

Occasionally, soft-tissue mobilisations such as massage can be helpful in the short term, but not in the long term. The use of analgesics or anti-inflammatory drugs should be avoided where necessary unless pain is severe.

Re-examination should be done every 4–6 weeks to monitor the condition and offer reassurance to the child and parents.

In some cases, bracing (to restrict further kyphosis) maybe necessary during aggressive episodes, but this should only be used sparingly and intermittently so that the child does not get used to wearing the brace. Specifically, bracing is considered when the kyphosis is between 55 degrees and 80 degrees, with promising results (Shanmugam & Maffulli, 2008).

Atypical Scheuermann's Disease

Atypical Scheuermann's disease is often seen in sports with repetitive flexion extension moments such as rowing and gymnastics. With excessive pressure on the lumbar spine combined with lower thoracic kyphosis, back pain is common. The excessive pressures can cause growth plate fractures and damage to the lower back discs such as disc bulges or even herniated discs (Birrer et al., 2002).

This is more common in males, thought to be potentially due to the nature of their aggressive and sometimes explosive growth spurts.

Management is normally conservative and similar to that of typical Scheuermann's disease. Even the teen with a spondylolysis or spondylolisthesis (without neurology) calms down with conservative management (as above). The long-term implications of a spondylolysis or spondylolisthesis is discussed later.

Adolescent Scoliosis

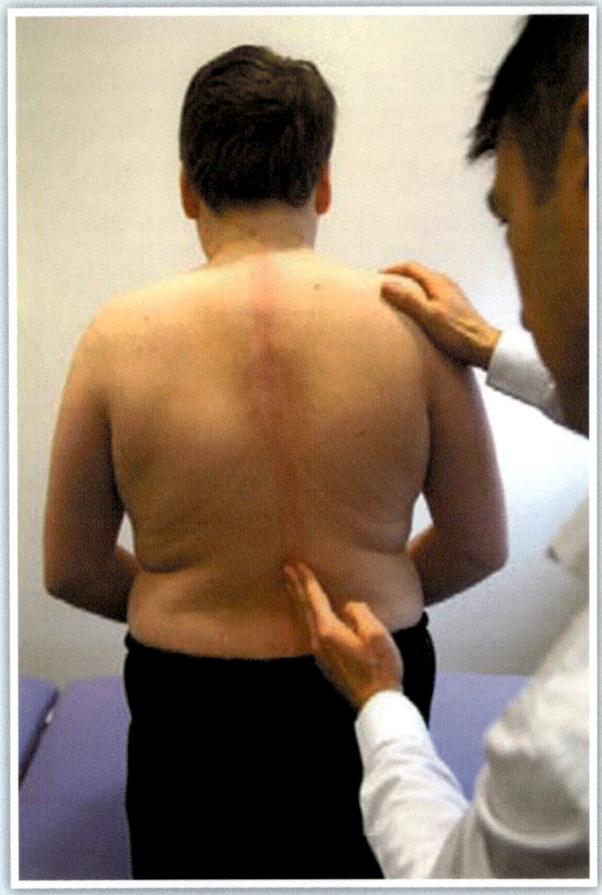

Scoliosis is simply a lateral curvature of the spine in adolescents and teens and is mostly asymptomtic. Arguably, some suggest this pathology is normal progression of the spine rather than a pathology (King, 1984). (See Fig. 5.4.)

Fig. 5.4 Spinal examination revealing a minimal scoliosis

The incidence of scoliosis of less than 10 degrees before the age of 16 is 2–3% and is normally not painful (Stanitski et al., 1994). The actual curvature is not normally found initially by the child or teen themselves, rather their parents or coaching staff.

The exact cause remains unclear, but is thought to multifactoral (Patel et al., 2009). If a severe scoliosis exists, this maybe attributed to congenital scoliosis, which maybe also associated with other pathologies such as renal and cardiac abnormalities (Stanitski et al., 1994).

Clinically, the scoliosis can be seen in standing position and when the child bends forwards into lumbar flexion or touches the toes. Severe deviation may require an orthopaedic consult, and in some cases, bracing may be needed.

Spondylolysis and Spondylolisthesis

Spondylolysis is defined as a fracture of the pars inticularis, part of the lamina bone on the vertebrae. It can be unilateral or bilateral and can lead to a spondylolisthesis, which is further slippage of the veterbae (due to the fracture) (Birrer et al., 2002). Spondylolisthesis is derived from the Greek words 'spondy' meaning vertebra and olisthesis meaning 'to slide down' (Lyle, 1984).

There are several known causes of a spondylolysis including congenital dysplasia, microtrauma (isthmic), and degenerative, pathological, and stress fractures (Carty, 1997; Patel et al., 2009; Shanmugam & Maffulli, 2008).

Spondylolysis defects have never been reported in newborn infants and are very rarely seen under the age of 5. Similarly, they are only seen in bipedal humans, revealing that axial pressures play an important role in the fracture (Stanitski et al., 1994).

After the age of 10, spondylolysis is the most common cause of back pain in the paediatric sports community (King, 1984). Certainly, it seems that active and aggressive growth spurts can exacerbate the pain.

It is more common in certain sports such as gymnastics, weightlifting, swimming, rowing, ballet, dance, fast bowling in cricket, volleyball, and sport involving extension and rotation (Patel et al., 2009). The incidence in the general childhood population has been reported to be 6% compared with occurrence in gymnasts which can be as high as 50% (Patel et al., 2009). However, not all authors agree; a study on 177 male high school athletes showed approximately 21% had radiographic evidence of spondylolysis (Stanitski et al., 1994).

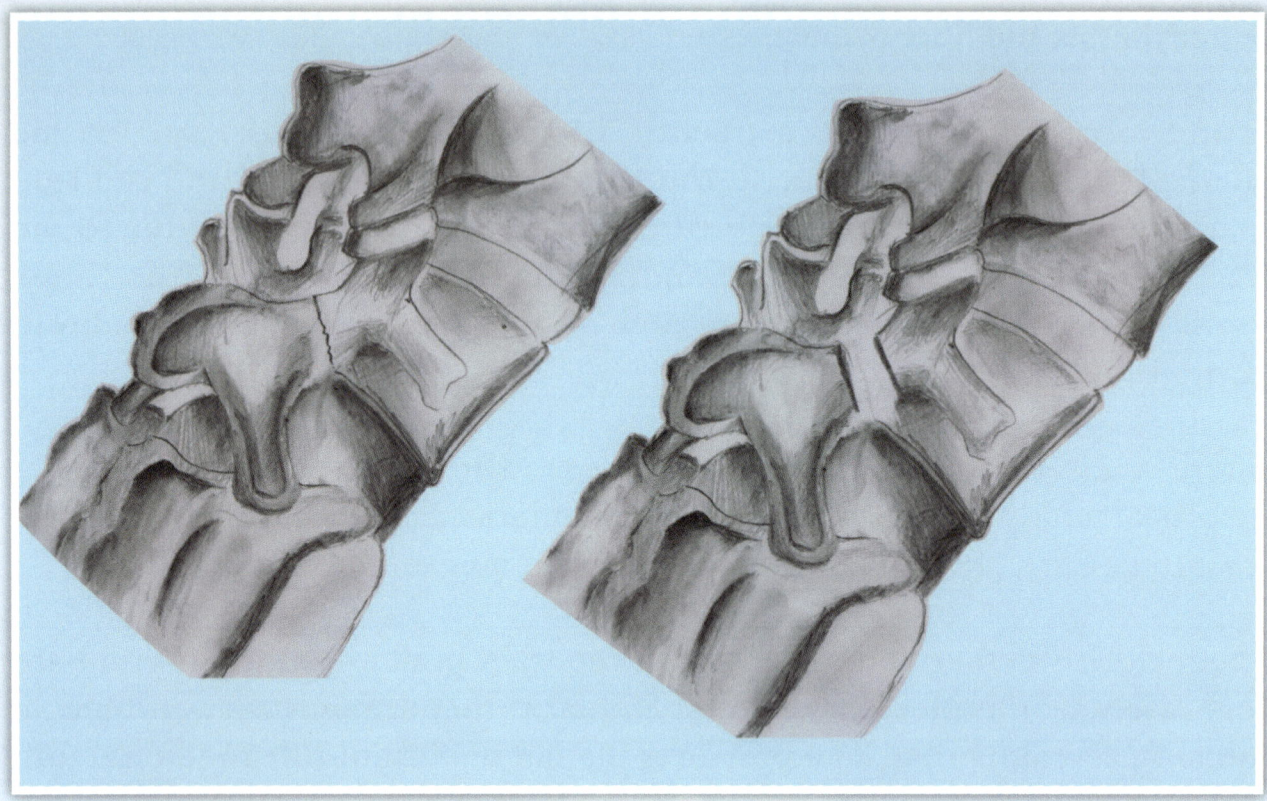

Fig. 5.5b Diagram to show (left) spondylolysis and (right) complete fracture of pars

The most common areas of the lumbar spine it seems to affect are L4 and L5 (Morita, Ikata, Katoh, & Miyake, 1995), and the onset of symptoms coincides with growth spurts in adolescents. Interestingly, Stanitski et al. (1994) report 20–50% of teens with spondylolysis may also have spina bifida occulta, which is 13 times more prevalent in teens than the found in general population. (See Fig. 5.5b.)

Most children who present with spondylolisthesis present with pain and/ or neurological symptoms, even though the latter is rarer. However, the actual slippage of bone is thought to be painless (Birrer et al., 2002). However, some teens are totally asymptomatic with both of these pathologies (Shanmugam & Maffulli, 2008).

Spondylolisthesis less than 25% slippage is defined as a grade 1 slippage, which is the most common. Within a range of 25–50% is a grade 2, and anything beyond 50% slippage is regarded as a grade 3 (Birrer et al., 2002).

The actual slippage is also twice as high in girls as opposed to boys, even though pars fractures are more common in males (Lyle, 1984).

Slippage of the bone by more than 30% is considered to be rare, and the majority of children and adolescent in sport with lower back pain, thought to be with simple back strains should have consideration to a spondylolysis, as this is one of the most misdiagnosed pathology in the spine in children.

Clinical Examination

Early diagnosis of this pathology can be advantageous for the success of conservative management and long-term prognosis.

Most of the time, the spondylolysis and spondylolisthesis are asymptomic at time of onset, but certain activities will aggravate the pathology (Birrer et al., 2002).

There can be unilateral or bilateral back pain with or without referred pain. Extension of the spine can be sore, often made worse with rotation.

Severe slippage will cause a modification of gait, often with a flexed hip and knee (Phalen & Dickson, 1961), but this remains rare. Extreme ranges of motion will be painful with more restriction on the pars side, if unilateral pars is involved. On palpation, the back may be sore if the pain has been recently exacerbated, and in some cases, a step-off maybe felt of the spinous process, but only in severe spondylolisthesis.

Tight hamstrings may also be present in 80% of children (Patel et al., 2009) with some positive neural tension (Phalen & Dickson, 1961). Provocation test for spondylolysis include lumbar extension with side flexion and rotation to the affected side. This will be more painful on the same side of movement if there is a postive pars fracture.

Tests

A single leg hyperextension test can also be tried (see Fig. 5.5c), involving the child standing on one leg and hyperextending the lumbar spine actively with the assistance of the clinician to ensure they do not hyperextend excessively. Pain on the weight-bearing side could be an indication of a positive test, thought to be the sheer amount of pressure on the pars fracture side (Birrer et al., 2002).

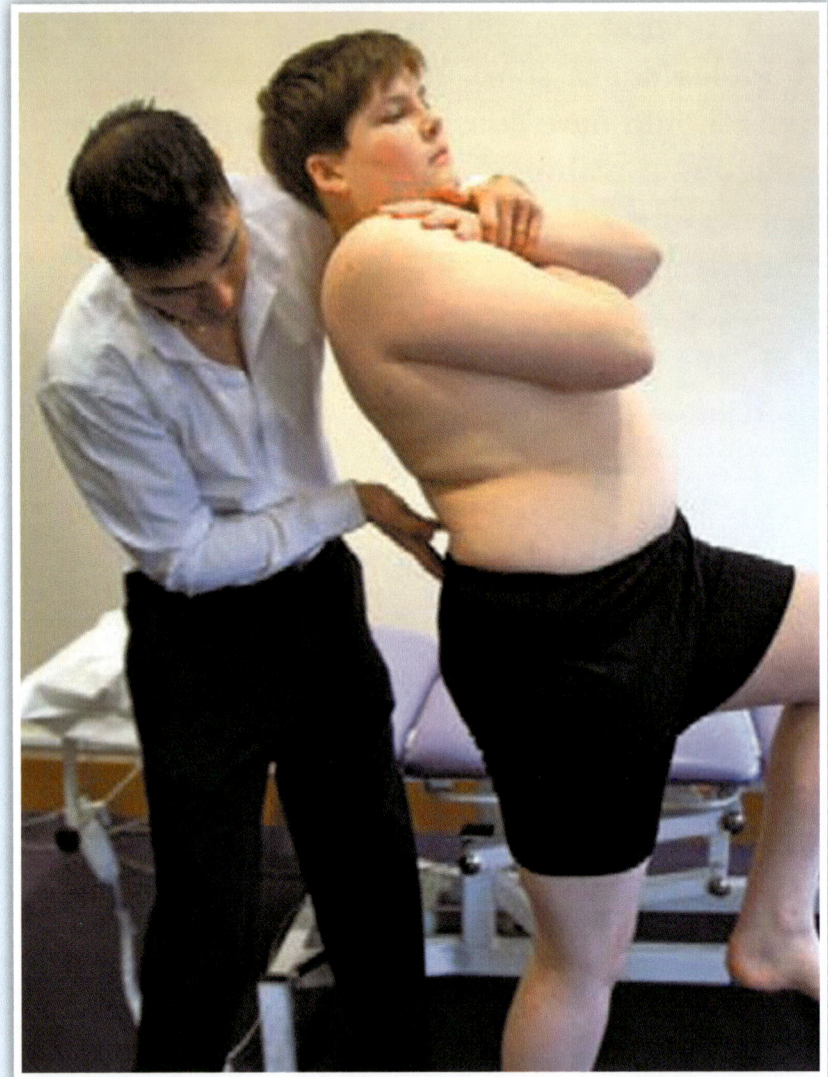

Fig. 5.5c Hyperextension test for spondylolisthesis

Radiographic imaging can confirm diagnosis, with anterior–posterior (AP), lateral, and more importantly, oblique view X-rays. Without an oblique view, 20% of spondylolisthesis can be missed, and suspicion of spondylolisthesis should always be on the referral X-ray form. Other scans which will confirm diagnosis include MRI scan, CT scan and a bone scan.

Treatment and Management

Treatment is normally conservative unless the spondylolisthesis is severe, diagnostically as well as symptomatically. Focus on symptom relief and allowing for any bone healing to occur should be the priority. Rest from sport and, in particular, extension movements is important, and this sometimes can be as long as a few months.

Analgesics should only be used to help manage the pain, but should not be used long term or consistently so that the athlete is unaware of the pathology. Some authors suggest the pathology should be treated like a stress fracture (Stanitski et al., 1994).

Bracing should always be a potential option, to restrict the child from activities. Telling a child to rest can be somewhat frustrating at times, as during growth spurts, many feel the need to exercise some energy. Bracing will help remind the child to be aware of what they are doing. However, the child should not get used to the brace either and become over-reliant, so care is required that the child does not wear the brace consistently throughout the day. Depending on the severity, activity-led rehabilitation can begin normally after 6–8 weeks, or following further scans/investigations.

Once the pain begins to settle with rest, gentle physiotherapy can be started to help restore muscle atrophy caused by pain inhibition and immobilisation. Core stability of the trunk muscles, abdominal strength, and paraspinal strength should be undertaken in a postural position, which can progress on to a more functional position. The rehabilitation should always be done in stages, so as to avoid any exacerbation of the injury. There is no set protocol, and research to investigate the best route back to sport varies amongst authors with inconsistent conclusions. Much of decision will be based on symptoms, updated X-rays/bone scans, and discussions with the player, parents and coaching staff.

In severe cases, where conservative treatment over a period of time fails to help the child, or where the spondylolisthesis is a grade 3 causing significant symptoms included neurology, surgery is sometimes indicated. Fusion or bone grafting are potential options, but this does depend on circumstances and the surgeon.

Infections of the Back
Discitis

Discitis is an inflammatory/infectious condition within the intervertebral discs common in 2–7 year age group. There still remains controversy about whether this pathology is indeed an infection or an inflammation. The exact mechanism remains unclear, but the infection is thought to be introduced into the disc via a rich blood supply. As the child matures, and certainly by adolescence, the amount of penetration from the blood vessels decreases and hence the risk of discitis in teenages and adults is far less (Birrer et al., 2002; Patel et al., 2009). Onset is often insidious, sometimes presenting as back pain or sometimes as vague abdominal pain (yet abdominal palpation is normal). The pain can be quite severe, even affecting gait. Range of motion is limited in the lumbar spine as the child feels unable to mobilise efficiently. Sometimes, fever is present or the child may of just recovered from an infection.

X-rays are normally inconclusive, but a bone scan will reveal increased uptake. Blood results do not show any significant increase in white blood cell count or blood erythrocyte sedimentation rate (ESR). However, an MRI scan will be able to differentiate discitis from osteomyelitis of the vertebrae, Scheuermann's disease, spinal abcess, and spondylolysis (Birrer et al., 2002).

Treatment is normally rest and antibiotics. In severe cases with abdominal cramps, intravenous antibiotics should be reviewed. Children can normally return to activity once pain has fully settled, within 4–6 weeks of treatment initiation.

Mechanical Injuries
Apophyseal Injuries

Children who are involved in repetitive flexion extension can sustain traction apophyseal injuries. These injuries are normally located in the lower thoracic spine and upper lumbar spine. They are rare injuries and more prevelant during growth spurts. Normally, rest with analgesics helps, and functional activity is restored once the spurts have calmed down.

Apophyseal Avulsion Fractures

An apophyseal avulsion fracture, also known as slipped vertebral apophysis, is simply an avulsion fracture of the cartilaginous apophyseal ring with a posterior displacement within the spinal canal (Birrer et al., 2002).

This condition affects children and teenagers, with a much higher incidence in teens (Patel et al., 2009). Between the vertebral bodies, cartilaginous rings separate the intervertebral discs and the bony vertebral body. These rings begin to ossify at the age 12 years and are fully fused by age 18. Repititive motions in flexion and extension can place stress on the rings which produces a chip fracture, which is normally displaced posteriorly, sometimes with disc involvement. In most cases, L4 and L5 are implicated, and it is common in wrestling and gymnastics (Patel et al., 2009).

This condition affects males more than females. This could be because boys take a longer time to mature and go through more aggressive growth spurts, making apophyseal rings more vulnerable to fracture. Neurological examination is normal, but movements of the lumbar spine are severely limited, more so in flexion and extension.

An X-ray should reveal avulsion fracture, but a CT scan, MRI scan or bone scan will be more reliable.

Treatment and Management

Treatment of this pathology is normally rest and non-steroidal anti-inflammatory drugs until the pain calms down. This can take anywhere between 4 and 12 weeks, depending on the severity and onset.

Once this settles, small extension exercises of the lumbar spine are helpful in increasing functionality. Improving core stability is important and addressing the potential cause, whether this be faulty technique or faulty biomechanics.

Strains and Sprains

As with the cervical spine, sprains and strains of the mid and lower back are common in the young athlete. Ligament strains and damage to the capsule of the intervertebral joints and facet joints can occur, especially during spurts or aggressive movements.

Soft-tissue injuries in children are never in isolation; they are found more so in combination with other structures (Lyle, 1984).

Strains like these will be more painful moving away from the pain, that is while stretching the damaged tissue. Normally, they begin to respond to rest within days, and analgesics are normally not necessary, unless the pain is very acute (Patel et al., 2009).

Hyperlordotic Back Pain

Hyperlordotic back pain tends to be more common in children who are of African (black) origin – who are naturally sway-backed – or children who are compensating, maybe with a high thoracic kyphosis due to posture or Scheuermann's disease. Hyperlordosis causes stress and strain on the ligaments and capsules. Normally, it is accompanied by muscle tightness,of the lower back and legs. It is more prevalent in extension-type sports such as gymnastics, swimming, and sprinting.

Clinical evaluation normally reveals hyperlordosis in standing position, but not necessarily in sitting position. Generalised stiffness and soreness is located at the lumbar spine. Rarely is there neurological deficit, and sometimes, the thoracic spine is hyperkyphotic.

Management normally consists of stretching any tight tissues and readdressing the posture. Occassionally, it may also be prudent to check their posture and the way they run (if they do) in their sport to ascertain any postural corrections that need to be done.

Facet Syndrome

Facet joint irritation remains rare in this age group, unless there is significant trauma or they have a juvenile arthritis.

The facet joints are held in place with a capsule and ligaments, both are rarely injured at this age group due to their flexibility (Osenbach, 1992).

The symptoms are similar to those of an adult with facet problems – localised back pain adjacent to the intervetebral disc joints which can refer pain down the leg and give redicular symptoms. The joint is usually tender on direct palpation. Neurological examination is normal in most cases.

Once the acute pain has settled, gentle rotational movements will encourage movement within the joint. Gentle flexion and extension exercises also encourage normal movement within the joint itself, so long as the exercises are graded over time.

Strength work should be focused around the paraspinal muscles and core and on ways to prevent the facet joint from being damaged again. Perhaps focusing on techniques (specific to sports) should be studied and it should be ensured that they are correct. Damage to most joints here in sport is due to incorrect or wrong technique, sometimes as a compensation for speed (Osenbach, 1992).

Herniated Discs

Disc herniation in children is rare, less than 3.2% (Patel et al., 2009), but it is more common in adolescents (Shanmugam & Maffulli, 2008). Their appearance is similar to severe muscle spasm and they don't normally give radicular symptoms, unlike adult's discs (Birrer et al., 2002).

The actual discs themselves are very strong in children and teens, so care must be taken if you suspect disc herniation, as they can also cause fractures of the end plates when the nucleus pulposus ruptures through the annulus (Moore, 1992).

A clear history of trauma is elicited in 40–50% of teens (Patel et al., 2009).

In children and teens, prolapsed discs normally occur *Posterolateral* rather than posterocentral prolapses due to a strong annulus and strong posterior longitudinal ligament. However, the thinnest membrane is posterior lateral, with L4 and L5 being some of the weakest. Therefore the signs and symptoms in children and teens tend to be different as opposed to adults, in that referred neurology or pain is not as common (Stanitski et al., 1994).

However, sometimes, neurology is implicated just like in adults. Other pathologies can also mimic these symptoms in teens, such as slipped vertebral apophysis or end plate fractures; therefore, good clinical evaluation and scans may be necessary (Stanitski et al., 1994).

Pain is normally referred into the buttock or hip rather than it being just a simple central low back pain. The pain worsens with vigorous exercise, including sneezing and coughing. There is normally a positive straight leg raise with hamstring tightness (Stanitski et al., 1994).

Flexion of the spine is limited, and extension may be sore. There may be a deviation away from the disc prolapse side during a Lumbar flexion movement, but this is more common in adults (Stanitski et al., 1994). An MRI or a CT scan is the best with suspicion of prolapsed intervetebral disc pathology. X-rays may show some joint space narrowing due to the fluid loss within the disc space.

Treatment is normally conservative. Reasonable rest and analgesics should be an option, but equally it is important for the child or teen to keep mobile to prevent stiffness and atrophy of other soft tissues.

Gentle stretching of tight neural structures and core stability muscles should begin. Graded exercises are important to help the disc adapt to pressures. Extension exercises of the spine can help, but education on sitting, standing, and other activities will be important. Reassurance is also important to the child and parents. Disc herniation takes time to heal, and allowance need to be applied accordingly.

Once pain settles to a reasonable level, increased activity can begin, from treadmill walking to treadmill incline walking; work the core muscles in tandem.

Sacroiliac Joint Pathology

Sacroiliac pathology (SIJ) is rare in children and is more common in females than in males (unless significant trauma is involved). Injury to the posterior or anterior sacroiliac ligaments (such as a fall on one side) will cause pain around the buttocks, normally unilateral rather than bilateral. Pregnancy in teens can also cause SIJ to be painful.

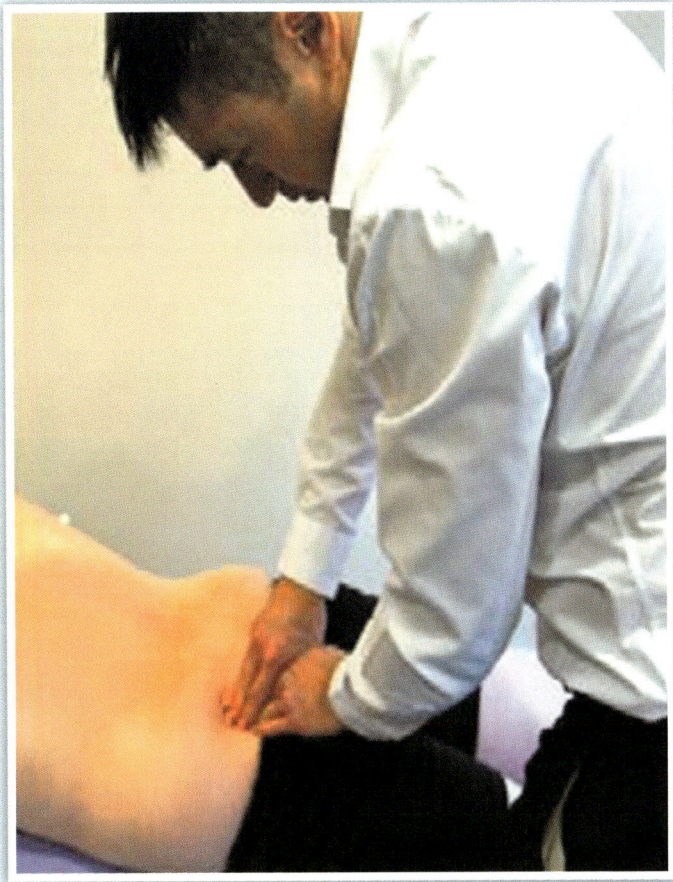

Fig. 5.6 Compression and palpation of the sacroiliac joint

Tenderness over the SIJ (see Fig. 5.6) is normally a good indicator in the absence of lower back pain (unless this has been involved in the trauma as well).

Treatment is normally rest from anything which increases the trauma through the SIJ (such as running) and working on the cause and prevention. Anti-inflammatory drugs can be helpful, along with physiotherapy to begin strength work. Biomechanical analysis maybe useful in non-traumatic SIJ pathology. Also, exclude pregnancy in girls.

Tuberculosis (TB) of the Thoracic and Lumbar Spine

TB of the thoracic and lumbar spine is the most common form of skeletal TB. The infection begins at the anterior margin of the spine, near the disc. TB eats away at the veterbral body and eventually causes wedge-compression fractures. Abcess formation can occur at the affected spinal level(Crawford & Hamblen, 1990).

Signs and Symptoms

Pain in the back with stiffness and weakness of legs. Spinal cord compression can occur in rare cases. Kyphosis is normally very prominent, and the child looks ill.

Confirmation can be done with X-rays or MRI scans.

Management includes immediate referral to a paediatrician.

Ankylosing Spondylitis

Ankylosing spondylitis is a chronic inflammation of the spinal and sacroiliac joints commonly seen in children aged 16–25 years. It causes pain and stiffness of the joints as the joints begin to fuse.

As the joints begin to fuse, the thoracic spine gets smaller and kyphosis develops. It eventually causes chronic pain of the spine and sacroiliac joint.

Blood tests confirm diagnosis, HLA b27 antigen positive (Crawford & Hamblen, 1990).

Treatment includes rheumotology option for symptom control and medical management.

Calves Vertebral Compression

Whereas Scheuermann's affects the whole spine in adolescents. Calves vertebral compression only affects the central bony nucleus of a vertebral body. It remains rare in children, but when present, it leads to eventual bony collapse, similar to wedge-compression fracture. It normally affects children aged 2–10 years (Crawford & Hamblen, 1990).

Pain in a localised area of the spine that worsens on weight bearing is a symptom. X-rays confirm diagnosis.

Management is orthopaedic consultant referral.

Visceral Causes of Back Pain

It is rare for visceral pathology to cause isolated back pain in children and teens. Kidney pathology, pneumonia, retrocecal appendicitis can refer.

Management of Back Pain in Children

Difference in training regime (duration, intensity, frequency), poor conditioning, reduced flexibility especially during growth spurts, improper technique, too much speed, poor equipment, biomechanical considerations, change in shoewear or camber, change in coaching staff, training pressures, and parental pressures have all been cited as potential causes of back pain in children (Patel et al., 2009). These causes should be addressed to prevent further re-injury.

Treatment of back injuries in children is more prolonged compared with other injuries they may sustain because of their constant growth (Stanitski et al., 1994).

Key Points

- Most common undiagnosed condition in lower back pain is spondylolysis.

- Complete ossification of vertebrae doesn't fuse till early twenties.

- Spondylolysis and spondylolisthesis is common secondary to Scheuermann's.

- Slippage of vertebrae in spondylolisthesis is not painful.

- Spina bifida occulta is common in 50% of children with spondylolysis.

References

Birrer, R., Greisemer, B., & Cataletto, M. (2002). *Pediatric sports medicine for primary care* (2nd ed.). Philadelphia, PA: Lippincott Williams & Wilkins.

Carty, J. (1997). Children's sports injuries. *European Journal of Radiology, 26,* 163.

Crawford, A., & Hamblen, K. (1990). *Outline of orthopaedics* (11th ed.). Edinburgh: Churchill Livingstone.

King, H. (1984). Back pain in children. *Pediatric Clinical North America, 31,* 1081–1085.

Loder, R. (1996). The cervical spine. *Lovell and winters pediatric orthopaedic* (4th ed.). Philadelphia, PA: Lippincott-Raven.

Lyle, J. (1984). *Pediatric and adolescent sports medicine* (1st ed.). Boston, MA: Little Brown and Company.

Moore, K. (1992). *Clinically orientated anatomy* (3rd ed.). Baltimore, MD: Williams and Wilkins.

Morita, T., Ikata, T., Katoh, S., & Miyake, R. (1995). Lumbar spondylosis in children and adolescents. *Journal of Bone and Joint Surgery, 77,* 620–625.

Osenbach, R. (1992). Pediatric spinal cord and vertebral column injury. *Neurosurgery, 30,* 385–390.

Patel, D., Greydanus, D., & Baker, R. (2009). *Pediatric sports medicine* (2nd ed.). New York, NY: McGraw Hill Medical.

Phalen, G., & Dickson, J. (1961). Spondylolisthesis and tight hamstrings. *American Journal of Sports Medicine, 24,* 94–99.

Stanitski, C., DeLee, J., & Drez, D. (1994). *Pediatric and adolescent sports medicine* (3rd ed.). Philadelphia, PA: W. B. Saunders.

Shanmugam, C., & Maffulli, N. (2008). Sports injury in children. *British Medical Bulletin, 86,* 33–57.

Wilberger, J. (1998). Athletic spinal cord and spinal injuries, guidelines for initial management. *Clinical Sports Medicine, 17,* 111–120.

CHAPTER 6

Hip, Pelvis, and Thigh Pathologies in Children and Adolescent Sport

Solomon Abrahams

Introduction

Hip injuries account for up to 10% of all sports injuries seen in children and teens, mainly stemming from apophyseal injuries, muscular strains, and contusions (Patel, Greydenus, & Baker, 2009).

The basic anatomy of the child's hip and pelvis is not too dissimilar compared with the adult's. The epiphyseal plates around the pelvis and hip fuse differently in each anatomical position, which may influence pathology at certain ages.

The lesser and great trochanteric epiphyses fuse between the ages of 16 and 18 years. The iliac crest, the anterior superior iliac spine (ASIS), and the anterior inferior iliac spine (AIIS) fuse between ages of 15 to 17, between ages of 21 to 25, and between ages of 16 to 18, respectively. The ischial tuberosity fuses quite late between ages 19 and 25 years. (Birrer, Greisemer, & Cataletto, 2002).

Soft-Tissue Injuries of the Hip and Pelvis

Soft-tissue injuries to the hip, pelvis, and thigh are common in children and teens. Contusions, abrasions, strains, and sprains are more common than bony injuries. Contusions of bony prominences is also common from direct trauma such as knocks to the ASIS, iliac crest, and trochanter of the hip.

Exclusion of apophyseal injuries should be assessed (later discussed) and relative rest, ice, and compression should be used initially. Following rest, and once pain has settled, gradual return to sport should be endorsed.

Sprains and Strains

Strain and sprains can be caused by excessive overstretching of tissues, strenuous contractions, and repetitive microtrauma. They are common and normally resolve within a few days of rest.

Soft-tissue strains are graded into three classifications: grade 1, a strain or damage of up to 25% of the fibres; grade 2, up to 50% strain or damage of the fibres normally accompanied by swelling and bleeding within the tissues; and grade 3, up to 75% strain or damage to the muscle fibres, with additional swelling in moderate to severe amounts (Patel et al., 2009).

Grade 1 strains are the most common in children and teens, and normally resolve within a couple of weeks with rest and ice.

Grade 2 strains normally take longer to recover, requiring more hands-on management including rest, ice, compression, and soft-tissue rehabilitation. They can normally take between 3 and 5 weeks to recover.

Grade 3 strains tend to be the most severest form of soft-tissue damage, apart from a complete rupture. These injuries are normally accompanied with intermuscular or intramuscular bleeding and swelling, causing severe pain on exertion. These injuries can take up to 3 months to make a full recovery (Cramer, 2004).

Upper Thigh Strains

Soft-tissue injuries of the thigh, hamstring, and adductors around the hip joint are common in children and teens.

Thigh Strain

Thigh strains normally affect the hip flexors (psoas, iliac, sartorius, and rectus femoris muscles) or the main kicking muscles of the hip. There is normally a mechanism of injury, and usually, a kicking action is involved.

Pain is normally aggravated with resistance against hip flexion. (See Fig. 6.1.)

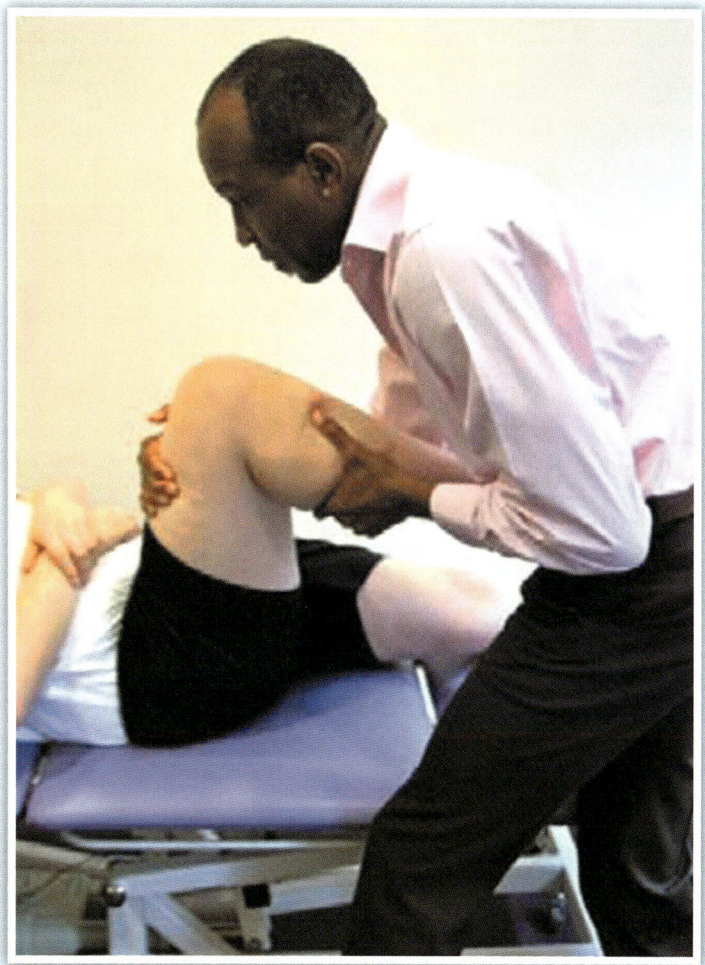

Fig. 6.1 Testing resistance against hip flexion

Treatment initially should be targeted at rest, ice, and compression. Gentle stretching of the tissue can begin after a few days and strengthening exercises can begin soon after.

Complications of Thigh Injuries

Partial or complete ruptures of the rectus femoris muscle and intramuscular haematomas are the two most common complications of a thigh strain.

Partial or Complete Rupture of Rectus Femoris Muscle

This can be a common complication in teens and is normally sustained during a kicking action. Pain is normally found in the upper 1/3 of the thigh muscle, and at first, the rupture – partial or full – is not normally seen due to the swelling around the area. (See Fig. 6.2.)

Signs and Symptoms

This should be managed with rest, ice, and compression and analgesics if necessary. After a few days, a slight dip may be found in the rectus femoris muscle, normally in the upper 1/3 of the thigh on contraction of the muscle, as seen in a straight leg raise. It is normally sore on resistance.

Treatment and Management

Normally rest for 6 weeks allows the rupture and resultant swelling and potential bleeding surrounding the muscle to calm down. Electrotherapy can be used along with gentle massages around the area. Gentle stretching can begin after a few weeks also, but it is unlikely that the rupture itself heals 100%. The body will try and add some scar tissue or 'glue' to the rupture, but often, this is not complete. However, function is rarely affected in the medium-to-long term as other muscles normally accommodate and adapt to the deficit.

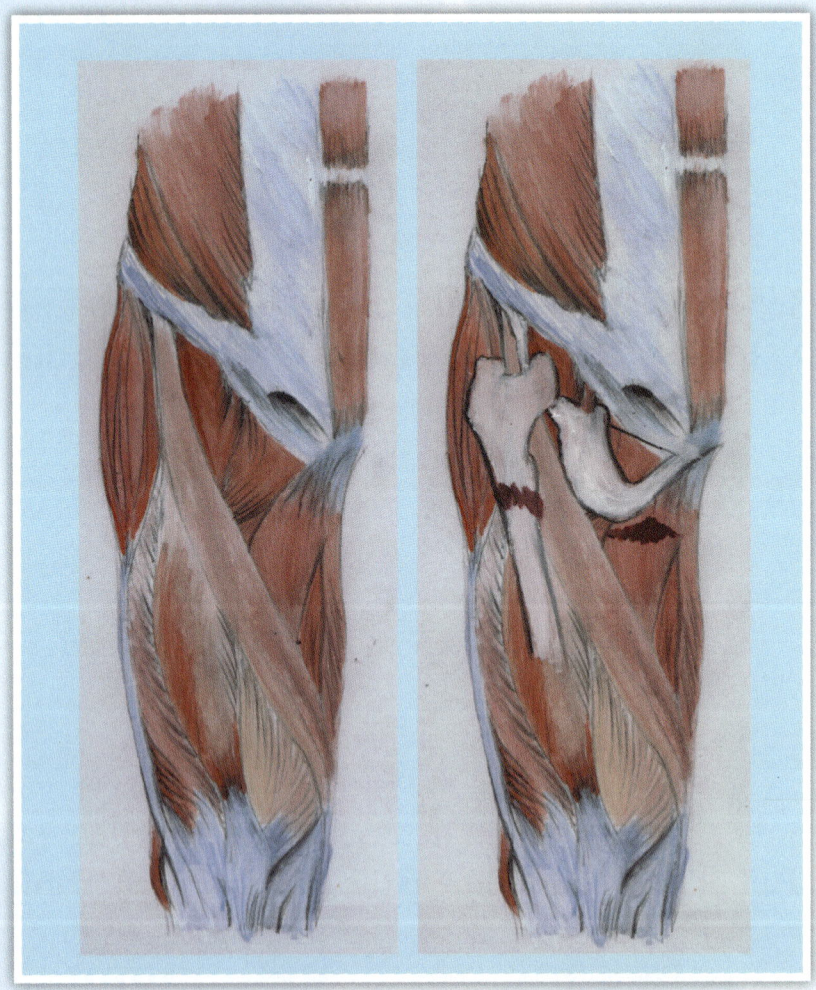

Fig. 6.2 Normal rectus femoris strain (left) and rectus femoris strain (right)

Intramuscular Haematoma and Myositis Ossificans (MOT)

At times, a direct impact on the thigh muscle can cause an intramuscular haematoma (sometimes called a dead leg). This is essentially an internal bruise within the muscle belly. If it does not resolve, it can manifest itself into an myostitis ossification. This simply means that the haematoma can ossify into a lump of solid bony tissue peripherally, which cannot be resolved easily. It interferes with the normal mechanism of the muscle; hence early diagnosis and management is essential (Lyle, 1984).

Myositis is present in 10–30% of all blunt traumas to the thigh muscle in children and teens (Birrer et al., 2002). Normally, the MOT is not detected until the scar tissue has solidified.

Signs and Symptoms

Initially, there is an ache and soreness which can get aggravated at night because of the oedema and bleeding that can create pressure within the thigh. After a few weeks, a palpable lump can be felt and the thigh is difficult to stretch out.

Test

On palpation, normally there is pain and a hard lump can be felt. Contraction of the quadriceps makes the thigh pain worse, and the thigh cannot be easily stretched without pain.

Treatment and Management

Treatment of the initial haematoma is with rest, ice, and compression initially. Massaging the soft tissues can help after a few days, along with stretching. Strength work is important as oedema or haematomas normally lead to muscle atrophy.

Treatment of a MOT is a little more vigorous. Identification can be done via an X-ray or by palpation. Deep massage, heat, and stretches can help break down the scar tissue. Electrotherapy can also help. This can take time to recover, anywhere between 3 and 6 months.

Hamstring Strain

Hamstring strains in children are uncommon, but they are more common in the older teens. Caused by excessive running and sprinting, or a change in acceleration or deceleration, the pain is felt immediately at the back of the thigh. Hamstring strains can be more common during growth spurts and should not be confused with an avulsion of the ischial tuberosity.

Signs and Symptoms

There is pain at the back of the thigh, commonly in the upper 1/3 of the upper posterior thigh. The teen will be unable to sprint without pain (Abrahams, 2009).

Test(s)

Resistance against knee flexion will be sore on a hamstring strain. MRI scan or diagnostic ultrasound scan can confirm. (See Fig. 6.3.)

Treatment and Management

Treatment initially should be rest, ice, compression, and elevation. After a few days, gentle stretching can begin. After a week or so, simple strengthening of the hamstring can begin, depending on the severity and grade of the injury. Gentle running can be started around week 2 (again depending on the grade and the severity), and from week 3, more aggressive exercises can be done, including small bursts of sprints (Abrahams, 2009).

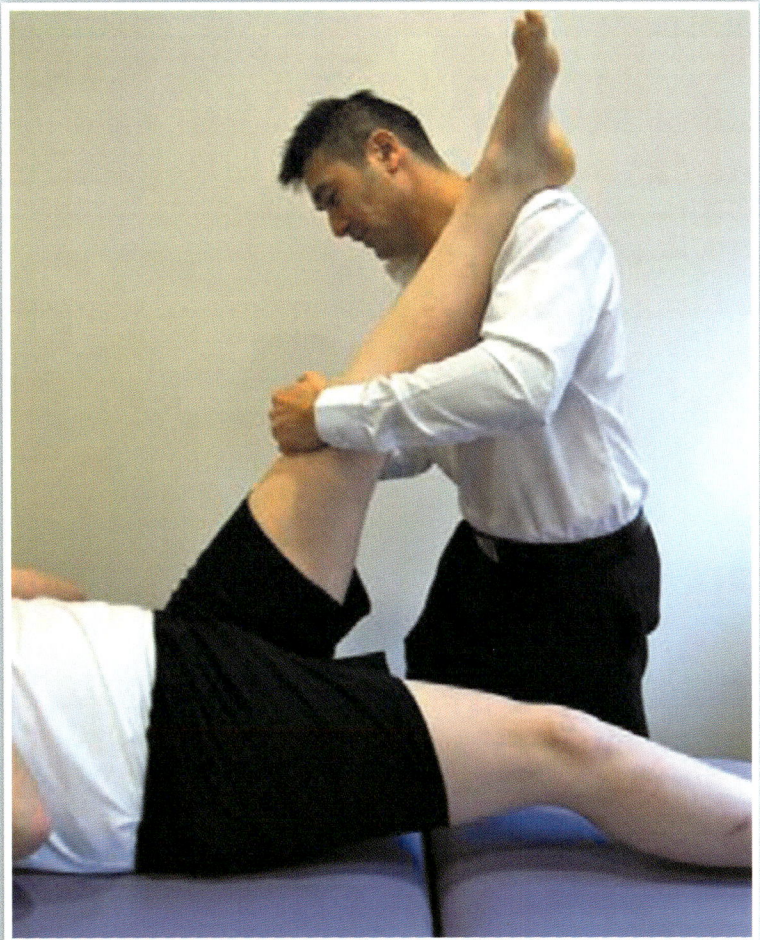

Fig. 6.3 Stretching of the hamstring

Adductor Strain (the Groin Strain)

Adductor strains are relatively uncommon in children and are more common in the older teens. Pain is felt on the inner groin, and it is common following any form of adduction of the thigh, such as seen in football when side-footing the ball. Pain is normally felt immediately.

Signs and Symptoms

Pain on the inner thigh, normally in the upper 1/3 of the groin, is the usual symptom.

Test(s)

Confirmation can be resistance against adduction of the thigh where pain will increase. An MRI scan will confirm extent of injury. The region can be sore on direct palpation.

Treatment and Management

Treatment initially should be rest, ice, compression, and elevation. After a few days, gentle stretching (see Fig. 6.4) can begin. After a week or so, simple strengthening of the adductor can begin, depending on the severity and grade of the injury. Gentle running can begin around week 2 (again depending on the grade and the severity) alongside adductor-strengthening exercises. Aggressive exercises, including side-footing a ball but with little power, can be done in week 3. As time progresses, during the week, this can increase steadily until full power is resumed (Abrahams, 2009).

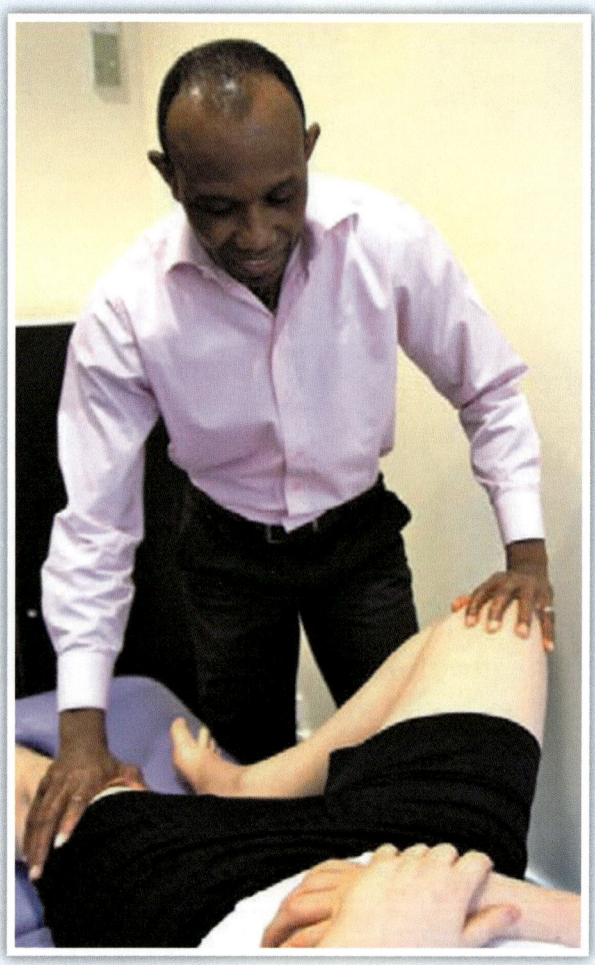

Fig. 6.4 Gentle stretching of the adductor longus tendon

Apophyseal Avulsion Fractures

Avulsion fractures at the apophyses of the hip and pelvis are common in adolescents, especially through growth spurts and around times of fusion of the plates.

The usual mechanism is a sudden force exerting eccentric or concentric action with acceleration or deceleration of the muscles which pulls the muscle away from the bone. Sometimes, there is no clear mechanism (Birrer et al., 2002).

Greater Trochanter

Greater trochanter avulsion fractures are rare in adolescents. The hip external rotators, such as obturators, gemelli, and gluteus medius and minimus attach to the greater trochanteric apophysis. An avulsion fracture can occur here with strong contraction of these muscles.

Signs and Symptoms

The pain is normally very localised to the greater trochanter and sometimes even walking and weight-bearing can be sore.

Test(s)

Pain can be reproduced through palpation, resisted hip abduction, or passive adduction.

Normally, an X-ray can confirm suspicions of fracture along with its severity and location.

Lesser Trochanter

The iliopsoas muscle attaches to the lesser trochanter, and strong hip flexion movements such as kicking a ball or even sprinting can cause an avulsion fracture.

Signs and Symptoms

Pain is normally felt in the anterior groin, and sometimes, a 'pop' or snapping sensation can be heard. (See Fig. 6.5.)

Test(s)

Pain is normally reproduced on palpation or against resisted hip flexion. Sometimes, in the sitting position, the child or teen cannot actively raise their thigh; this is known as Ludloff sign (Birrer et al., 2002).

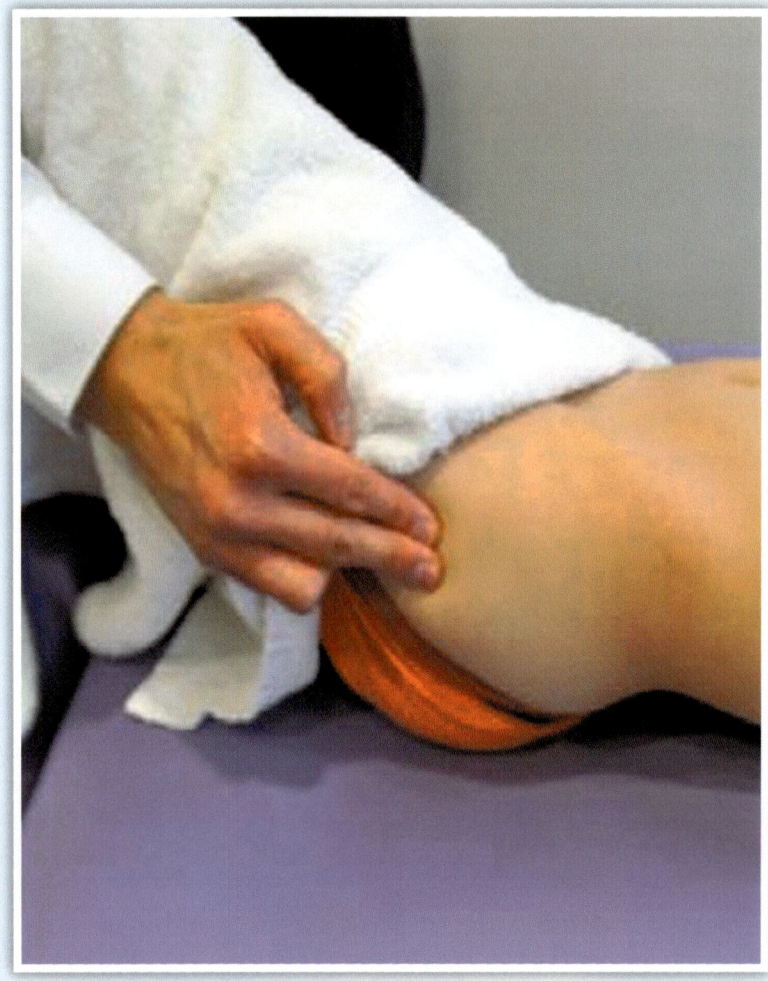

Fig. 6.5 Palpation of the lesser trochanter

X-ray or bone scan or MRI scan can confirm diagnosis.

Ischial Tuberosity

The hamstring muscles attach to the ischial tuberosity, and strong contraction from an acceleration or deceleration, mainly under eccentric control, can cause an avulsion fracture.

Signs and Symptoms

Acute pain is normally felt at the origin, and the child or teen is unable to run or sprint.

Test(s)

Pain is very localised to the ischial tuberosity, and even sitting down can sometimes be sore. Pain can occur on resisted knee flexion or resisted hip extension. Stretching the hamstring rarely gives any short-term relief. Pain can also be reproduced upon a straight leg raise (Cramer, 2004).

X-ray, bone scan, or MRI scan can confirm diagnosis, severity, and likely prognosis.

Anterior Superior Iliac Spine (ASIS)

The tensor fascia lata muscle and sartorius attach to the front of the pelvis, at the ASIS, and movements involving repetitive hip flexion can sometimes cause an avulsion fracture at this site if contractions are strong enough. Again, this tends to be more common in adolescents, during growth spurts (Atanda, Shah, O'Brien, 2011).

Signs and Symptoms

Pain is normally felt at the ASIS and is very localised. There is pain on hip flexion movements.

Test(s)

Any form of kicking is normally sore and palpation of the ASIS, or slightly below it, is very sore.

X-ray normally reveals an avulsion fracture.

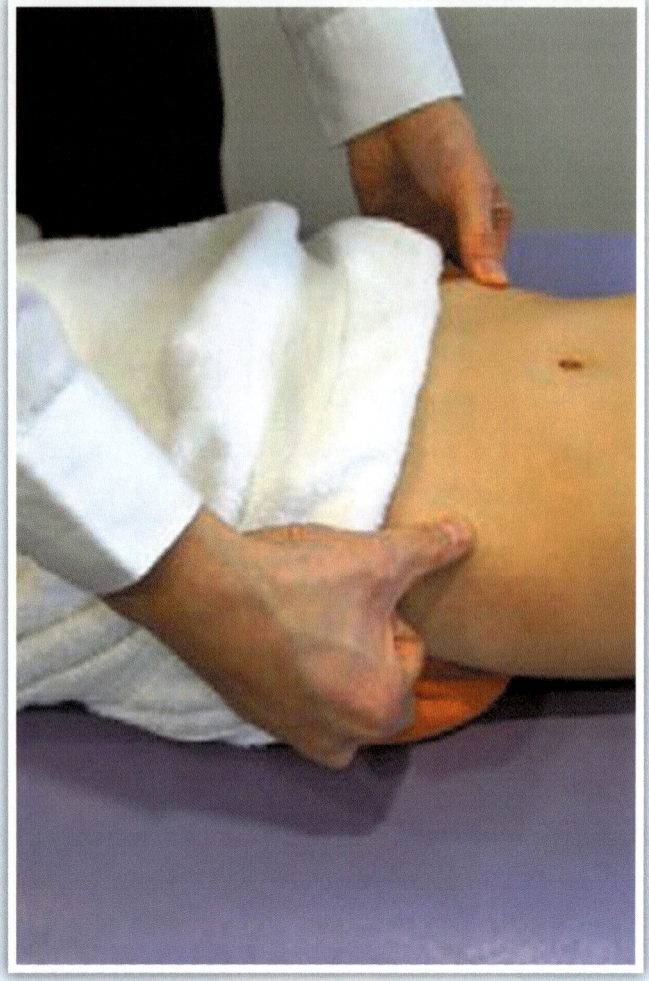

Fig. 6.6 Palpation of the ASIS

Anterior Inferior Iliac Spine (AIIS)

Rectus femoris, a strong hip flexor and kicking muscle, attaches to the AIIS. Repetitive flexion movements, such as seen in sprinters, or kicking actions can sometimes fracture away from the AIIS.

Signs and Symptoms

Pain is normally felt directly at the AIIS. Care must be taken not to confuse this with a sartorius fracture, which is only 2–3 cm superior to the AIIS.

Test(s)

Pain is localised to the AIIS, and rarely is the pain referred.
X-ray can also be used to confirmed.

Iliac Crest

The iliac crest has many attachments of muscles which can fracture away. Latissimus dorsi, gluteus maximus, gluteus medius, tensor fascia lata and obliques all attach to this area.

Aggressive twisting movements of the back can cause a fracture here.

Signs and Symptoms

Pain is normally localised anteriorly, posteriorly, or laterally, depending on which muscle pulls away from the bone and how aggressive the action is.

Test(s)

An X-ray normally confirms the fracture. Pain on palpation. (See Fig. 6.7.)

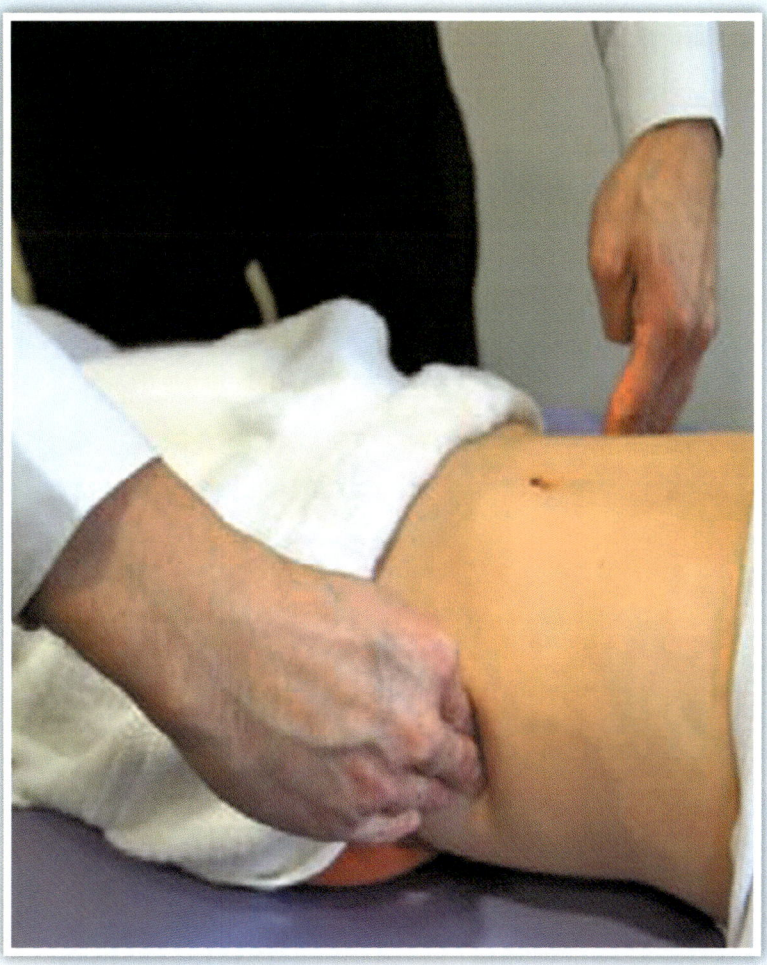

Fig. 6.7 Palpation of the iliac crest(s)

Treatment and Management of Apophyseal Injuries

In the initial stages, rest, ice, and compression of the injured area is essential to reduce and limit further damage. Analgesics can be used, but anti-inflammatory drugs should be avoided for a few days and should only be used if necessary.

Stretching of the tissues or any aggressive mobilisation should not be done at this point, as this may aggravate the condition. It is important to educate the parents and the child about the condition and the need for rest. An X-ray should be done to confirm diagnosis and to see how bad the injury is. Reassurance is also important to ensure good prognosis and to comfort over anxious parents and teens.

Once the condition settles, gentle stretching and soft-tissue work can begin on and around the injured site. Massages (gentle) can help to alleviate any muscle tension and soreness around the area and help to remove any remaining inflammation or swelling which maybe present (Patel et al., 2009).

Strength exercises concentrically and isometrically should be done after a few weeks, progressing on to eccentric exercises, and then functional exercises. If exercises are graded and regular stretching is done on a daily basis, this should hopefully not re-aggravate the teen, unless they continue to undergo an aggressive growth spurt.

Some surgeons recommend surgical intervention in large fractures, but this should be avoided where necessary (Birrer et al., 2002).

Fractures and Dislocations of the Hip

Apart from apophyseal fractures, normal fractures can affect children and teens in sports. Normally, these are much more traumatic and direct contact is normally involved.

Femoral Neck Fractures and Femoral Stress Fractures

Fractures of this kind in children are rare (see Fig. 6.8), and other pathologies (such as osteosarcoma) should be suspected with fractures of the neck of femur (NoF), especially if the trauma is not severe. Femoral stress fractures are more common in military recruits or in late teens who simply overtrain (Patel et al., 2009).

If fractures do occur, pain is extreme in weight bearing and a noticeable limp is present. Most cannot weight bear. The leg is normally shortened and externally rotated. If a fracture is suspected, the child should be taken to hospital to reveal the extent of fracture and pathology.

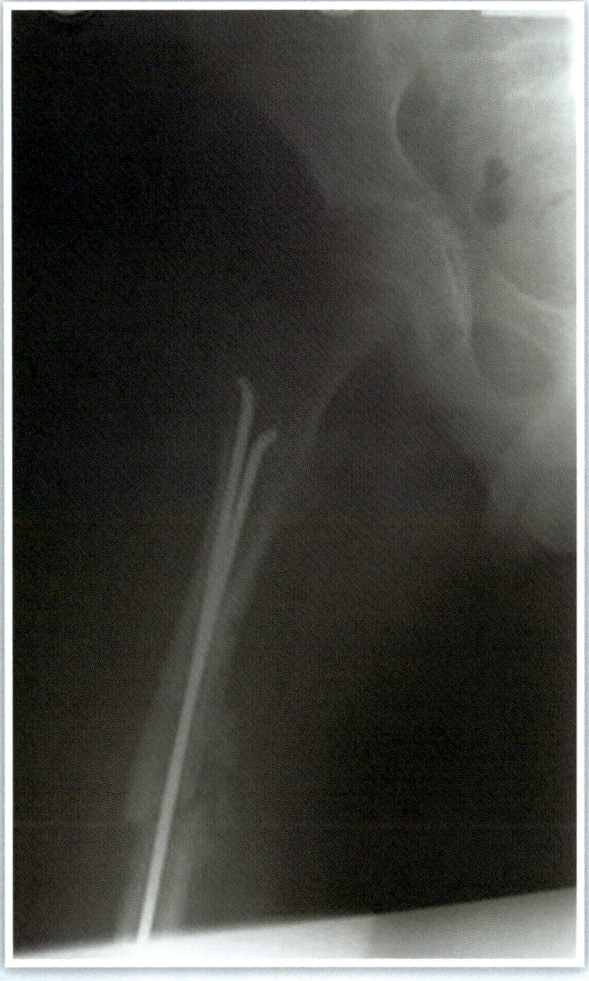

Fig. 6.8 Mid-shaft fracture (with internal fixation of two nails) of 15-year-old

Stress fractures react slightly differently. They are normally sore, but pain is relieved with rest. Weight bearing is normally fine following relative rest, but continued running aggravates the pain again. There is a vague pain, which is quite hard to identify unless a bone scan is done (Patel et al., 2009).

Treatment for stress fractures is rest for 6 weeks and a re-scan, and once cleared, to restart training slowly but progressively. Also, trying to identify the exact cause which will help prevent re-exacerbation, such as shoewear, overtraining, camber, duration, and sudden changes in intensity and frequency of running (Patel et al., 2009).

Pelvic Fractures

Pelvic fractures, apart from apophyseal fractures, are rare in teens and children and are normally seen as a result of severe trauma. Fractures of the pelvic ring, interior pubic rami, and acetabulum can occur and have been reported with direct trauma. In rare cases, stress fractures of the inferior pubic ring can occur; they are similar in symptoms to stress fractures of the neck of the femur and follow similar patterns in diagnosis and management. Anatomically, the pain will be directly on the inferior pubic ring, just inferior and lateral to the pubic synthesis, or slightly superior to the insertion of the adductor longus tendon in children.

Hip Dislocation

Hip dislocations are more common in children than in teens. They are even more common than fractures in adolescents (Birrer et al., 2002). Certain sports such as skiing, snowboarding, motorcross, and gymnastics have been implicated in this traumatic injury (Patel et al., 2009), with a 12% incident rate in child and teen skiers (Patel et al., 2009).

The most common dislocation is a posterior dislocation, normally when the hip is flexed and in adduction. Sometimes called a 'dashboard-type' injury, this dislocation is caused by severe trauma where the leg is driven backwards on the pelvis. The dislocation may cause avascular necrosis, and unless this dislocation is reduced within 6 hours of injury, avasular necrosis is likely (Atanda et al., 2011; Birrer et al., 2002).

Signs and Symptoms

Apart from seeing the initial trauma, extreme pain is felt in the buttock, pelvis, and posterior thigh, and the child or teen is unable to move their leg or hip. They are unable to weight bear and the affected leg is normally shortened (Patel et al., 2009).

No reduction should be attempted until an X-ray is done to exclude fracture dislocation. However, this is treated as an emergency due to the risk of avascular necrosis, and emergency services should be called in any event.

Treatment and Management

Once reduction is performed, relative rest and possible traction is applied to reduce the risk of any further potential avascular necrosis. Following a period of partial weight bearing after a week or so (or depending on how serious the injury is, it could be longer), full weight bearing should be gradually increased. Re-X-ray should also be done after a few weeks, normally after 3–6 weeks, to ensure that the joint is stable.

Once weight bearing has been re-established, exercises can begin in the form of concentric exercises, followed by more functional exercises. Full return to sport should not be resumed at least for 6–8 weeks to allow the injury to fully repair (Birrer et al., 2002).

Stress Fractures

Stress fractures of the femoral shaft, femoral neck, and pelvis remain rare in children and teens but can be caused by repetitive microtrauma. Constant running, athletics, or pounding sports can cause these type of injuries (Birrer et al., 2002).

Stress fractures can also be caused by a change in training intensity, duration, and frequency. Change in shoewear, camber, or training type can also be a precursor. These injuries are more common in females, in particular in those at risk of amenorrhea – such as seen in girls taking part in gymnastics or long-distance running from a young age.

Signs and Symptoms

Pain is normally localised to where the stress fracture is. Around the groin is a common place where the area becomes painful during activity, and the pain continues to worsen as activity increases until it becomes unbearable. Once the activity stops, the symptoms reduce slowly after a few days, or until the activity restarts.

Tests

Confirmation of diagnosis can be by an X-ray initially, but seldom does this pick up acute stress fractures. A bone scan is more reliable.

Treatment and Management

Once diagnosis is confirmed, sports should stop and rest imposed. The child or teen is still able to be mobile and doesn't normally require crutches or immobilisation, but they should not be encouraged to do anything that places extra stress or pressure on the hips.

Stress fractures in children normally take 4–6 weeks to fully recover, and within this time, the children are still able to do some activity; they are just unable to run. The likely cause (whether this be intensity of training or shoewear) should be assessed, and where necessary, steps should be taken to prevent further injury.

Pathologic Fractures

Any suspected fracture in children and teens should be X-rayed. Pathology such as osteogenic sarcomas, malignant neoplasms, and osteiod osteoma, even though rare, can cause fractures of bones in children and teens (Birrer et al., 2002).

Osteitis Pubis

Osteitis pubis is uncommon in children but may present in an older adolescent. It is inflammation of the pubic synthesis and is caused mainly by traction of the adductors or hip flexors/abdominals during twisting movements or by the trauma of pounding during running. It is more common in recreational long-distance runners, hockey players, and footballers (Abrahams, 2003).

Finding the cause is essential. Normally, a change in running style, frequency, intensity, or duration should be checked. Similarly, change in running shoes, camber/surface can also be potential causes.

Signs and Symptoms

Pain in one or both the groins can be common. There is localised pain on palpation of the pubic synthesis itself. The pain can sometimes refer down the groin in severe cases and is exacerbated by running.

Test(s)

Clinical examination reveals local tenderness, with pain on resisted adduction and hip flexion (Abrahams, 2003).

Confirmation is usually by an X-ray, but a bone scan or a CT scan is more reliable.

There is little reliability with orthopaedic testing (Abrahams, 2003).

Treatment and Management

Treatment includes rest, ice, and compression if necessary. Addressing the cause is important to prevent re-exacerbation and help settle the diagnosis. Painkillers or analgesics can be used.

Once the inflammation and the pain settle, rehabilitation can start slowly and progressively. Running should be left to last, as this is normally the main aggravator (Birrer et al., 2002).

Iliotibial Band Syndrome (ITB)

ITB syndrome is inflammation of the ITB tendon as it frictions across the lateral epicondyle of the knee or across the greater trochanter in running or cycling, which can be seen in teens. Repetitive flexion and extension movements cause friction between the tendon sheath and the epicondyle or greater trochanter, causing localised pain on the lateral portion of the knee or, indeed, the lateral portion of the hip joint (Abrahams, 2009).

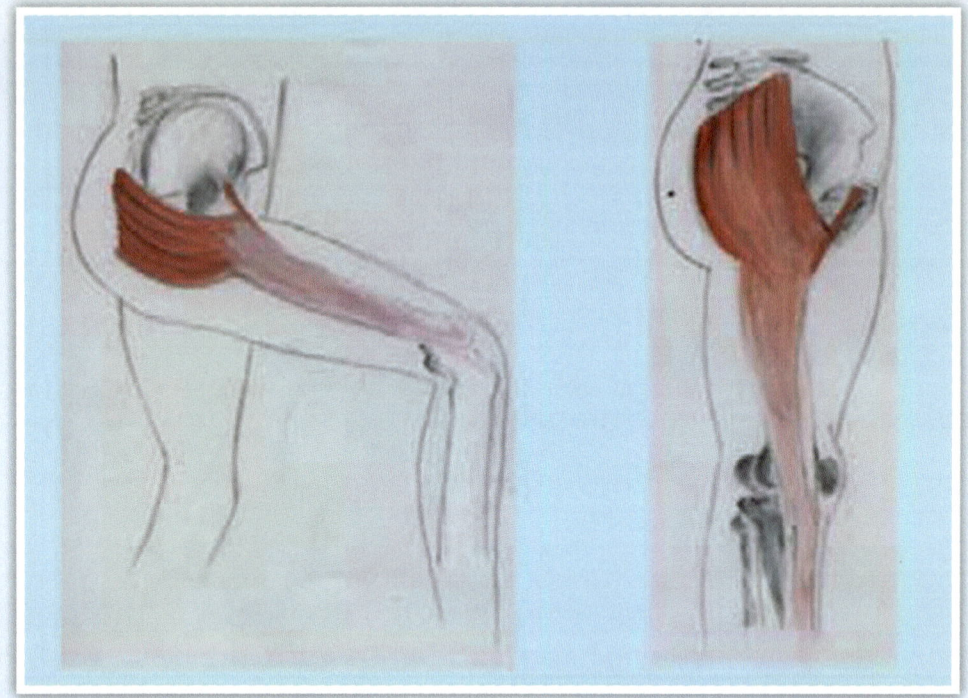

Fig. 6.9 The ITB muscle

There are normally different causes or triggers for ITB syndrome, ranging from change in training such as more hill running, or change in shoewear, camber, bicycle, or change in intensity of training. (See Fig. 6.9.)

Signs and Symptoms

Pain localised to the lateral epicondyle of the knee or lateral trochanter of the hip is a symptom. The pain worsens on flexion and extension movements and on running downhill or at fast speed (Abrahams, 2009).

Test(s)

An MRI scan or a CT scan should reveal and confirm ITB syndrome.

Treatment and Management

Management should initially be rest, ice, and compression. Trying to find the cause is equally important so as not to re-aggravate the pathology. Close attention needs to be paid to shoewear, biomechanics, duration, frequency, and intensity of training in runners, and in cyclists, the bicycle itself, seating, and pedals should be checked (Abrahams, 2009).

Stretching of the ITB to the surrounding tissues is important; massage, deep friction-massages, and electrotherapy can also be used.

Once pain settles with rest, restart exercise training at a low grade and build up slowly and progressively (Birrer et al., 2002).

Trochanteric Bursitis

Trochanteric bursitis is rare in children and teens. It is simply an inflammation of the trochanteric bursa, located on the lateral potion of the hip joint (see Fig. 6.9b). It is normally caused by excessive friction of the ITB (as above) but the friction is higher up on the hip joint. It can be traumatic as well, with teens sustaining a direct trauma, such as a fall on the hip (Abrahams, 2009).

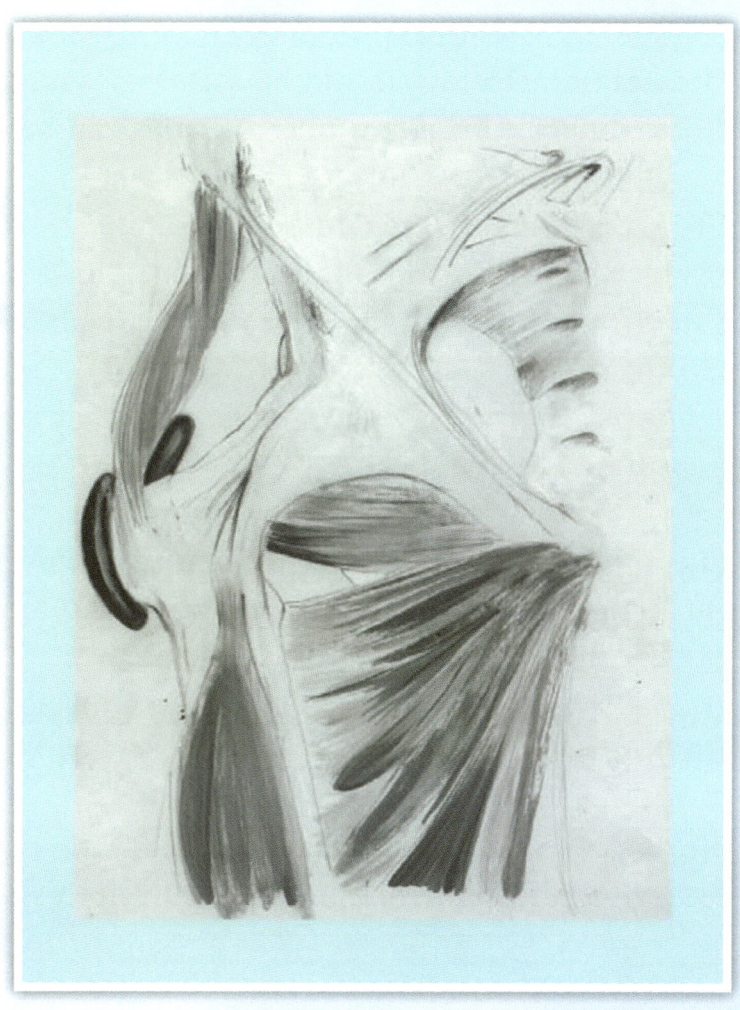

Fig. 6.9b trochanteric bursa(s)

Signs and Symptoms

Tenderness is seen over the greater trochanter, and lying on the side (affected side) is more painful. Running and walking over long distances make the pain worse.

Test(s)

There is soreness on direct palpation. MRI scan confirms the condition.

Treatment and Management

Treatment includes rest from the aggravating factor, ice, and compression if necessary. Addressing the cause (such as any change in type of training or change in shoewear) is important to ensure avoidance of re-exacerbation. Direct compression should be avoided (such as lying on the affected side), and stretching for the surrounding tissues can be done.

Progressive exercises can be done, and training should be slow and gradual over weeks. Speedy rehabilitation of this bursa can re-aggravate the pain. Injection of steroid to the joint can also help, but this is uncommon in children (Abrahams, 2009).

Snapping Hip Syndrome

Hip noises and clicky hips are common in children and adolescents. Much of this is normal for the developing child and tends to be non-pathological. Causes of the 'click' can be the ITB snapping over the greater trochanter, psoas tendon over the psoas bursa, acetabular tears, instability, hypermobility, or dysplasia of the hips.

Normally, clicking stops spontaneously. Strength exercises around the hip can help re-stabilise the hip, and core strength should be addressed

Piriformis Syndrome

Piriformis syndrome in children is rare but may be slightly more common in adolescents. It is where the sciatic nerve becomes inflamed as it pierces through the piriformis muscle. This is caused by excessive friction of the nerve within the muscle itself.

Care must be taken to ensure that pain in the buttock is not mistaken for an indication of a prolapsed disc, which can refer pain into the buttock, mimicking symptoms similar to piriformis syndrome.

Meralgia Paresthetica

Meralgia parathesia in children and teens is rare. It simply is compression of the lateral femoral cutaneous nerve as it exits the top part of the thigh muscle (Patel et al., 2009).

Direct compression of this area, normally from trauma, can cause numbness and tingling on the outer part of the thigh. In most cases, it recovers by itself.

Legg– Calvé–Perthes disease (Osteochondritis Juvenilis)

Legg–Calvé–Perthes disease is an avascular necrosis of the femoral head and is the result of an interruption in blood supply that can lead to deformation of the head of the femur. It is unclear as to whether the deformation is the result of a singular vascular occlusion or multiple occlusions over a longer period of time.

Legg–Calvé–Perthes disease is one of the most common causes of lower limb pain in children, normally in the 4–8 years range, and is more common in males. The disease is 5 times more common in males as opposed to females, and can occur bilaterally (in both hips) in 10% of cases (Birrer et al., 2002).

Because the resulting limp is liable to cause biomechanical changes, pains can refer elsewhere (Cramer, 2004).

Signs and Symptoms

Pain in the groin, with occasional slight limp, is a symptom of this disease. A lack of rotation at the hip and a stiff hip will be noticed. It maybe painful with running or increased weight bearing. This pathology can be asymptomatic for a long time, or the pain can present as a long history. Normally, something upsets the condition.

Tests

Diagnosis is made by X-rays, although it is normal to notice a limp or a change in the gait of the child first. An MRI scan or a CT scan is more reliable. (See Fig. 6.10.)

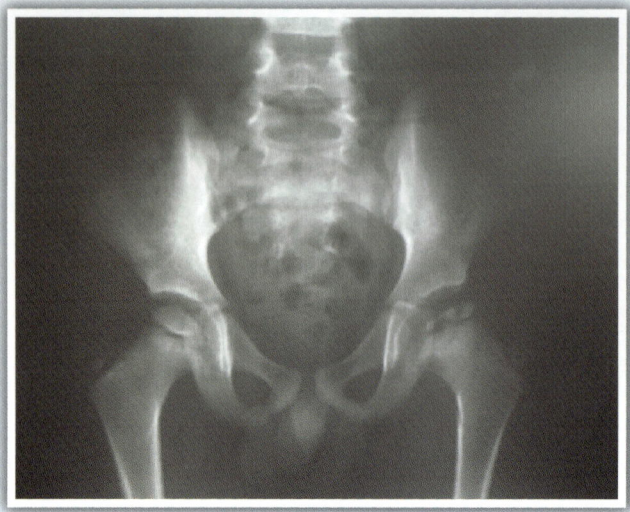
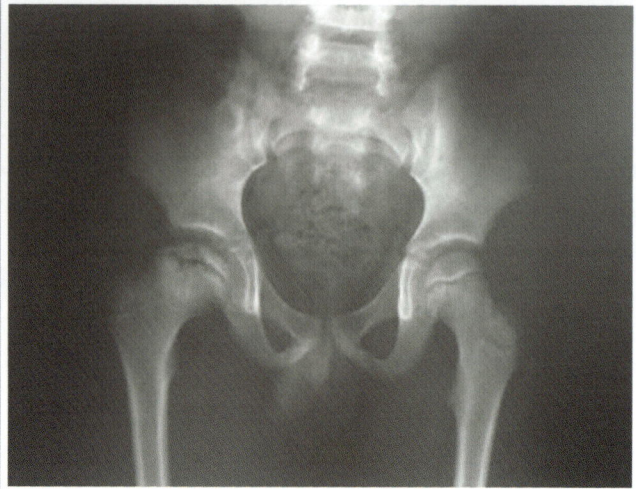

Fig. 6.10 Perthes in a 14-year-old

Treatment and Management

Initial therapy aims to minimise weight bearing, protect the hip joint, and maintain good range of motion (ROM). Abduction and external rotation of the femur allows the femoral head to be positioned in the rounded part of the acetabulum and prevent deterioration. This position can be achieved by wearing a brace or by surgery. The goal of the treatment is to reduce the risk of degenerative joint disease or arthritis in later life (Crawford & Hamblen, 1990).

If this pathology is left alone, it can lead to long-term problems such as premature osteoarthritis.

Sometimes, surgery is indicated if Perthes is severe hence X-rays, and an orthopaedic consult should always be done on diagnosis of this pathology.

Slipped Capital Femoral Epiphysis (SCFE)

The *British Medical Association (BMA) Illustrated Medical Dictionary* defines slipped capital femoral epiphysis (SCFE) as 'A displacement of the upper epiphysis of the femur'. Even though this type of displacement is rare, it occurs more often in boys and obese children; normally it affects children aged between 11 and 13 years (Page, 2007).

Here, at the upper growing end plate of the bone, there is a separation of the thigh bone from the ball of the hip joint (Fish, 1984). In other words, the upper or capital epiphysis of the femur slips in relation to the rest of the femur. This condition is seen as one of the most important paediatric and adolescent hip disorders detected in the medical profession (Larson, Yu, Peterson, Stans, & Melton, 2010; Lehmann, Arons, Loder, & Vitale, 2006; Phillips, Griffiths, & Clarke, 2001).

Causes

Rapid growth is the main cause as this condition affects children in their early adolescent period when they grow rapidly. And with this rapid growth comes an increase in the force and stress placed on the upper part of the femur, which may pull or twist it if the forces are great enough.

Overweight or obese children may put an extra strain on the femur's upper area, which is why this condition normally affects obese children.

A slip can occur from a fall or an injury, and repetitive actions over a long period of time can cause the slip. Genetic predisposition, medications such as long-term steroids, chemotherapy, radiotherapy, and bone problems related to kidney disease can also be factors (Clarke & Kendrick, 2009; Fish, 1984; Houghton, 2009; Loder, Aronson, Dobbs, & Weinstein, 2000; Wabitsch et al., 2012).

Prevalence

In the United Kingdom, in every 100,000 children, 1 in 7 get SCFE. In the States, of every 100,000 children, this condition represents 10.8 cases. The condition is more common in overweight and/ or obese children, as mentioned earlier. As obesity increases, the shear force around the proximal growth plate in the hip also increases.

Left hip is affected more often than the right. To a lesser extent, the condition also affects tall and thin children. It affects 3 times more boys than girls, particularly girls between the ages 11 and 13 years and boys between 13 and 15 years (Uglow & Clarke, 2004).

SCFE can affect children with known hormonal disorders, kidney failure, or a history of radiotherapy. It is also often seen in patients younger than 10 years of age (Page, 2007; Phillips et al., 2001; Uglow & Clarke, 2004; Wabitsch et al., 2012).

Patients with SCFE have an unusually widened epiphyseal growth plate as hypertrophy occurs during a growth spurt. (See Fig. 6.10b, 6.11.) This affects the organisation of a normal cartilaginous column, allowing slippage to occur as a result of a less-ordered column and a more weakened area. Increased stresses across a weakened physis causes SCFE, with biomechanical and biochemical factors contributing to the slip. The direction of the deforming force determines the displacement (Dwek, 2009; Fish, 1984; Kocher, Bishop, Hresko, et al., 2004; Murray & Wilson, 2008).

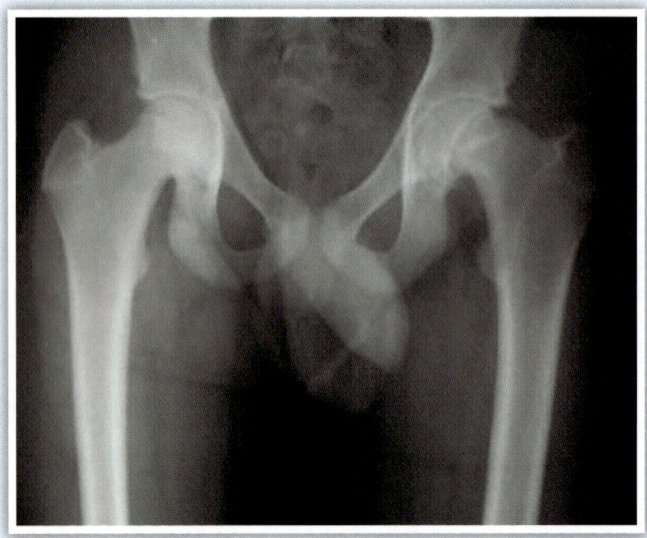

Fig. 6.10b Slipped capital epiphyses in a 12–year–old boy

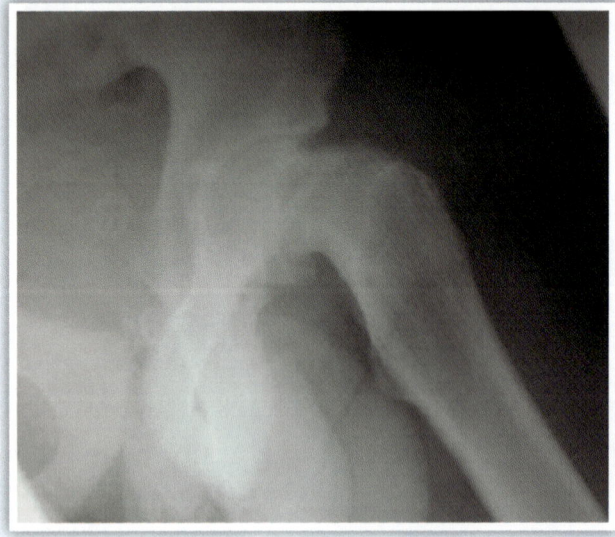

Fig. 6.11 Slipped captial epiphyses (Lateral view)

Signs and Symptoms

There is pain in the hip or knee, and the child may present with a limp. Pain in the knee may be referred from the hip via the obturator nerve. There may be a decrease in passive internal rotation of the hip or pain on internal rotation of the hip (or both).

There is rotation and abduction of the lower extremity with gently positive hip flexion. If the condition is severe, the patient is unable to weight bear and to sit with knees straight (knees tend to be externally rotated) (Lehmann et al., 2006; Page, 2007; Thacker & Clarke, 2009; Witbreuk, Bolkenbaas, Mullender, Sierevelt, & Besselaar, 2009).

Tests

Like any other illness or injury, a complete medical history should be taken, and physical examination should be done.

An X-ray of the hip or an MRI scan should be taken.

A radiograph of the hip, containing two views, should be taken. From the radiograph, a Klein line can be used on the anteroposterior (AP) view to see the degree of displacement of the femoral head.

Blood test is done in rare cases

Treatment and Management

Initial hospitalisation may be an option or complete bed rest to avoid further necrosis of the femoral head is advised.

In some cases, an operation to stabilise the epiphysis and stop it from moving any further may be performed.(Fish, 1984; Maeda, Kita, Funayama, & Kokubun, 2001; Phillips et al., 2001; Rhoad, Davidson, Heyman, Dormans, & Drummond, 1999).

Rehabilitation

Long-term follow-up is advised for SCFE, especially if surgery is performed and pinning was done in one or both hips, as there is oftentimes controversy about the value of the surgery in terms of its timing and the differential illnesses that may follow.

Immediately after surgery, patients are placed on crutches for weeks to months.

X-rays are taken to keep an eye on the growth plate, and sports and certain activities are avoided until the growth plate closes.

Modalities such as heat, ice, ultrasound, or electrical current may be used to assist with decreasing any pain associated with the surgery.

Crutches and a non-weight-bearing status are standard following surgery for SCFE, but within 3–5 days, most patients will be able to start putting some weight down while standing or walking (Aronson & Carlson, 1992; Kocher et al., 2004; Larson et al., 2010; Uglow & Clarke, 2004).

Advise that patients keep walking with either one or two crutches until limping ceases. Improper gait can lead to a host of other pains in the knee, hip, and back, so it is prudent to continue on crutches until near-normal walking can be achieved. Gait re-education is important.

- Normalise any deficits that may have developed in the range of motion and strength of your child's lower limb joints.

- Stretch the child's limb or lower back whilst at the clinic and, if necessary, 'mobilise' the joints of your child. This hands-on technique encourages the stiff joints to move gradually into their normal range of motion.

- Address any strength deficits.

- Introduce activities and exercises for the patient to regain coordination, balance, and proprioception in order to assist in the patient's return to normal activities.

Sports Hernia

A sports hernia is defined as a weakness of the posterior wall of the inguinal canal. It is rare in the general population but more common in sports like football, hockey, and rugby. Unlike a normal inguinal hernia where you can visually see a lump in the inguinal region, a sports hernia does not show this (Abrahams, Chadwick, & Zirpin, 2013). It remains rare in children, but can be more common in older adolescents.

Signs and Symptoms

There is pain following sports, which can last for up to 24 hours. It is a generalised ache in the groin rather than a sharp pain. The pain settles after 24 hours and does not re-exacerbate unless the sport is played again. Coughing and sneezing is sore within the 24-hour-period of the sport (Abrahams et al., 2013).

Test

Currently, the only reliable confirmation test is laparoscopy.

Treatment and Management

Laparoscopy is currently the best form of treatment for this pathology. Post-op physiotherapy remains controversial, but core stability and a progressive exercise programme should be encouraged (Abrahams et al., 2013).

Nerve Entrapments

Nerve entrapments in children and teens remain rare in the hip. Obturator nerve entrapment causes weakness and numbness of the adductors and groin area. Referral should be made if one suspects this pathology (Patel et al., 2009).

Congenital Dislocation of the Hip (CDH)

CDH itself rarely affects the older teen but can present with sudden subluxation and pains of the hip joints. CDH is congenital and is simply dysplasia of the hip joints at birth. The actual cause remains unclear, but it is normally seen in Cesarean-section babies or breech deliveries. Even though this is managed conservatively at birth, it can lead to joint laxity and instability of the hip joints, which later on can be a precursor to hip joint impingement, osteoarthritis (OA) changes, and cluncky hips. It normally affects girls more than boys (Crawford & Hamblen, 1990).

Signs and Symptoms

Dislocation itself is very rare, but instability or hypermobility can lead to pains, clicky hips, giving way, and sharp pains.

Tests

X-rays normally reveal hip dysplasia

Management

Physiotherapy entails strength and core stability of the hip joints. Avoid excessive weight bearing through the joints such as uneven running or increased shock through the joints. Because the condition can lead to arthritic changes in the adult, precautions should be taken to manage the condition.

Other Pathologies Affecting the Hip Joint

Urinary tract infections, ovarian cysts, endometriosis, ectopic pregnancy, inguinal hernia, testicular torsion, sexually transmitted diseases, neoplasms can all refer pain in teens into the groin area.

Other rare pathologies such as osteogenus imperfect (see Fig. 6.12), which is simply fragile bones and rickets (Vitamin D deficiency) can also present in children.

Osteosarcoma tumours and other such nasties can occur in teens and children in the hip area and femur bone, but this is rare.

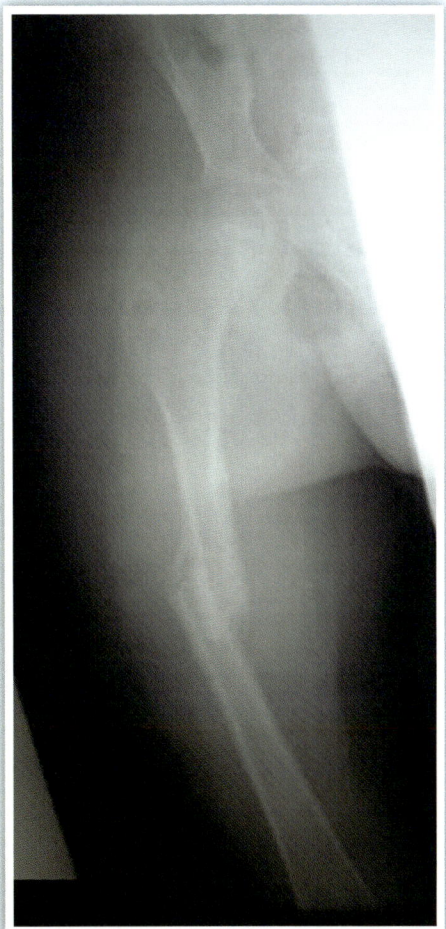

Fig. 6.12 Osteogenus imperfecta (mid-shaft femur fracture)

However, any complaint which doesn't follow a normal mechanical pattern of signs and symptoms should be investigated further.

Key Points

- Myositis ossificans is a complication of an intramuscular haematoma.

- Apophyseal fractures occur at over six places on the pelvis.

- Fractures of the femur should always be treated as suspicious as there could be an underlying cause.

- Posterior dislocation of the hip is more common than fractures of the hip.

- Perthes and slipped capital epipyses can present as anterior knee pain.

References

Abrahams, S. D. (2003). Atypical groin pain, The sportsmens hernia. *Critical Reviews in Physical & Rehabilitation Medicine, 15*(1), 41.

Abrahams, S. D. (2009). Five most common running injuries. *Health & Fitness Professional Journal,* EZ Articles.

Abrahams, S., Chadwick, S., & Zirpin, S. (2013). Sportsmens hernia. *British Journal of Sports Medicine for General Practitioners,* 5, 12, 97-99.

Aronson, D. D., & Carlson, W. E. (1992). Slipped capital femoral epiphysis. A prospective study of fixation with a single screw. *American Journal of Bone & Joint Surgery, 74*(6), 810–819.

Atanda, A., Shah, S., & O'Brien, K. (2011). Osteochondrosis: Common causes of pain in growing bones. *American Family Physician, 83*(3), 285–291.

Birrer, R., Greisemer, B., & Cataletto, M. (2002). *Pediatric sports medicine for primary care* (2nd ed.). Philadelphia, PA: Lippincott Williams & Wilkins.

Clarke, N. M., & Kendrick, T. (2009). Slipped capital femoral epiphysis, *British Medical Journal, 339*(6), 44-49.

Cramer, K. (2004). *Pediatrics* (pp. 44–50). New York, NY: Lippincott Williams & Wilkins.

Crawford, A., & Hamblen, K. (1990). *Outline of orthopaedics* (11th ed.). Edinburgh: Churchill Livingstone.

Dwek, J. R. (2009). The hip: MR imaging of uniquely paediatric disorders. *Magnetic Resonance Imaging Clinics of North America, 17*(3), 509–529.

Fish, J. (1984). Cuneiform osteotomy of the femoral neck in the treatment of slipped capital femoral epiphysis. *American Journal of Bone and Joint Surgery, 66*(A), 1153–1168.

Houghton, K. M. (2009). Review for the generalist: Evaluation of paediatric hip pain. *Pediatric Rheumatology Online Journal* [online]. Retrieved from http://www.ncbi.nlm.nih.gov/entrez/query.fcgi?cmd=Retrieve&db=PubMed&dopt=Abstract&list_uids=19450281 [accessed on 1/11/2012].

Kocher, M. S., Bishop, J. A., Hresko, M. T. (2004). Prophylactic pinning of the contralateral hip after unilateral slipped capital femoral epiphysis. *American Journal of Bone & Joint Surgery, 86A*(12), 2658–2665.

Larson, A. N., Yu, E. M., Peterson, H. A., Stans, A. A., & Melton III, L. J. (2010). Incidence of slipped capital femoral epiphysis: a population-based study. *Journal of Paediatric Orthopaedics, 19*(1), 9–12.

Lehmann, C. L., Arons, R. R., Loder, R. T., & Vitale, M. G. (2006). The epidemiology of slipped capital femoral epiphysis: an update. *Journal of Paediatric Orthopaedics, 26*(3), 286–295.

Loder, R. T., Aronson, D. D., Dobbs, M. B., & Weinstein, S. L. (2000). Slipped capital femoral epipysis: An instructional course lecture. *American Journal of Bone Joint Surgery, 82-A,* 1170–1188.

Lyle, J. (1984). *Pediatric and adolescent sports medicine* (1st ed.). Boston, MA: Little Brown and Company.

Maeda, S., Kita, A., Funayama, K., & Kokubun, S. (2001). Vascular supply to slipped capital femoral epiphysis. *Journal of Paediatric Orthopaedics, 21,* 664–667.

Murray, A. W., & Wilson, N. I. (2008). Changing incidence of slipped capital femoral epiphysis: A relationship with obesity. *British Journal of Bone & Joint Surgery, 90*(1), 92–94.

Page, M. (2007). *The British Medical Association illustrated medical dictionary* (2nd ed., pp. 224–229). London: Dorling Kindersley.

Patel, D., Greydenus, D., & Baker, R. (2009). *Pediatric sports medicine* (2nd ed.). New York, NY: McGraw Hill Medical.

Phillips, S. A., Griffiths, W. E. G., & Clarke, N. M. P. (2001). The timing of reduction and stabilisation of the acute, unstable, slipped upper femoral epiphysis. *British Journal of Bone Joint Surgery, 83*(B), 46–49.

Rhoad, R. C., Davidson, R. S., Heyman, S., Dormans, J. P., & Drummond, D. S. (1999). Pretreatmentbone scan in SCFE: A predictor of ischaemic and avascular necrosis. *Journal of Paediatric Orthopaedics, 19,* 164–168.

Thacker, M. M., & Clarke, M. S. (2009). Slipped capital femoral epiphysis [online]. Retrieved from http://emedicine.medscape.com/article/1248422-overview [accessed 1/11/2012].

Uglow, M. G., & Clarke, N. M. (2004). The management of slipped capital femoral epiphysis. *British Journal of Bone & Joint Surgery, 86*(5), 631–636.

Wabitsch, M., Horn, M., Esch, V., Mayer, H., Moss, A., Gunther, K., et al. (2012). Silent slipped capital femoral epiphysis in overweight and obese children and adolescents. *European Journal of Pediatrics, 171*(10), 1461–1465.

Witbreuk, M. M., Bolkenbaas, M., Mullender, M. G., Sierevelt, I. N., & Besselaar, P. P. (2009). The results of downgrading moderate and severe slipped capital femoral epiphysis by an early Imhauser femur osteotomy. *Journal Children Orthopaedics, 4, 9,* 12-18.

CHAPTER 7

Knee and Leg Pathologies in Children and Adolescent Sport

Solomon Abrahams

The Knee

The knee joint in children and adolescents is very similar to that of adults.

The epiphyses of the proximal and distal femur (see Fig. 7.1) are present at birth. The proximal fibula epiphyses and the patella ossification centre are, however, not present until age 4 years.

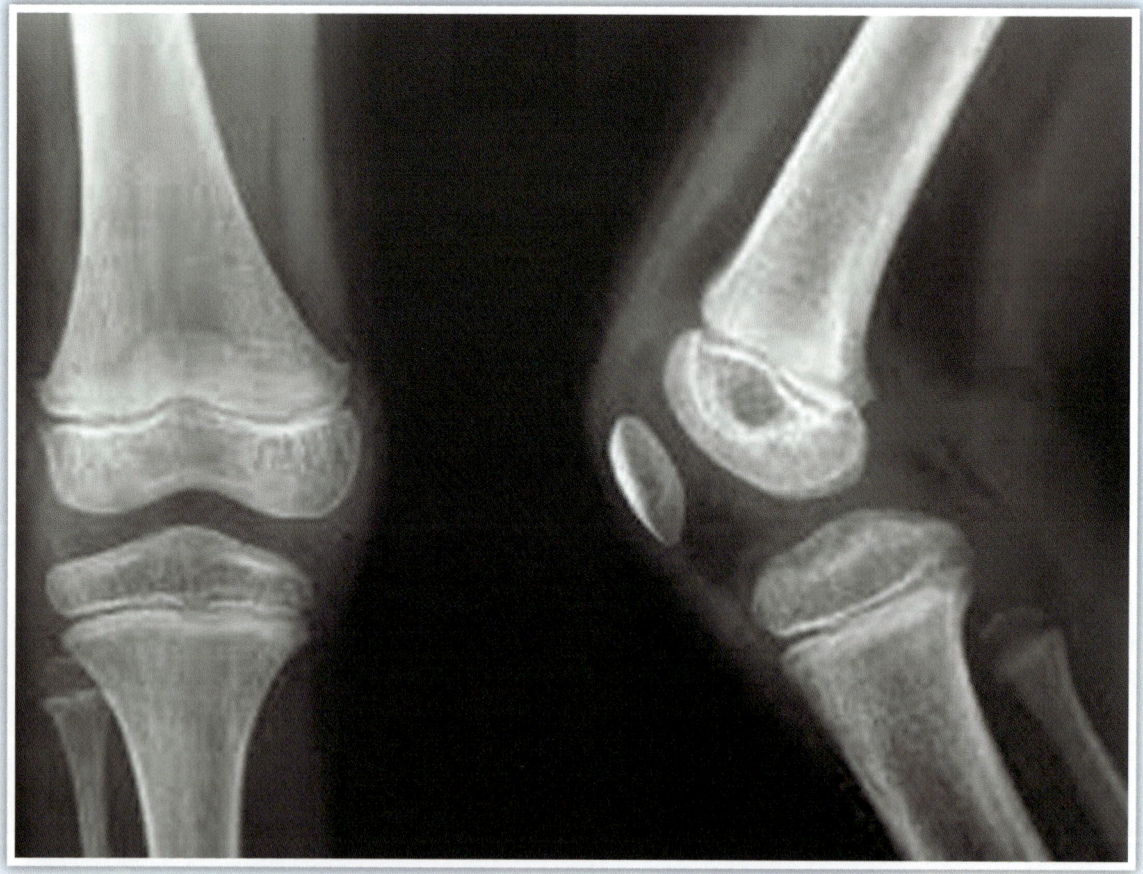

Fig. 7.1 Growth plates of the knee joint in a child

As with the adult knee, ligaments and a relatively strong capsule surround the knee to give it stability. This comprises mainly of the medial collateral ligament (MCL), lateral collateral ligament (LCL), anterior cruciate ligament and posterior cruciate ligament (ACL and PCL), and arcuate ligament.

The distal femoral epiphysis acts as an attachment for the proximal MCL and blends in with the capsule and the medial border of the medial meniscus, as in adults. The LCL remains extracapsular.

The ACL resists anterior displacement of the tibia on the femur, and the PCL acts as resistance to the posterior displacement of the tibia on the femur.

The ligaments in general do tend to be more lax in the young athlete compared with the adult, mainly due to the high elastin content and also the very well-hydrated connective tissue and ligament structure. This should be considered during an examination of a child, and this laxity should not be mistaken as an injury to the ligaments (Houghton, 2007).

The blood supply to the menisci is tenuous in adolescents, with the outer 1/3 of the menisci vascularised, whist the inner 2/3 remains unvascularised.

Knee injuries in children are common, accounting for over 1/3 of all injuries sustained in recreational sports and by far the most common joint to be injured (Abrahams et al., 2006; Birrer, Griesemer, & Cataletto, 2002).

Numerous studies have shown that young females tend to be more prone to knee injuries, obviously depending on the sport being played. Some authors suggest that this is due to hormonal influences, making the joints more loose. Others suggest that the knee injuries in females could be as high as 44% more than in males (Birrer et al., 2002).

History of Knee Injury

Knee history is always important to determine injury. In children, mechanism of injury is equally important, but because some children have difficulty explaining how it happened, it can be useful to also speak to the parents or the coaching staff, who could have observed how the injury occurred.

Acute swelling or haemarthrosis could indicate an intra-articular pathology such as an ACL tear, fracture, or patella dislocation. Episodes of instability could indicate a meniscus pathology, ACL rupture, or patella instability. Catching or locking sensations could indicate a loose body, menisci pathology, patella instability or Plica syndrome (Abrahams, 2001).

Family history along with the child's history, is also relevant in children, as it may indicate menisci or patella pathology. In case there is a sibling who had Osgood–Schlatter disease, it is more likely to indicate the same in the patient.

Knee Injuries

Anterior Cruciate Ligament Injuries (ACL)

ACL injuries in children are rare, but they are more common in adolescents. They remain, as they do in adults, serious knee injuries. Mechanism of injury is a twist on the weight-bearing knee, normally when nobody else is around, with a popping sensation being heard in 72% of cases (Birrer et al., 2002; Malanga, Andrus, Nadler, & McLean, 2003). ACL injuries are 6 times more common in females as opposed to males (Patel et al., 2009).

As with adults, ACL tears can be associated with further meniscus damage, and early diagnosis is important so that cartilage repair can be an option as soon as possible in order to provide a better long-term prognosis. ACL ruptures in children are more likely to avulse from the femoral condyle than be midsubstance tears (Patel et al., 2009). Similarly, a study of 62 children with ACL tears revealed that over 80% were avulsion fractures of the tibia or femoral bones in children under 12 years (Shanmugam & Maffuli, 2008). This may have implications to prognosis and management.

Signs and Symptoms

Pain and a giving way of the knee is commonly felt. There could be swelling of the knee within an hour, and possibly a haemarthrosis within 10 minutes. Sometimes, they are unable to weight bear immediately after the injury, and the knee remains sore. Sometimes, there is a limitation of movement for a few days. The knee can give way or even lock (Houghton, 2007).

Tests

Sometimes, in the acute stage, young adolescents will not allow their knees to be examined, as they remain clearly painful in the initial stages.

Lachman's test can be used to identify any instability of the knee, but a clearer understanding will be given by an MRI scan (Patel et al., 2009). Other tests include Apley's draw test and pivot shift.

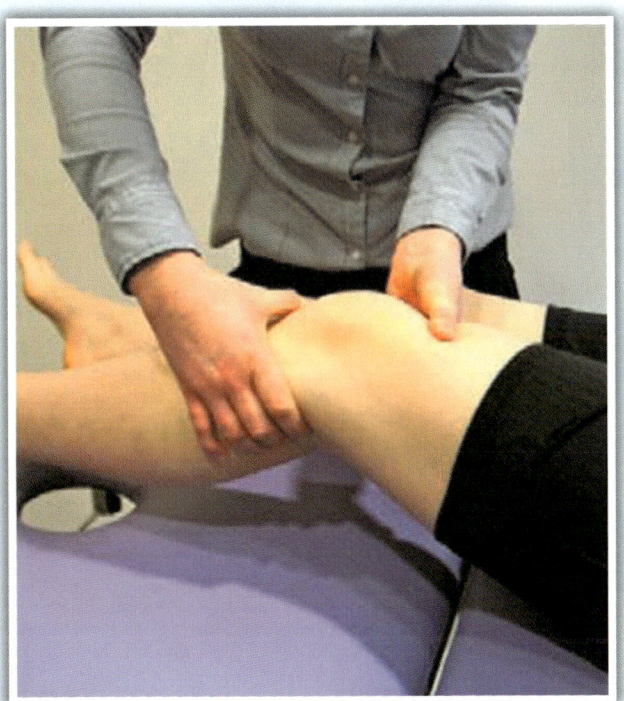 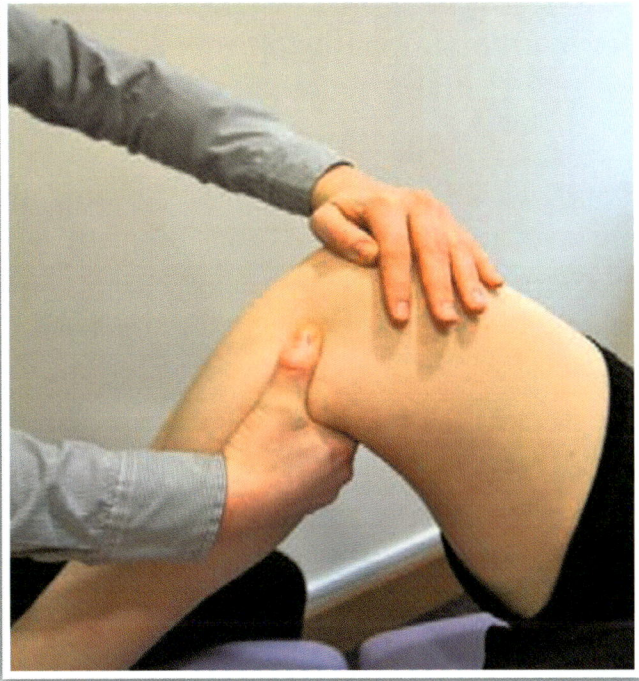

Fig. 7.2 Lachman's test (left) and Apley's drawer test (right)

Lachman's test is a simple test and arguably the most utilised test to examine the laxity of the cruciate ligament. Here, the knee is stabilised at 30 degrees of flexion, and with the examiner holding the thigh muscle to stabilise the femur, the tibia is translated forwards and backwards andthe laxity is compared with the other knee (Malanga et al., 2003).

Apley's test is conducted with the knee bent at 90 degrees flexion and the tibia drawn forwards on the femur. A more lax knee is compared with the opposite side.

It is important also to check the pulses in the leg, including the popliteal pulse and dorsalis pedis pulse just to ensure that a dislocation/subluxation of the joint has not encroached on the blood vessels (Patel et al., 2009).

Treatment and Management

Surgery is the last resort, and for midsubstance tears in adolescents, rehabilitation should be tried first, if the ACL has an isolated tear. For tears which also involve meniscus tears, surgery is normally indicated so that the meniscus can be repaired.

Pivoting sports which involve weight bearing is more likely to cause problems where surgery is not indicated. However, if the young adolescent plays at a good level, an orthopaedic consult should always be considered.

Rehabilitation should consist of hamstring and quadriceps strengthening exercises and weight-bearing exercises, but twisting in full weight bearing should be avoided initially. Rehabilitation of a non-ACL tear in children normally responds more quickly, and if pain or giving way persists after a few months, repeat scans should be considered (Houghton, 2007).

Posterior Cruciate Ligament Injury (PCL)

Injury to the PCL is rare. Most injuries are dashboard-type injuries, where a child's knee smashes against the dashboard, forcing the tibia posteriorly on the femur. This can happen if a child falls off a bike or in similar incidents.

Signs and Symptoms

Symptoms can be somewhat vague as most PCL injuries are relatively asymptomatic unless grossly unstable or an additional pathology is present. If symptomatic, pain tends to be on the posterior lateral side of the knee.

Tests

A Lachman's test (as described above) is mainly for the ACL, but it can be used to determine any anterior posterior instability of the knee and, arguably, can be used for excessive translation posteriorly of the knee. An Apley's test (as described above) or a posterior sag test can also be used. An MRI scan is more reliable (Malanga et al., 2003).

In the posterior sag test, the patient lies with the knee at 90 degrees, and the tibial tuberostity sags backwards. This is not a very reliable test (Malanga et al., 2003).

Treatment and Management

Treatment and management is normally non-surgical. Prognosis for PCL tears is good with conservative management as the PCL is not the main stabiliser of the knee. Working on quadriceps and hamstrings helps the dynamic stability of the knee.

Medial Collateral Ligament Strain (MCL)

The normal medial collateral ligament is more lax in children and adolescents. Injury, however, can occur from a direct blow or a valgus shunt. Ligament strains can vary in seriousness; grade 1 strains are normally stable and recover well. Grade 2 strains are slightly more lax but normally demonstrate instability of no more than 1 cm. Grade 3 strains tend to be more serious, with more than 1 cm laxity, and normally there is damage to the menisci as well (Patel et al., 2009).

Signs and Symptoms

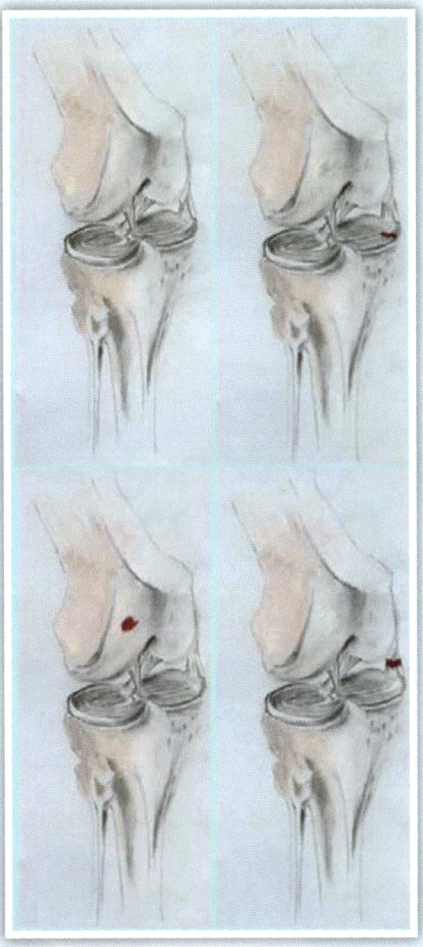

Pain is normally isolated to the medial side of the knee. Weight bearing, unless it is a grade 3 strain, is normally fine, but a valgus strain can increase pain and sometimes there is a soreness on twisting. If the ligament is damaged severely as seen in a grade 3 strain, flexion, as well as end-range extension, can be sore. (See Fig. 7.3.) Swelling is rare unless the ligament is damaged badly, and if there is severe damage, sometimes the medial menisci is implicated.

Fig. 7.3 Knee injuries
Top left: normal knee, top right: medial menisci damage, bottom left: femoral condral defect,
bottom right: medial collateral ligament

Test

A valgus stress test normally can identify a strain and there can be soreness and sensitive on palpation. The knee is held in 30 degrees of flexion (see Fig. 7.4), and a valgus force is applied from the lateral side of the knee, thereby stressing the medial side. Any pain elicited on the medial side may indicate an MCL strain (Malanga et al., 2003).

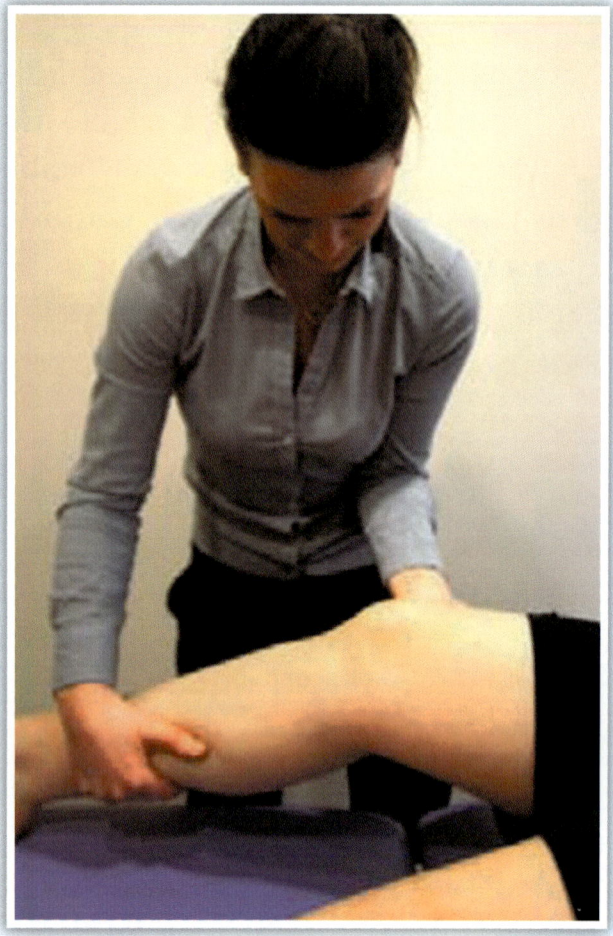

Fig. 7.4 Valgus stress test

Treatment and Management

Treatment of grade 1 and grade 2 strains is normally rest, ice, and compression in the initial stages. Following a relative time of rest, weight-bearing exercises should be encouraged but without twisting. Quadriceps strengthening helps support the knee, and proprioception should begin. After 2 weeks, running can begin again, which needs to be steadily increased.

Grade 3 strains sometimes require bracing if the knee is unstable. Exercises should be encouraged along with weight bearing in particular, which will make the knee more functional quickly. Bracing normally takes 4–6 weeks by which time, scarring of the MCL should have made the ligament more stable; hence, more activity can commence.

Lateral Collateral Ligament (LCL) Strain

LCL injuries in children and adolescents remain rare. Management and symptoms are similar to that of the MCL and are graded similarly to that of an MCL strain.

Menisci Injuries of the Knee

Meniscus injuries in children are rare but are more prevalent in adolescents. The menisci play an enormous role in the stability of the knee, in particular in children and adolescents where the ligaments are more lax. In a study of young children and adolescents who underwent arthroscopy and meniscectomy, 71% reported persistent pain, 54% reported swelling, and 41% reported giving way (Birrer et al., 2002). The most common menisci tear in adolescents is the medial meniscus, mainly in the posterior section, giving knee pain on the medial side and at the back of the knee (Patel et al., 2009).

As in adults, the vascular supply of the outer meniscus is good, but the inner 2/3 remains limited and, therefore, does not repair too well with a large tear or bucket-handle tear (Malanga et al., 2003).

Signs and Symptoms

Clicking, pain, giving way, locking, and swelling are all indications of a potential menisci pathology.

Tests

McMurray's test remains arguably the most commonly used orthopaedic test to determine a menisci tear, normally used to identify a 'bucket handle' or larger tear of the meniscus. Sometimes, if there is a tender joint line, the Thessaly test and Apley's test can be used (Patel et al., 2009).

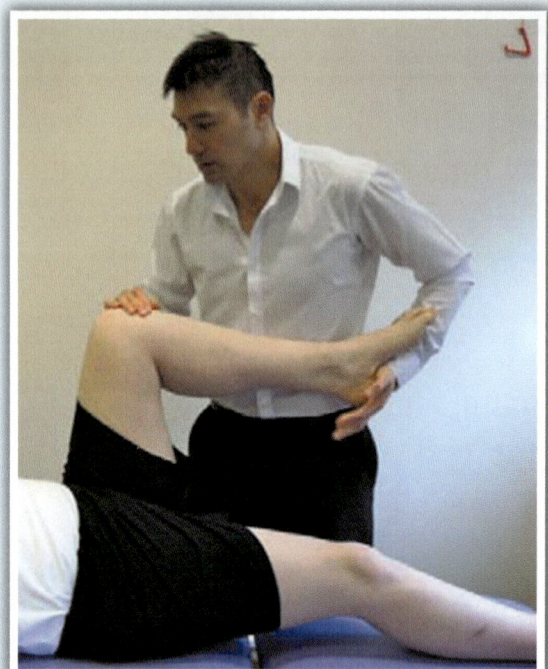 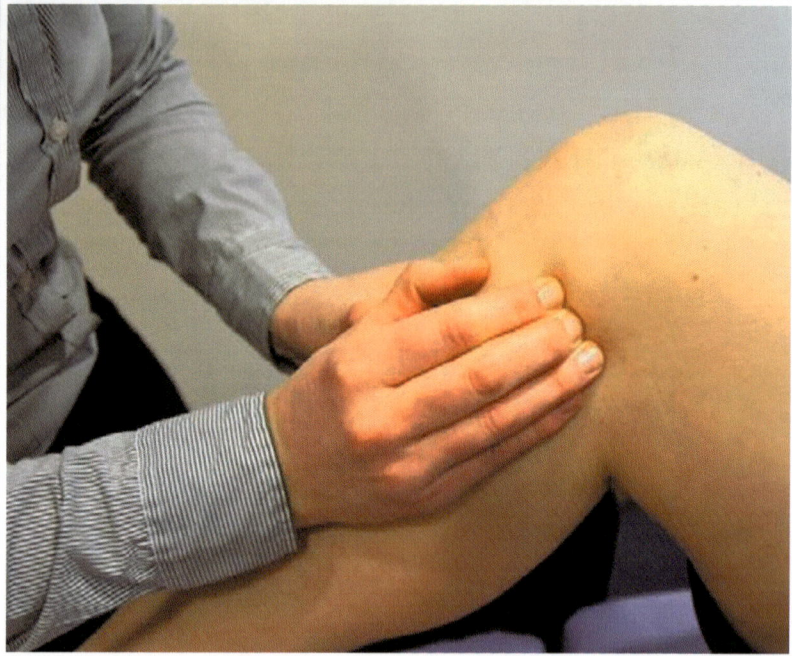

Fig. 7.5 McMurray's test (left) and joint line tenderness (right)

McMurray's test is conducted by placing the knee in full flexion. For the medial meniscus, the leg is externally rotated and adducted, and holding the leg in the position, the knee is fully extended. A clunk maybe indicative of a bucket-handle meniscus tear. For the lateral menisci, the above procedure is repeated but the leg is held in medial rotation and abduction (Malanga et al., 2003).

Palpation of the joint line (see Fig. 7.5) is another test for a peripheral meniscus tear. Tenderness on one side could represent a small tear (Malanga et al., 2003).

MRI and CT scans can be used, and even though they are not 100% reliable, they are a good indicator of menisci pathology.

Treatment and Management

Conservative management should always be considered first. Quadriceps strengthening is vital for the stability of the knee, and hamstring strengthening is equally important. Weight-bearing exercises without twisting should be always encouraged and should be considered within the first 6 weeks of rehabilitation.

Posterolateral Corner injuries

The posterolateral corner of the knee in children and adolescents is normally weak and can get damaged very easily, in addition to the structures which support it such as the hamstrings, capsule, cruciate ligaments, and lateral meniscus (Patel et al., 2009).

Signs and Symptoms

There is pain at the posterolateral corner of the knee and a sense of instability and even giving way. Sudden rotation of the knee can be more sore, and hyperextension of the knee is uncomfortable.

Treatment

The LCL, cruciates, and menisci should all be checked for instability. Bracing is sometimes required to help stabilise the knee and allow the capsule to regain some of its integrity. Strengthening of the hamstring is important and avoiding sudden twisting for the first few months is equally important. Sometimes, surgery is indicated in extreme circumstances.

Patella Dislocation

Patella dislocation in children can be common during certain sports. It normally affects the 9–15-year-old age group and is more common in girls than in boys. It is caused by twisting movements where the foot is planted into the ground. Various causes also include faulty biomechanics, such as patella alta, pes planus, and modified Q angle (Shanmugam & Maffuli, 2008).

Signs and Symptoms

Physical dislocation can be seen. The child is unable to flex the knee (due to reflex inhibition), and the pain at the time is excruciating.

Test(s)

X-rays clearly show dislocation.

Treatment and Management

Once the dislocation recedes into its correct position, rest, ice, compression, and elevation should be employed. Sometimes, immobilisation of the knee with a brace is required for 3–6 weeks, depending on the severity. Once out of the brace, gentle strengthening exercises should begin, particularly weight bearing, which can speed the knee recovery (Shanmugam & Maffuli, 2007). Normally, full running shouldn't resume for at least a few months, and addressing biomechanical problems is essential.

Patellar Instability

Patellar instability and dislocation is more common in female adolescents than in male adolescents. Normally, it is caused by trauma unless the patella is hypermobile, in which case it can be unstable anyway. Most instability is lateral because of the tighter structures (see Fig. 7.6) that have a tendency to pull the patella laterally (Abrahams & Ellis, 2006).

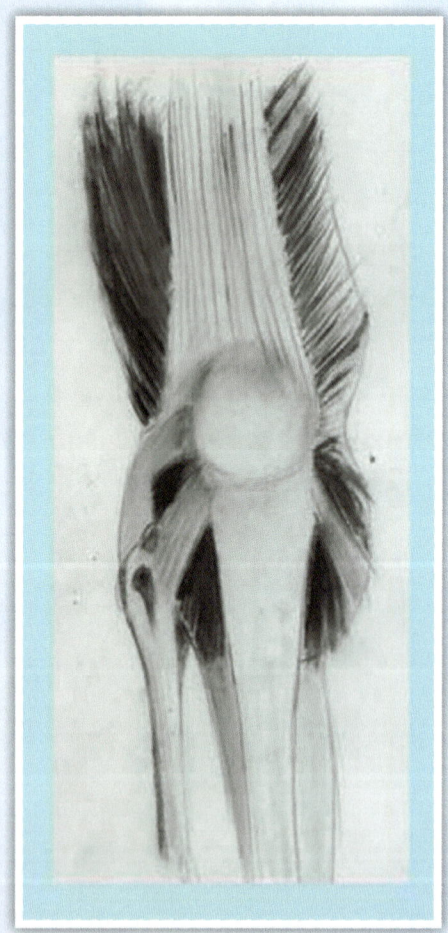

Fig. 7.6 Patellofemoral joint with tight lateral structures

Signs and Symptoms

Anterior knee pain, the feeling of giving way, and clicking sensations are all indications of patella instability. Sometimes, there maybe biomechanical abnormalities seen, such as femoral anteversion or valgus knees (Abrahams e al., 2006).

Tests

Patellar apprehension testing is a simple way of assessing instability. X-rays (bird's eye view) can see if the knee is tracking laterally, and MRI scans may depict pathology at the patellofemoral joint.

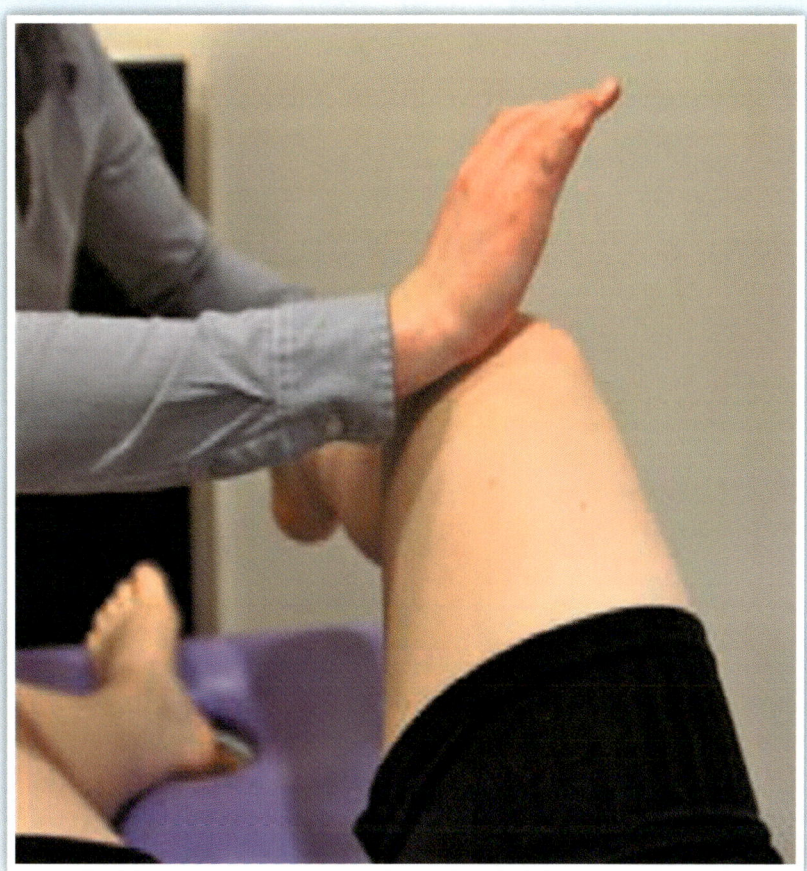

Fig. 7.7 Patella apprehension test

The patella apprehension test (see Fig. 7.7) is performed with the knee in flexion, and with a varus stress placed on the medial border of the patella, the knee is extended passively. Apprehension of the knee is normally felt at 30 degrees of flexion, where the child will apprehend any further extension to avoid the patella from dislocating (Malanga et al., 2003).

Treatment and Management

Treatment includes the strengthening of quadriceps, bracing if the condition is grossly or persistently unstable, and sometimes surgery. Assessing the biomechanics can be useful, and sports which involve excessive twisting are to be avoided (Abrahams & Ellis, 2006).

Patellofemoral Knee Pain

Anterior knee pain is arguably the most common complaint amongst adolescents and children, more so in females than males. It is triggered mainly by overuse and presents normally as pain at the front of the knee. It can have various causes, including patella alta, patella maltracking, abnormal Q angle, hypermobility, patella laxity, genu varus and valgus, flat feet, and tight muscles (Abrahams et al., 2006; Patel et al., 2009).

Signs and Symptoms

The onset of pain is normally insidious, as a dull ache. Stair climbing, especially coming down the stairs, aggravates the pain. Prolonged sitting, or sitting on the knees also aggravate the pain. Kneeling and squatting can be more sore. Normally, swelling is minimal, but giving way of the knee can sometimes happen. Occasionally, clicking can be problem (Abrahams & Ellis, 2006).

Tests

Clark's compression test can be used, but X-rays and MRI scans normally reveal where the inflammation is.

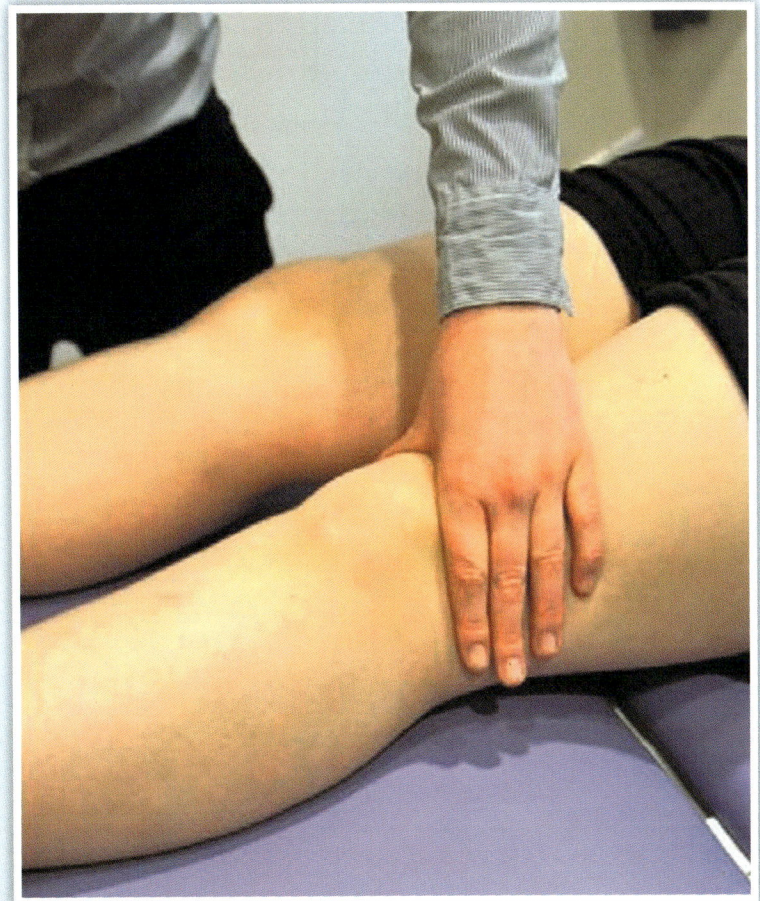

Fig. 7.8 Clark's compression test

Clark's test (see Fig. 7.8) is performed with the knee in full extension and the web of the hand of the examiner placed around the superior border of the patella. The child is asked to brace their knee into full extension actively, and an apprehension or pain could be indicative of patellofemoral knee pain (Malanga et al., 2003).

Treatment and Management

Treatment should be geared at reducing the inflammation and pain. This can be achieved with rest and ice and removing the aggravating factors. The next step is to identify the cause, whether this be faulty biomechanics, or whether there is tightness in some muscle groups such as hamstrings, calves, and quadriceps. Improving strength around the knee is also important. Working on the vastus medialis oblique muscle (VMO) helps to stabilise the kneecap (Abrahams & Ellis, 2006).

Sometimes, simple training methods or a change in training methods may trigger the pain. Change in intensity, duration, and frequency of training may trigger the anterior knee pain. Similarly, change in shoewear and camber can be blamed.

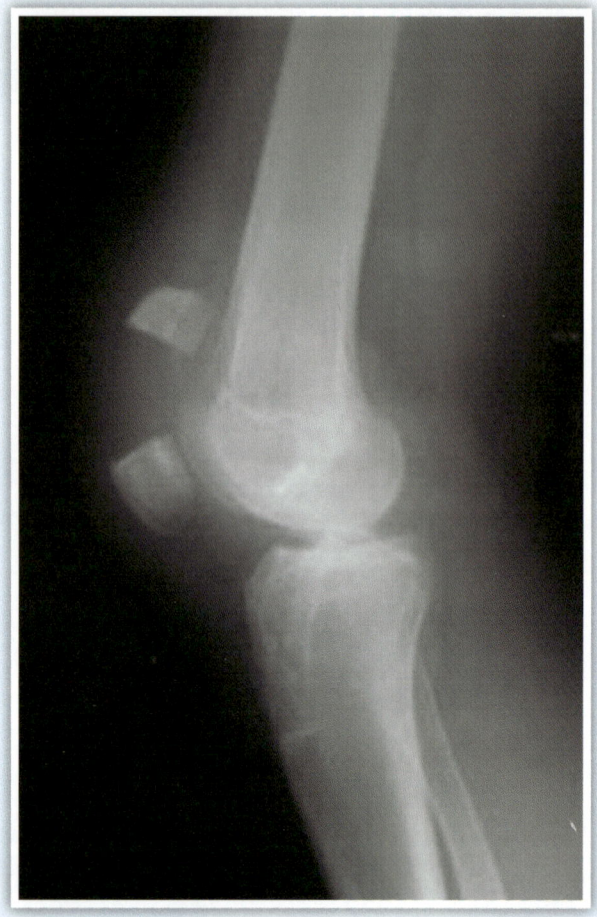

Fig. 7.9 Other patella pathologies include patella fracture in 15-year-old male

Osgood–Schlatter Disease (Traction Apophysitis)

Osgood–Schlatter disease is a traction apophysitis of the quadriceps tendon from the tibial tuberosity (see Fig. 7.10). Its incidence can be as high as 13% in the general population but is much higher in sporting adolescents.

This is an overuse injury, with sport being an aggravator. Normally, it occurs more in males than in females, at ages of an adolescent spurt (Gholve, Scher, Khakharia, Widmann, & Green, 2007). If it does affect girls, it tends to occur at an earlier age than boys, typically 11–13 years of age. Boys normally present with this between ages 12 and 15 (Stanitski, Delee, & Drez, 1994).

The actual cause of OSD is unknown, whether it is a lesion of micro tears of the tendon or stress fracture of the physis (Gerbino, 2006).

Signs and Symptoms

Pain at the inferior part of the patellofemoral knee joint, directly and around the tibial tuberosity, is a symptom. Pain worsens with activity such as going down the stairs, running, kneeling, and sitting for long periods.

Test

Pain is felt on direct palpation of the tibial tuberosity with an X-ray, confirming diagnosis.

Treatment

Most cases of Osgood–Schlatter disease do calm down with rest. Ice and compression can be useful. Analgesics can be used in severe pain but are not always necessary. Once the pain does calm down, then treatment should be aimed at prevention of recurrence. This may include stretching of tight muscles; reducing training intensity, frequency, and duration; and wearing appropriate shoewear.

Osgood–Schlatter disease very seldom causes long-term problems and normally fully resolves by itself with rest.

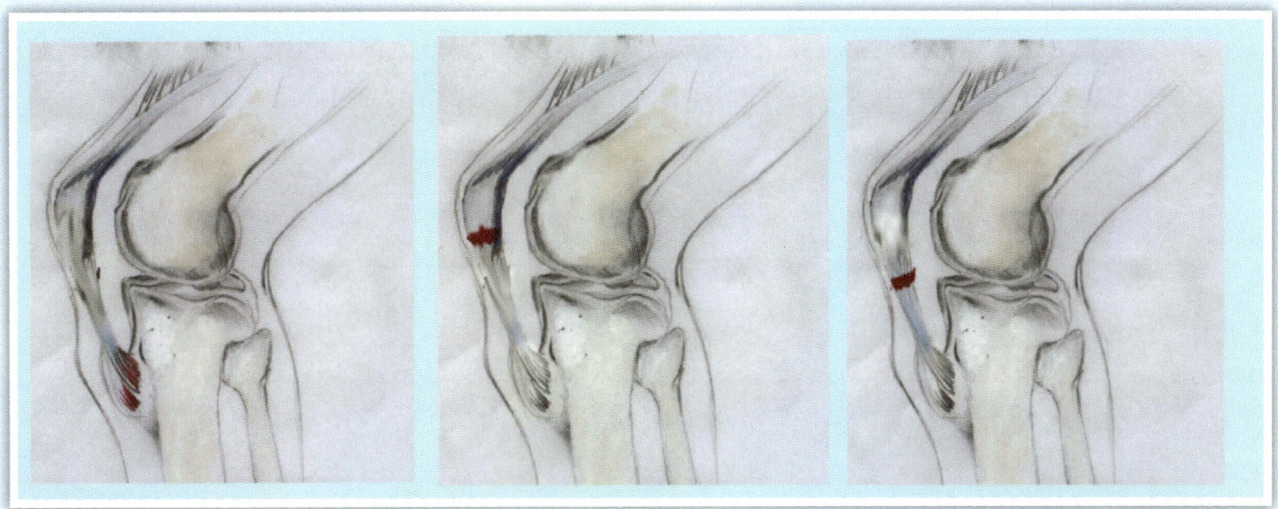

Fig. 7.10 Left: Osgood–Schlatter disease, middle: Sindig Larsen, and right: tendonitis of patella tendon

Sindig Larsen Johansson Disease (Traction Apophysitis)

Sindig Larsen Johansson disease (see Fig. 7.10) is another traction apophysitis of the interior pole of the patella and the patella tendon. This is also known as jumper's knee, common in players of basketball, netball, or sports which involve a lot of running, jumping, or kicking. The actual tendon is not the pathology, rather it is the avulsing bone from the inferior patella itself; hence there is pain on palpation (Shanmugam & Maffuli, 2008).

Signs and Symptoms

Pain is normally localised to the inferior pole of the patella, which can be aggravated with jumping and continuous running.

Test

Direct compression of the inferior pole of the patella or contraction of the quadriceps can be sore. X-rays will confirm diagnosis (Malanga et al., 2003).

Treatment

Rest and ice are advised in the first instance. This tendon pathology does normally take time to settle.

Afterwards, stretches of the quadriceps, hip flexors, calf muscles, and hamstring muscles should be done. Rest can be quite prolonged with this pathology, possibly up to 3 months.

Tendonitis

Tendonitis can affect adolescents at the patella tendon and iliotibial band (ITB). Both are rare in children and early adolescents. Pain is due to overuse and generally related to running. Pain is normally at the site of anatomical pathology, and both can be managed conservatively with rest and ice. Generally, there is a cause which makes the pain worse, and identifying this cause and correcting it can be instrumental in the successful return to sport.

Osteochondritis Dissecans (OCD)

OCD normally involves a cartilage fragment avulsing from the medial femoral condyle (occasionally the lateral), which can then float within the knee joint. Sometimes, there can be a mechanism, but at times, the onset can be insidious (Birrer et al., 2002).

Signs and Symptoms

Pain can be quite diffused and unlocalised. It can also change from side to side. Clicking, clunking, and giving way can also be evident, and the soreness is normally related with weight-bearing activities with twisting.

Test

Most orthopaedic test remains unreliable. MRI scans and X-rays should be used.

Treatment and Management

Most of these pathologies, if large enough, require arthroscopy and removal of the debris. Conservatively, quadriceps strengthening and hamstring strengthening is vital to maintain functional stability of the knee joint.

Plica Syndrome

Plica syndrome is quite simply an irritation and inflammation of the patellofemoral joint due to a hypertrophied ridge between the patella and femoral condyle, causing pain and clicking (Abrahams et al., 2002). When parts of the capsule in the embryo are not fully fused together, repeated trauma of the fusion line forms a ridge. Plica can be normal, causing the occasional click, but it can become more troublesome with pain if continually irritated. (See Fig. 7.11.)

Signs and Symptoms

Pain and clicking are present, mainly on the medial side of the patellofemoral joint. Swelling is rare, but using the stairs, squatting, and kneeling can be more sore (Abrahams, 2001).

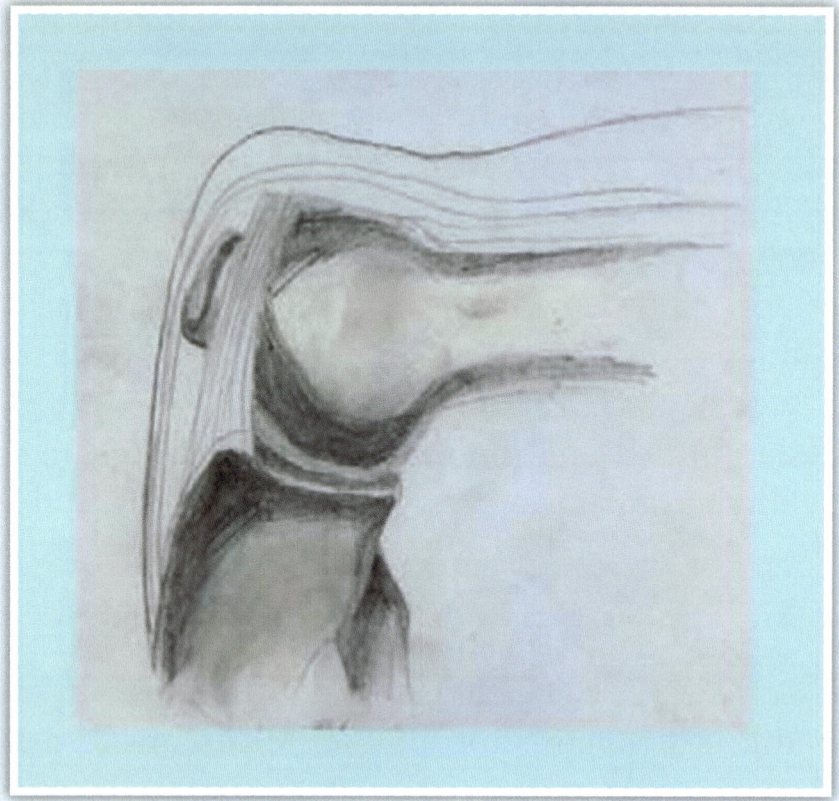

Fig. 7.11 Medial plica

Test

Medial plica test can be performed, but an MRI is more reliable.

The knee is fully flexed, and the lateral border of the patella is pushed into medially. With this push, the knee is gradually extended passively, and a click at 30 degrees of flexion could indicate a medial plica (Abrahams, 2001).

Treatment

Treatment is normally surgical if the pain is consistent and not helped with conservative management, which may include anti-inflammatory drugs and removal of the aggravating factors. Surgery may remove the plica.

Leg Injuries

Solomon Abrahams

Leg injuries remain rare in children and adolescent sports, apart from lacerations and bruising.

The most common pathologies of this area remain 'shin splints' or, more specifically, medial tibial stress syndrome (MTSS), stress fractures, and compartment syndrome.

Medial Tibial Stress Syndrome (MTSS)

MTSS occurs on the medial and distal lower 1/3 of the tibia (see Fig. 7.12). It is an inflammation of the fascia attachment from the soleus to the inner

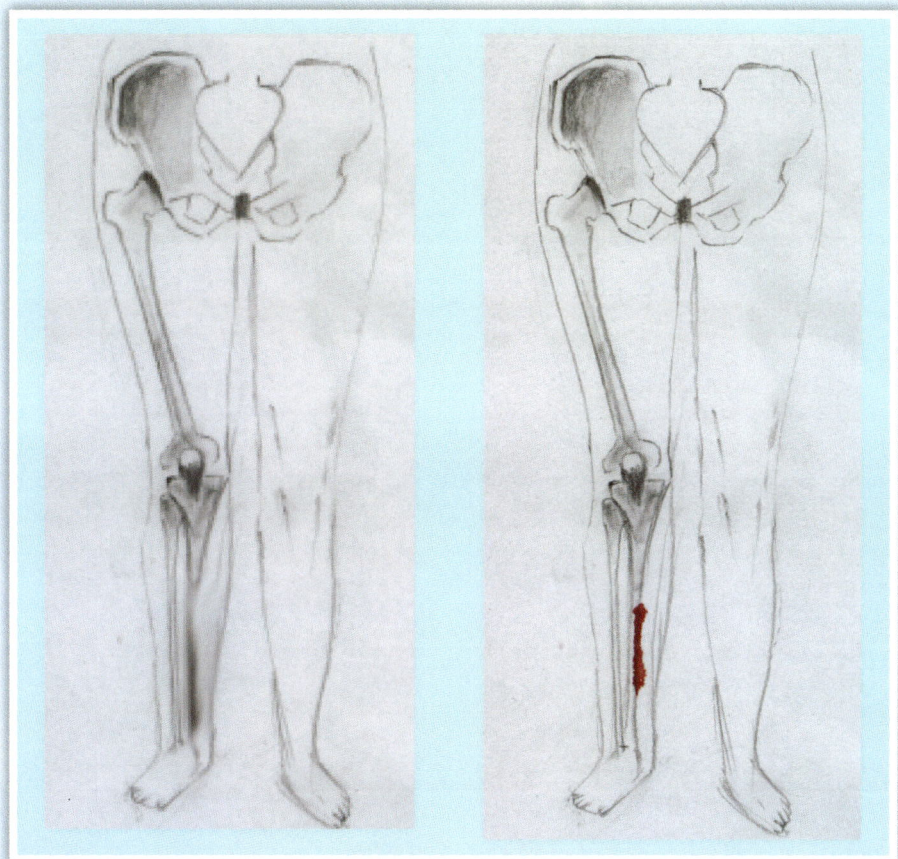

border of the tibia; sometimes it is also known as periostitis (Birrer et al., 2002). It is common in long-distance runners (Patel et al., 2009).

Intrinsically, pronation of the feet, tight Achilles and calf muscles, excessive tibial torsion, femoral anteversion, and midfoot pronation can cause MTSS.

Fig. 7.12 Medial tibial stress syndrome in the biomechanically compromised adolescent

Extrinsically, training errors; camber; shoewear; training duration, intensity, and frequency; and overuse can cause or trigger MTSS.

Signs and Symptoms

There is pain on the medial inner tibia, along the distal or lower 1/3 tibia. Pain materialises during activity and becomes an ache. The pain does not worsen with continued activity, but the patient remains uncomfortable. Rest does help. It is normally triggered with a change in training, which needs further probing on subjective examination (Abrahams et al., 2006).

Test

The medial 1/3 distal shin is sore on palpation, normally after the run (see Fig. 7.12b). Bone scan is reliable.

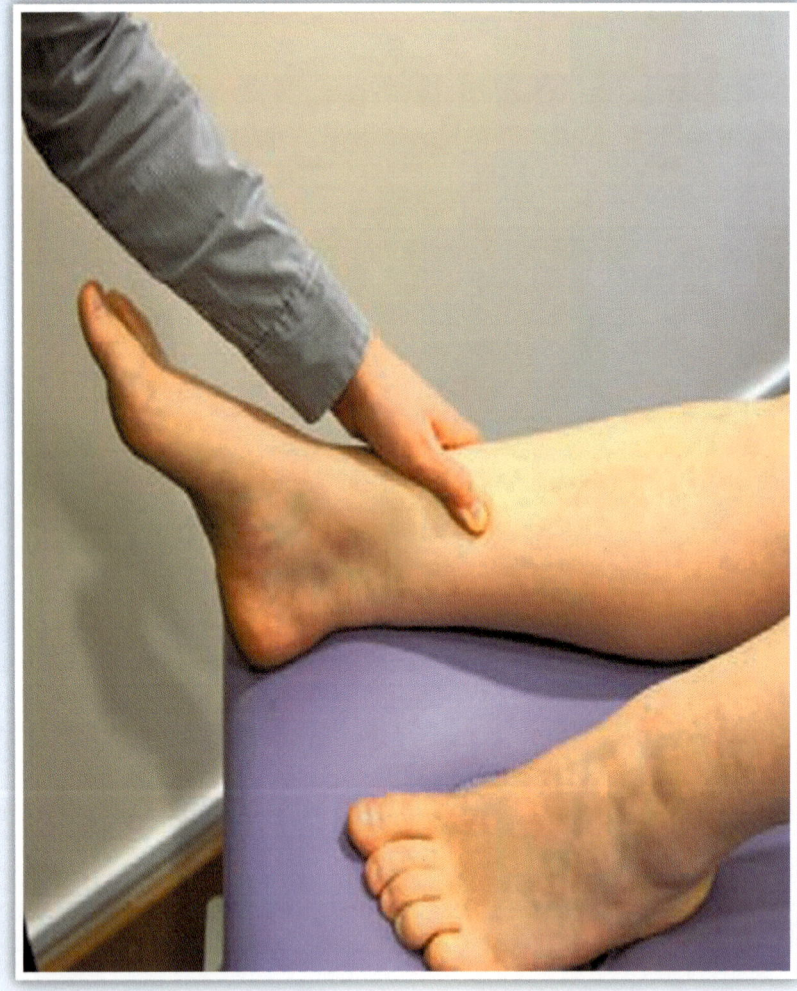

Fig. 7.12b Palpation of the lower 1/3 of the medial tibia

Treatment and Management

Treatment involves calming down the condition with rest, ice and compression. Trying to investigate the cause will help prevent re-exacerbation. Review of biomechanics, shoewear, and camber and training modification will help. A slow build-up to running again should be advised.

Stress Fracture

Stress fractures in children are rare, but they can occur in mature adolescents. They are caused by repetitive microtrauma to the tibia. Excessive loading, faulty biomechanics, and changes in training and shoewear can also cause trauma through the shin. Stress fracture and MTSS are similar in pathophysiology and symptoms, but stress fractures tend to be more localised. A study of 320 children with stress fractures showed that 49% were lower tibia fractures, presenting as lower leg pain (Shanmugam & Maffuli, 2008).

Signs and Symptoms

Pain is localised to specific area of the shin. Pain is extreme on palpation, after a prolonged run. Sometimes, it does take alot of activity to aggravate the condition, so adolescents may be quite asymptomatic when they come in for assessment. In which case, they need to go and aggravate the pain and then come back and see the examiner.

Pain increases on running and worsens with prolonged running until the adolescent has to stop due to the intensity of pain, whereas with MTSS, the adolescent can still continue running.

Test

A bone scan or an X-ray and palpation of the inner tibia following a long run will confirm the diagnosis. Point tenderness is normally a good indicator.

Treatment and Management

Rest from the activity is advisable. No immobilisation is required for stress fractures but rest from activity that makes it worse is essential. Correcting the cause is also important, and most likely the biomechanics, change in camber, and change in duration, frequency, and intensity of training are paramount.

Chronic Compartment Syndrome (CCS)

CCS is characterised by an inadequacy of the musculofascia compartment size, producing chronic recurring pain on exertion. It is very rare in children, but it can occur in late adolescents. Increase in muscle bulk from excessive training increases the blood flow, which sometimes is unable to penetrate through to its distal point due to the pressure build-up of muscle hypertrophy/ fascia. This then causes an ischemic pain, tingling, and numbness in the distal component (Patel et al., 2009).

Pain is normally localised to the calf muscle, where it can affect different compartments.

Signs and Symptoms

Pain is normally caused by continued running, which leads to such pain that the athlete eventually has to stop. Tingling and numbness can add to the symptoms. When the running stops, the pain dissipates away and becomes the leg becomes asymptomatic quickly and cannot be re-exacerbated unless running restarts. Pain tends to be more vague, unlike pain in MTSS or stress fracture (Abrahams et al., 2006).

Test

Compartment pressure testing can be done by specialists in sports medicine.

Treatment and Management

Treatment varies depending on the individual. Biomechanics, orthotics, and stretching of calves and hamstrings can sometimes control the pathology. However, fasciotomy, which is curative in over 90% of adolescents, is an option (Birrer et al., 2002).

Gastrocnemius Strain (Calf Strain)

Acute strains of the gastrocnemius occur during ballistic activities or a change in speed. They can be slight strains, partial-thickness tears, and full tears. (See Fig 7.14.)

Signs and Symptoms

There is pain in the calf muscle and an inability to go on tiptoes. Running makes the pains worse, and sprinting is very painful.

Test

Pain against resistance (plantarflexion) is sore (see Fig 7.13), and stretching the muscle in the acute stage is sore. Standing on tiptoes (Fig. 7.13) can be very painful.

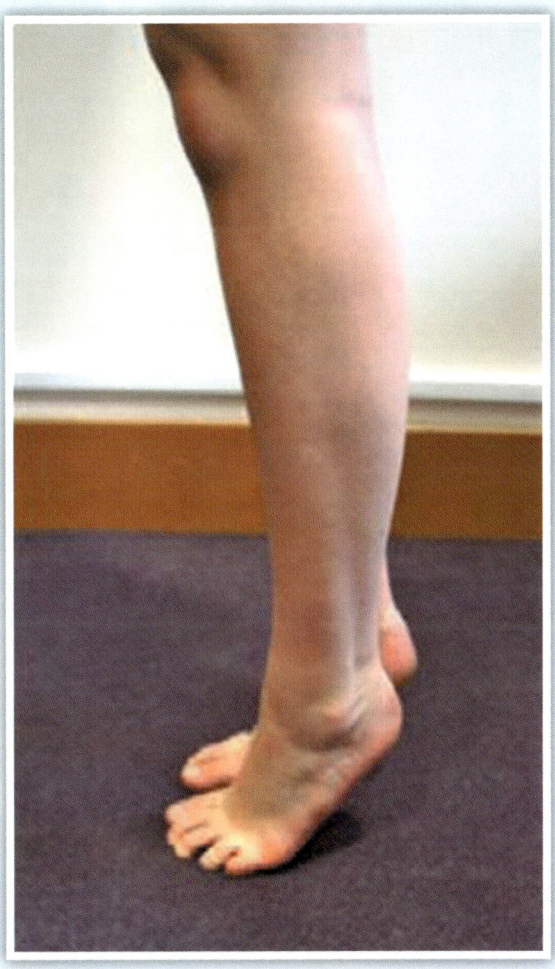

Fig. 7.13 Calf raise to test for calf strain

Thompson's test can be applied if there is any implication of rupture of a lower muscle or a tendon. Here, the patient lies in the prone position and the calf is squeezed passively. A positive test for a rupture is when the foot does not plantarflex on squeezing. A normal response is when the calf is squeezed and the foot does plantarflex (Patel et al., 2009).

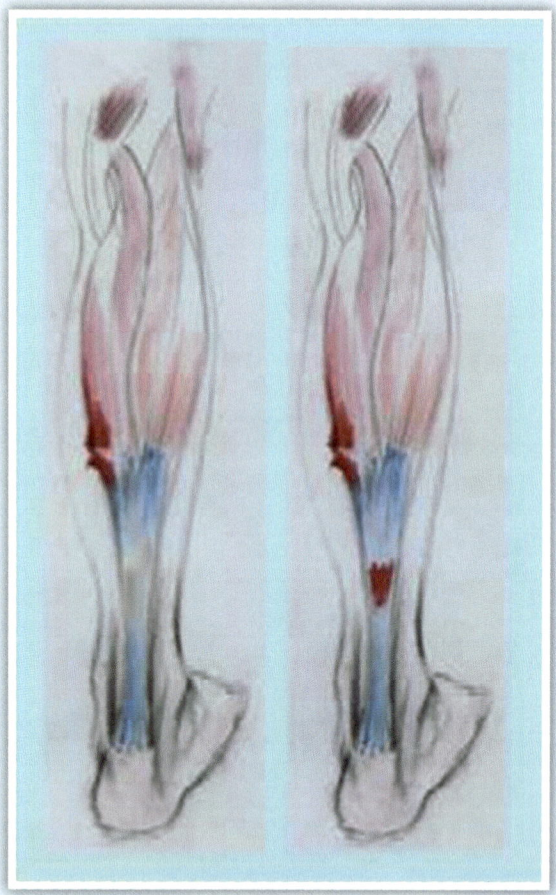

Fig. 7.14 Medial calf strain and (right) Achilles strain

Treatment and Management

In the first instance, rest, ice, compression, and elevation should be advised. When the pain settles, normal gait should be encouraged and gentle stretching should be applied. When the calf becomes more pain-free, active and resisted exercises should begin, if possible in weight bearing. Normally, and obviously depending on severity, the child can restart gentle running after 3 weeks.

Other Potential Causes of Lower Leg Pain

Other potential causes of leg pain in adolescents, which is non-mechanical, include thrombophlebitis, osteomyelitis, cellulitis, deep vein thrombosis, tumour, and intermittent claudicaiton.

Key Points

- ACL tears tend to avulse from femoral condyle rather than midsubstance.

- Knee pathology is 6 times more likely in females.

- Ligaments and capsule are more lax in children.

- Pain is not an indicator in McMurray's test.

- Posterior lateral corner is the weakest region in children.

References

Abrahams, S. D. (2001). Anterior knee pain. *Plica Syndrome, Physiotherapy, 87*, 10.

Abrahams, S., Demetriou, P., Nicolas, D. (2002). The treatment of Osteoarthritis of the knee, Journal of Orthopaedic Medicine, 2, 4, 32-40.

Abrahams, S., & Ellis, R. (2006). Patellofemoral instability of the knee. *Journal of Orthopaedic Medicine, 28,* 3.

Abrahams, S., Gulliford, D., Korkia, P., & Prince, J. (2006). The influence of leg postioning in exercises for the patellofoemoral joint pain, Journal of Orthopaedic Medicine, 25, 3, 107-113.

Birrer. R., Griesemer, B., & Cataletto, M. (2002). *Pediatric sports medicine in primary care* (2nd ed.). Philadelphia, PA: Lippincott, Williams and Wilkins.

Gerbino, P. G. (2006). Adolescent anterior knee pain. *Operative Techniques in Sports Medicine* [online] *14*(3), 203–211. Retrieved from http://www.sciencedirect.com/science/article/pii/S1060187206000426 [accessed on 10/11/12].

Gholve, P. A., Scher, D. M., Khakharia, S., Widmann, R. F., & Green, D. W. (2007). Osgood–Schlatter syndrome. *Current Opinion in Pediatrics* [online] *19*(1), 44–50. Retrieved from http://www.ncbi.nlm.nih.gov/pubmed/17224661 [accessed on 7/11/12].

Houghton, K. M. (2007). Review for the generalist: evaluation of anterior knee pain. *Pediatric Rheumatology Online Journal* [online]. Retrieved from http://www.ncbi.nlm.nih.gov/pmc/articles/PMC1887528/?tool=pubmed [accessed on 7/11/12].

Magee, D. (2002). *Orthopedic Physical Assessment* (3rd ed.). Ed, WB Saunders.

Malanga, G., Andrus, S., Nadler, S., & McLean, J. (2003). Physical examination of the knee: A review, *Archives Physical Medical Rehabilitation, 84,* 592–600.

Patel, D., Greydanus, D., & Baker, R. (2009). *Sports Medicine* (2nd ed.). McGraw Hill Publishing.

Shanmugam, C., & Maffuli, N. (2008). Sports injuries in children, *British Medical Bulletin, 26,* 33–57.

Stanitski, C., Delee, J., & Drez, D. (1994). *Pediatric sports medicine* (3rd ed.). Philadelphia, PA: W. B. Saunders.

CHAPTER 8

Ankle Pathologies in Children and Adolescent Sport

Solomon Abrahams

The Ankle

Ankle joint problems in children and adolescents are common, because the ankle joint is the ossification centre and the most weight-bearing joint in the body.

Normal range of motion in a child at the ankle is up to 25 degrees in dorsifleixon and up to 55 degrees in plantarflexion. If the child is hypermobile, these ranges will be more (Patel, Greydanus, & Baker, 2009).

The closure of the epiphyseal plates has a bearing on where the injury occurs. Specifically in children, fusion of the tibial epiphyseal plate begins in the central portion of the physis and spreads medially. The lateral tibial physeal is the last to fuse, where complete fusion takes 18 months. This makes the distal tibia a common area for fractures in children and adolescents due to the differences in strength across the epiphyseal area of the ankle, as seen in juvenile Tillaux and triplane fractures (Birrer, Griesemer, & Cataletto, 2002).

The ligaments of the child remain flexible and extensible compared with those of an adult. The anterior talofibular ligament is the weakest and most commonly damaged ligament. Also commonly injured, and arguably the most undiagnosed pathology in the child, is the syndesmosis. The ankle syndesmosis between the tibia and fibula is composed of the anterior tibiofibular ligament and the posterior tibiofibular ligament and the interosseous membrane.

Ankle Sprains

Ankle sprains remain the most common lower limb injury in children and adolescents. There are traditionally three major sprains of the ankle: medial, lateral, and anterior.

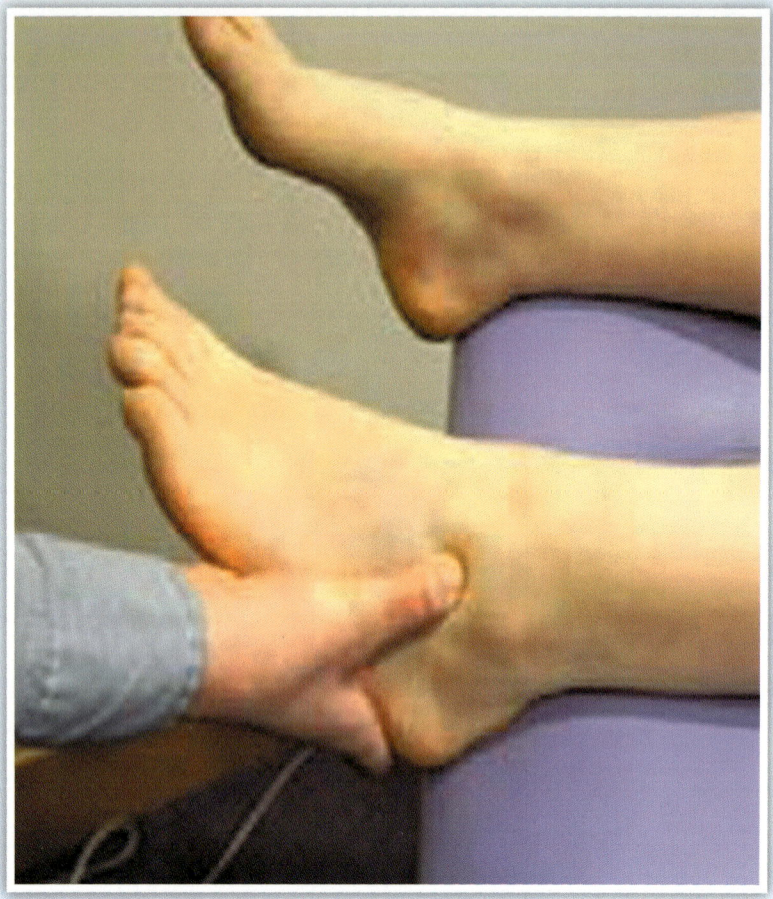

Fig. 8.1 Palpation of the anteriortalofibular ligament

Damage to the lateral ligaments of the ankle – in particular the anterior talofibular ligament (see Fig. 8.1, 8.2) as it is the weakest – is common on excessive inversion (85%). Damage to the medial deltoid ligaments of the ankle is normally caused by an eversion injury. (See Fig. 8.2b.)

The other sprain is the syndesmosis sprain (10%), mainly due to high impact or a caudal load as seen in landing from a height (see Fig. 8.5). Here, the membrane and ligaments (normally anterior tibiofibular ligament and posterior tibiofibular ligament) are damaged due to excessive dorsiflexion. This can leave the ankle unstable, so testing needs to be done to confirm diagnosis.

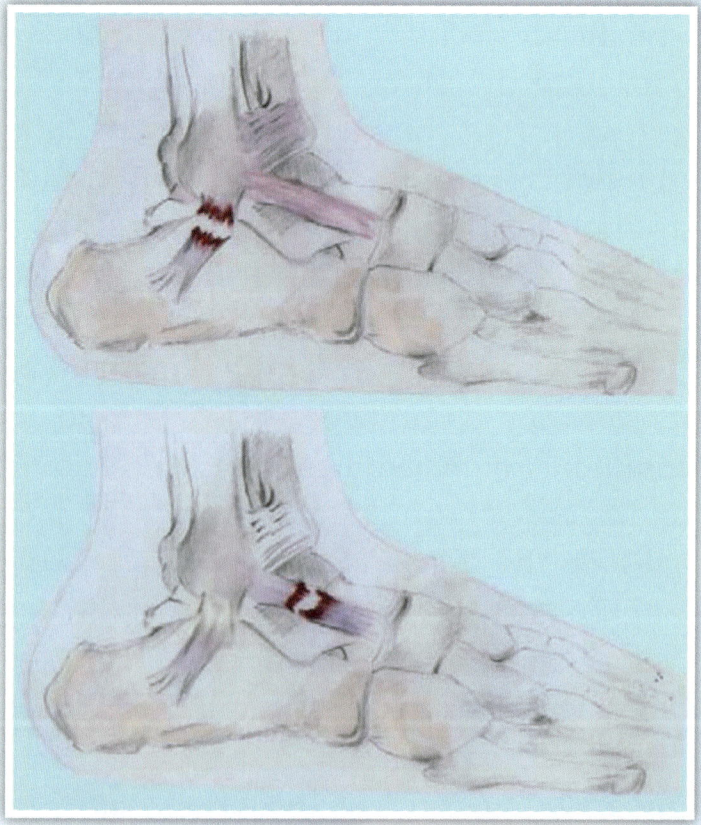

Fig. 8.2 Top: calcaneofibula, middle: ligament strain, and bottom: anterior talofibular ligament strain

Presentation

Ankle sprains vary according to the severity: grade 1, 2, and 3 (as discussed in the earlier chapter). Pain and swelling accompany the more severe ankle sprains, but the child is still normally able to weight bear.

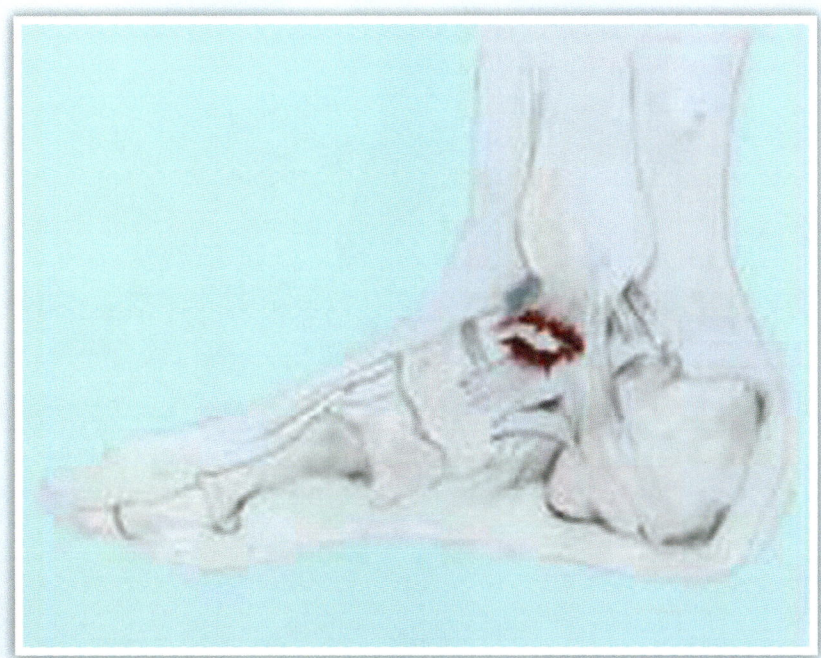

Fig. 8.2b Detoild (medial) ligament ankle strain

Examination

Gross swelling of the capsule should be noted as this may indicate potential damage to the syndesmosis or talus in children. End feel of plantarflexion and dorsiflexion should also be observed. Normal end feels should be soft and springy; empty end feels may indicate ligamentous laxity/rupture, and hard end feels may indicate bony pathology such as chrondral fracture within the ankle joint (Birrer et al., 2002).

Tests
Anterior Draw Test

The anterior draw test (see Fig. 8.3) is specifically designed to test the integrity of ligamentous instability. With the patient in the supine position and with the ankle at the end of the bed, the examiner should hold the lower leg just above the ankle with one hand, and with the other hand, he should cup the heel and draw the foot forwards on the tibia. If one ankle feels more lax (i.e. draws forwards more) compared with the non-injured side, a positive test may be indicated. Alternatively, movement in excess of 5 mm maybe clinically significant (Birrer et al., 2002). This test is not 100% reliable and is a mechanical test for the integrity of the anterior talofibular ligament.

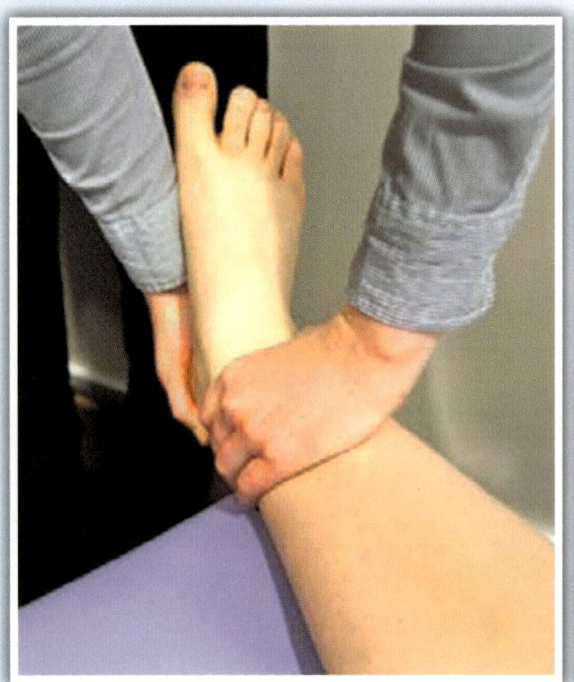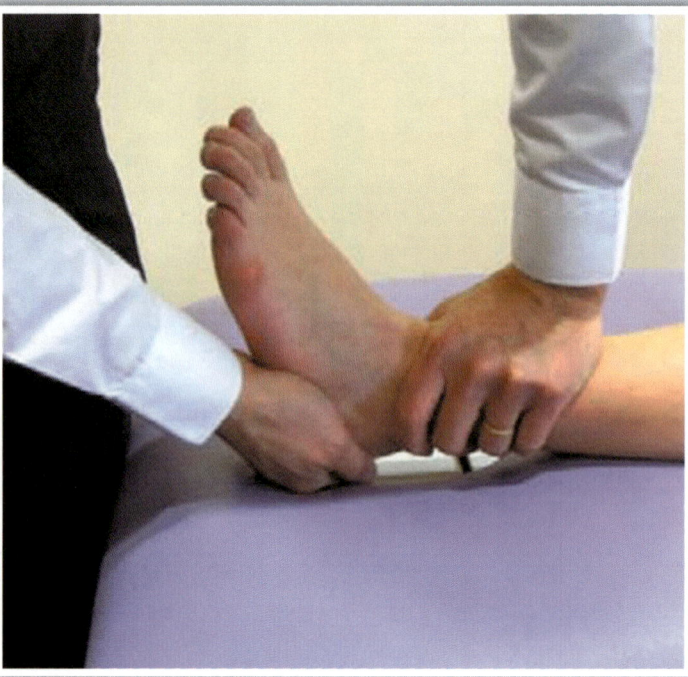

Fig. 8.3 Anterior drawer test of the ankle

Talar Tilt

This test is an instability test of for the calcaneofibular ligament on the lateral side and mid-deltoid ligament on the medial side. The patient should be supine with the patient's foot at the end of the bed; the ankle should be placed in slight dorsiflexion so that the ankle is 90 degrees to the foot. One hand should be placed on both malleoli and the other hand should cup the heel. The ankle should then be inverted and everted, and any pain or laxity may indicate ligament damage to the specific side. Any laxity compared with the uninjured side should also be noted.

Squeeze Test for Syndesmosis

This is a simple test which involves the patient lying supine with the foot at the end of the bed (see Fig. 8.4). The child's ankle is dorsiflexed, and both malleoli are compressed. Pain at ankle may indicate a sprain or instability of the syndesmosis.

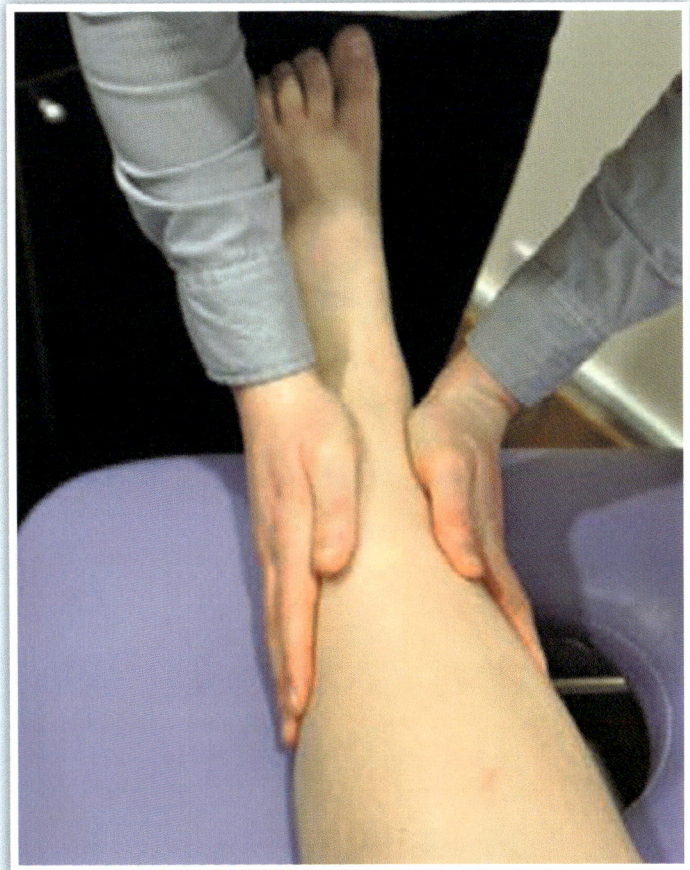

Fig. 8.4 Squeeze test of the ankle

Treatment and Management

Most ankle sprains can be handled with conservative management, whereas fractures or suspected fractures should receive an orthopaedic consult due to proximity of growth plates.

Rest, ice, and compression should be utilised with any acute strain. Sometimes, when the ankle is very painful and may be swollen, diagnostic tests (apart from suspected fractures) may have to wait for a few days so that the acute inflammation can settle.

Once the pain has settled, early weight bearing and normal gait should be encouraged as soon as possible, along with active exercises. After a week or so, proprioception and resistance exercises can begin. Weight-bearing exercises and functional exercises should begin as soon as the pain allows.

Depending on the grade of sprain, grade 1, 2, or 3, a gradual increase to sport should be encouraged.

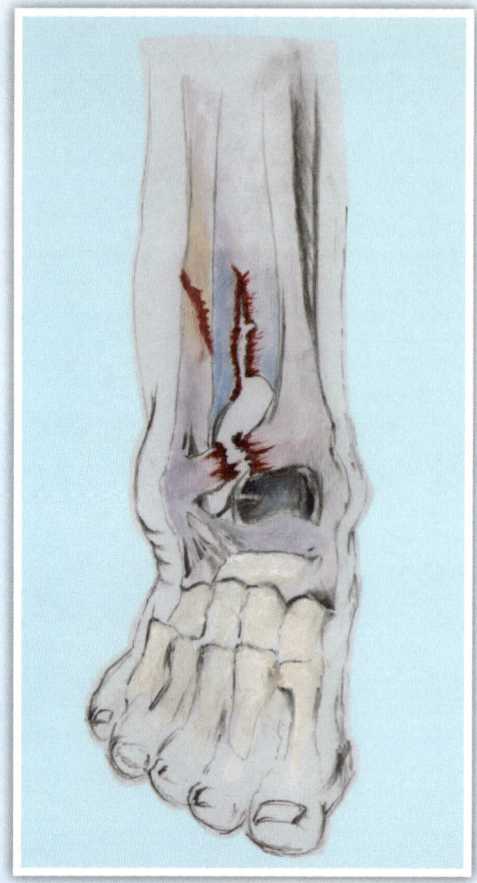

Fig. 8.5 Damage to the syndesmosis and anterior inferior tibiofibular ligament

Sever's Disease
(Calcaneal Apophysitis)

Sever's disease, first described by James Sever in 1912 (Sitati & Kingori, 2009), is a common cause of heel pain (Hosgören, Köktener, & Dilmen, 2004). It involves inflammation of the calcaneal apophysis during childhood (Scharfbillig, Jones, & Scutter, 2008) and is common in adolescent boys and girls (Sitati & Kingori, 2009).

Induced by repetitive use of the calf muscles that formulate the Achilles tendon, it causes a pull on the apophysis during plantar and dorsiflexion, thus creating painful inflammation (Hendrix, 2005). 'It frequently occurs before or during the peak growth spurt and often shortly after a child begins a new sport' (Hendrix, 2005).

It is a common cause of heel pain in athletes aged 5–11 years (Cassas & Cassettari-Wayhs, 2006). It is 75% more common in physically active boys (Frush & Lindenfeld, 2009). Approximately 60% of the cases are bilateral (Soprano, 2005). 'The condition develops earlier in females as opposed to males due to gender differences in skeletal development' (Hunt, Stowell, Alnwick, & Evans, 2007).

Signs and Symptoms

The most common sign of Sever's disease is pain at the base of the Achilles tendon (Cassas & Cassettari-Wayhs, 2006). Often it is so severe that after physical activity, the child will limp to take weight off the heel (Scharfbillig et al., 2008). Ankle dorsiflexion is limited (Scharfbillig et al., 2008) and painful due to tight heel cords (Frush & Lindenfeld, 2009).

Tests

The main form of diagnosis is compression of the medial and lateral calcaneus – 'squeeze test' – or direct palpation of the back of the heel (see Fig. 8.6). Pain indicates calcaneal apophysitis (Cassas & Cassettari-Wayhs, 2006; Frush & Lindenfeld, 2009; Hunt et al., 2007; Scharfbillig et al., 2008).

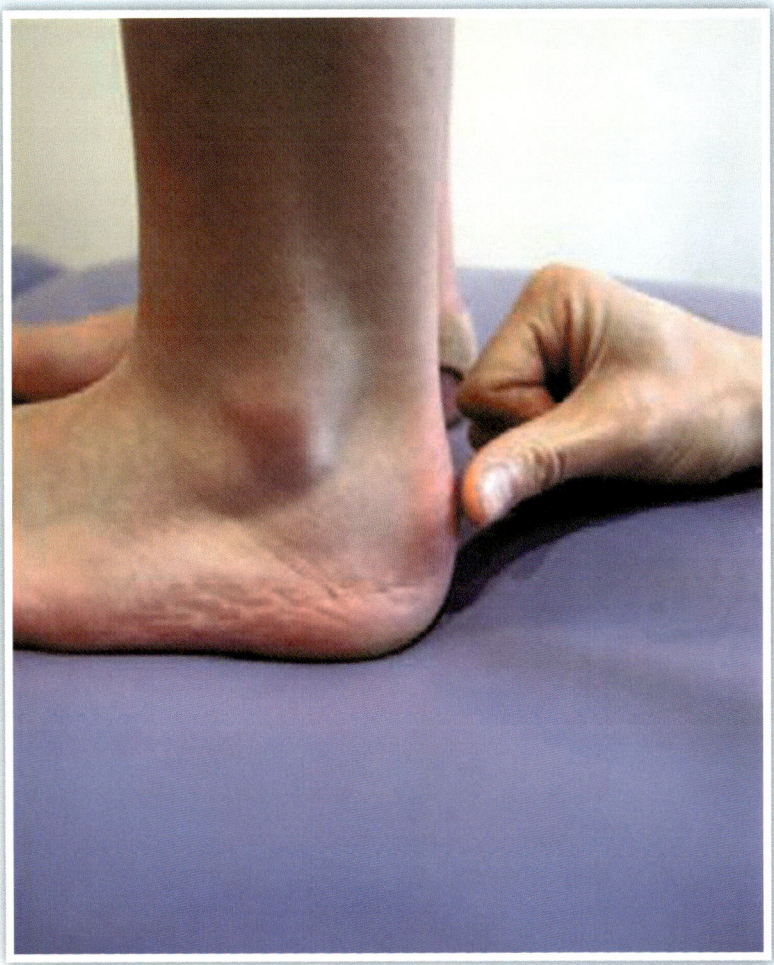

Fig. 8.6 Squeeze test for Sever's disease

X-ray is normally reliable.

If the apophysis has already fused, then the diagnosis for calcaneal apopysitis should be reconsidered as this pain could be a result of ankle or midfoot discomfort (Frush & Lindenfeld, 2009). It's also common to find a tight Achilles tendon (Soprano, 2005).

Treatment and Management

Treatments includes ice, compression, heel lifts, and analgesic medications, if necessary (Cassas & Cassettari-Wayhs, 2006; Frush & Lindenfeld, 2009; James, Williams, & Haines, 2010).

Rest with limited sports is prescribed until all symptoms have resolved (Hunt et al., 2007). Arch-taping helps reduce the effects of Sever's disease during sporting activities (Hunt et al., 2007). Immobilisation in a short leg cast can provide the quickest resolution of symptoms in roughly 2 weeks but should only be considered in severe cases (Frush & Lindenfeld, 2009; Soprano, 2005).

Rehabilitation

Rehabilitation must take place once all symptoms have gone. Stretches for the gastrocnemius and soleus complex, increasing the flexibility of the Achilles tendon, can be repeated daily (Cassas & Cassettari-Wayhs, 2006; Frush & Lindenfeld, 2009).

The individual can also strengthen the muscles involved with dorsiflexion (tibalis anterior) (Frush & Lindenfeld, 2009). Young athletes tend to be non-compliant with stretching exercises, which slows the recovery (Frush & Lindenfeld, 2009).

Achilles Tendon Rupture

Achilles strains and tendon ruptures are rare in children and adolescents. (See Fig. 8.8.)

Acute strains of the Achilles tendon occur during ballistic activities or a change in speed. They can be slight strains, partial thickness tears, and full tears. They follow the same management as for a severe calf strain or rupture.

Signs and Symptoms

A visible limp may be indicated. There is pain directly at the Achilles tendon, and the patient is unable to go on tiptoes. Running makes the pains worse, and sprinting is very painful. Sometimes, swelling is visible.

Test

Pain against resistance is sore, and tenderness is observed on palpation of the tendon.

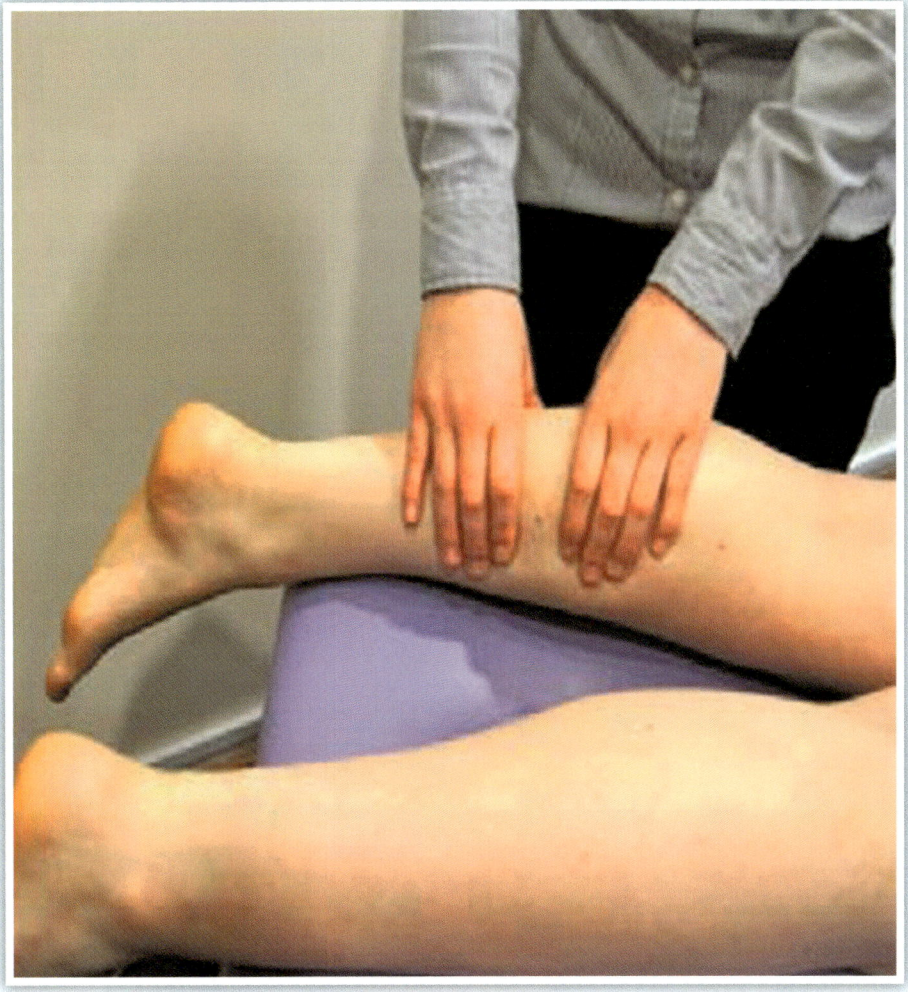

Fig. 8.7 Thompson's squeeze test for rupture

Thompson's test can be applied if there is any implication of a muscle or tendon rupture. Here, the patient lies in prone and the calf is squeezed passively. A positive test for a rupture is when the foot does not plantarflexed on the Thomson's squeeze test. A normal response is when the calf is squeezed and the foot does plantarflexed (Patel et al., 2009).

Treatment and Management

In the first instance, rest, ice, compression, and elevation should be prescribed. When the pain settles, normal gait should be encouraged and gentle stretching should be applied. When the calf becomes more pain-free, active and resisted exercises should begin, if possible in weight bearing. Normally, and obviously depending on severity, the child can restart gentle running after 3 weeks.

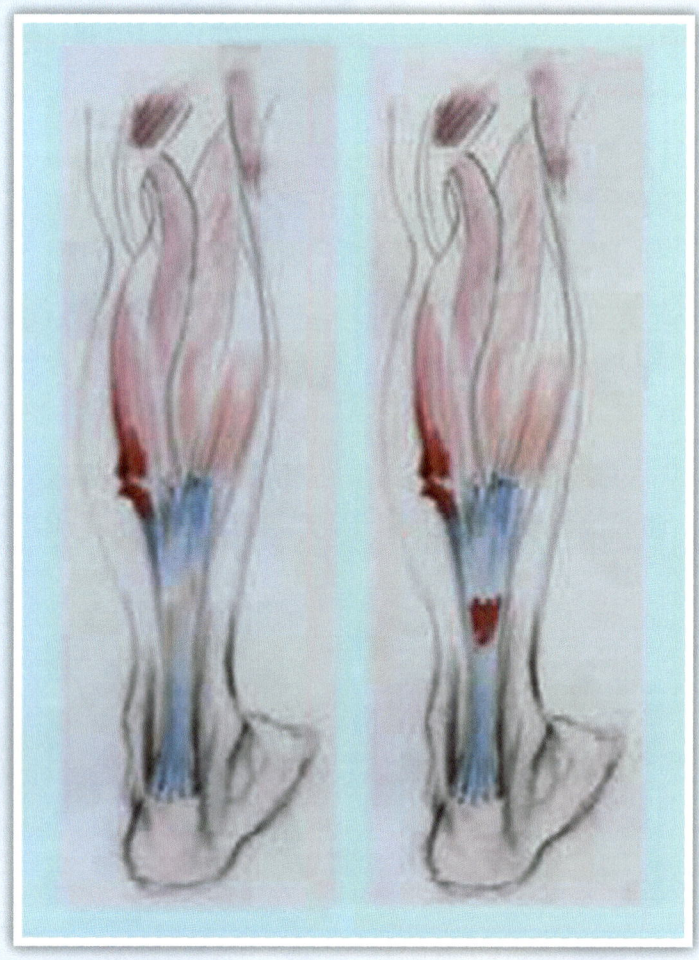

Fig. 8.8 Partial Achilles rupture and medial calf strain

A ruptured Achilles will require an orthopaedic consult.

Ankle Fractures

Physeal Fractures

Paediatric ankle fractures are classified according to the Salter and Harris classification of fractures, consisting of five different classes. This system is the most widely accepted classification system (Birrer et al., 2002).

Tibial physeal fractures, including distal and proximal, are the most common fractures in the lower limb in the growing child. Fibula physeal fractures are also quite common. Both physes are essential for tibia growth and contribute up to 45% of the total length of the tibia.

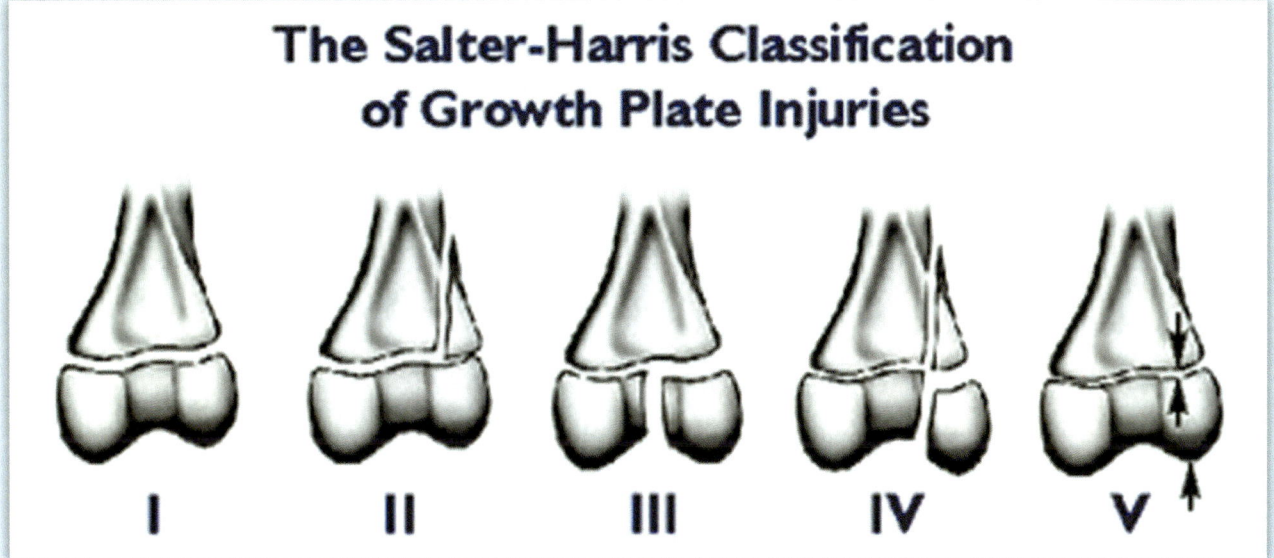

Fig. 8.8b Classificaiton of Salter-Harris fractures

- (I)   Fracture through growth plate

- (II)   Fracture through the growth plate and metaphysis

- (III)   Fracture through growth plate and epiphysis

- (IV)   Fracture through growth plate, metaphysis and epihysis

- (V)   Compression fracture through growth plate

Salter-Harris Type 1 Fracture
Tibia

Type 1 fractures of the distal tibia are rare in adolescents but are more common in children below age 10 years. These fractures are commonly mistaken for simple ankle sprains.

Pain and swelling is common, but physical deformity is rare. Full range of motion is possible. X-rays can reveal normality, but closer inspection may reveal more separation of the tibial physis.

Fibula

Type 1 fractures of the distal fibula are the most common in children. They are also the most common mis-diagnosed fractures, often mistaken for a sprain ligament.

Pain and swelling are localised to the lateral malleoli, specifically at the physis. X-rays may show widening of the physis plate, but patient responds well to rest and immobilisation for 3–4 weeks.

Salter-Harris Type 2 Fracture
Tibia

This is the most common fracture of the distal tibia in children but is normally accompanied by fracture of the distal fibula (non-physis).

This ankle fracture causes more swelling and pain than a type 1, and normally a physical deformity is apparent. Management normally consists of immobility for 3–4 weeks.

Fibula

Type 2 Salter Harris fractures of the fibula are rare and are managed similarly to a type 2 tibia fracture.

Salter-Harris Type 3 Fracture
Tibia

There are two kinds of this fracture, medial and lateral. The distal tibial physis closes centrally to medially, and laterally last.

The medial type 3 fracture normally occurs in children where the medial physis has not closed. Pain is normally localised to the medial malleoli, and if the fibula is fractured, lateral malleoli is painful as well. The gap of this physis is normally

2 mm when fully open, so fractures which increase the gap more may require surgical intervention; otherwise, growth of the bone may be affected (Birrer et al., 2002).

The lateral type 3 fracture of the tibia physis (also known as juvenile Thillaux fracture) occurs in children whose medial physis has closed but lateral remains open. This fracture is normally complex as there is normally damage to much of the soft tissue as well.

Pain is normally localised to the anterior lateral joint line, but swelling tends to be minimal. Normally, the fracture is a small avulsion fracture and healing is normally good. If the fracture is more than 2 mm, then open reduction may be an option.

Fibula

Salter type 3 fractures of the fibula are rare.

Salter-Harris Type 4 Fracture
Tibia

Salter-Harris type 4 fractures are similar to type 3 fractures, affecting the medial and lateral side.

Fracture of the medial side is rare. Sometimes the medial portion's avulsion is small and can be easily missed on X-ray. This fracture can stunt growth of the tibia if not diagnosed; therefore, bone scan may be necessary.

Lateral type 4 fractures are also known as triplane fractures (see Fig. 8.9). These fractures occur in the younger age group, normally under the age of 10 because fewer physeal plates have closed and the fracture plane may have longer to travel along the physis until it reaches a portion that is closed. Triplane fractures normally produce 2 bone fragments in adolescents and 3 in children. As these plates are near closing, these fractures do normally heal well if managed correctly.

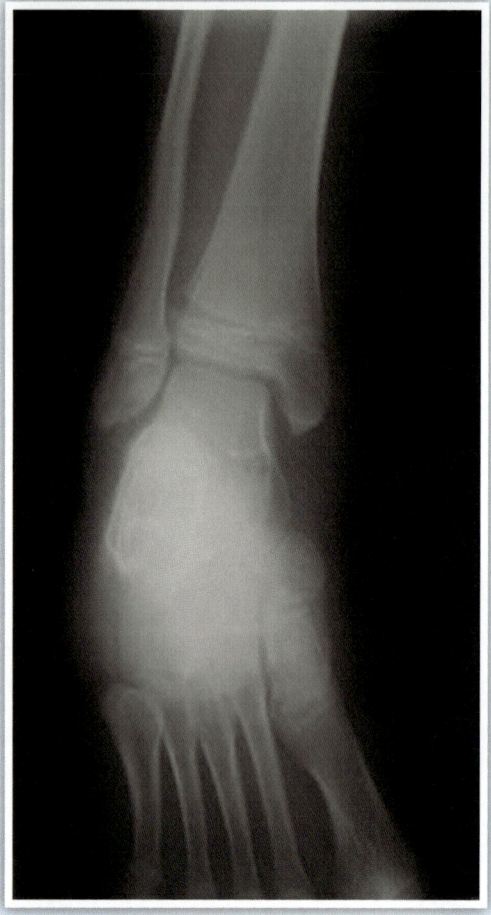

Fig. 8.9 Triplane fracture in a 15–year–old girl

Fibula

These fractures are rare.

Salter-Harris Type 5 Fracture

These fractures are very rare and normally result in crush-type injuries with high impact.

Non-physeal Fractures of the Distal Lower Leg

Four common fractures affect the distal lower leg, which include non-displaced lateral malleoli fracture, displaced lateral malleoli fracture, bimalleoli fracture, and trimalleoli fracture (see Fig. 8.6).

The non-displaced lateral malleoli fracture is normally immobilised for 4–6 weeks. The displaced fracture of the lateral malleoli sometimes requires open reduction. Normally, return to sport is slow.

Bimalleoli fractures are more uncommon, but if they do happen, they tend to be unstable, requiring surgical opinion. These injuries normally take months to heal, as damage to other structures can prolong the recovery.

A trimalleoli fracture is a fracture of both malleoli and the posterior portion of the tibial plafond. These fractures are also unstable, normally requiring surgical intervention.

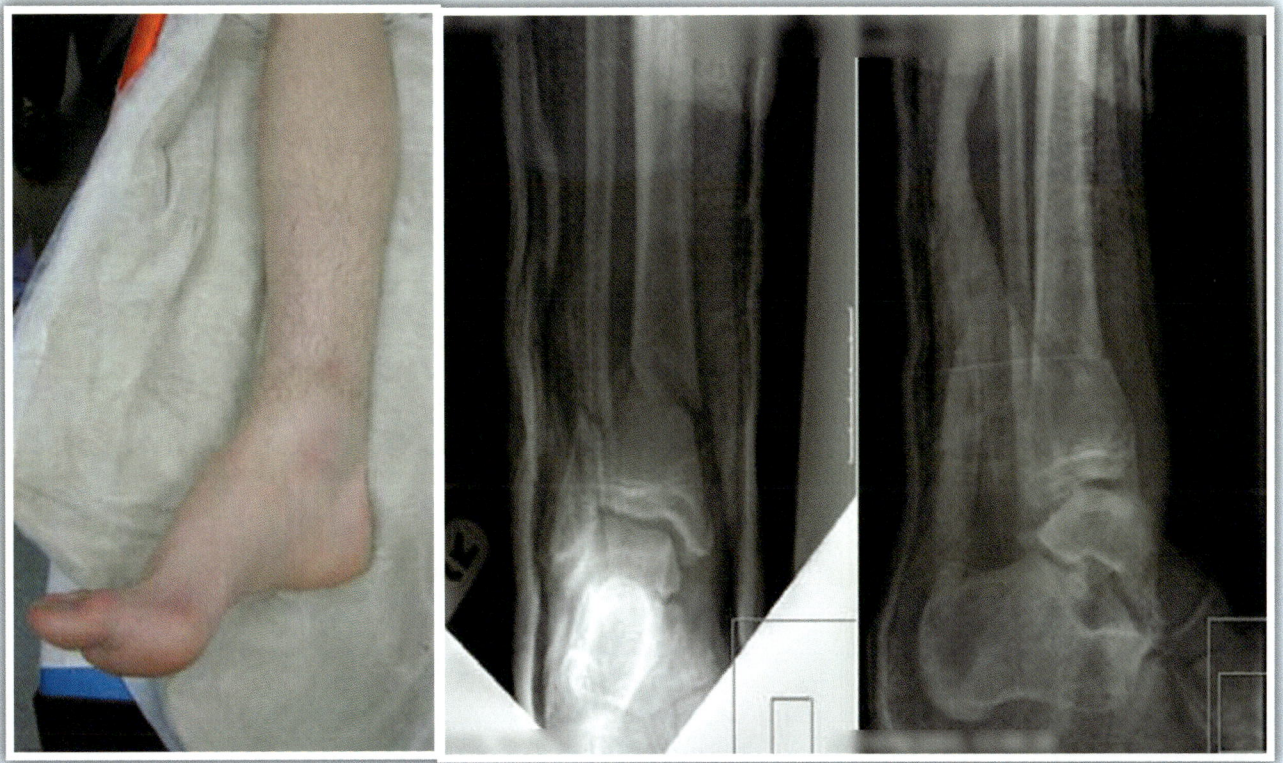

Fig. 8.10 Tibia and fibula fracture in 17-year-old male

Suspected Fracture Examination

If a fracture is suspected in the ankle of a child, some general rules may help. If you suspect a fracture, some basic anatomical landmarks should be palpated, which apply to common areas of fractures in children and adolescents.

These include

- Children with open growth plates that are painful compared with the opposite side,

- Pain on the distal 6 cm of the posterior 1/3 of either malleoli,

- Pain over the navicular bone,

- Pain over the base of fifth metatarsal,

- Unable to weight bear (Birrer et al., 2002).

These are a modified version of the Ottawa ankle rules, and even though they used to apply to adults only, more clinicians are using these rules regardless of the fact that the growth plates remain open in children. The comparable is determining if the pain is more on the injured side than on the uninjured or non affected side on palpation.

Osteochondral Dissecans (OCD) of the Talus

OCD of the talus is uncommon, but normally it follows a severe sprain or is accompanied with a fracture of the ankle. OCD is an injury of the articular cartilage of the underlying subchondral bone.

44% of OCDs of the talus follow a severe inversion sprain of the AFTL.

Signs and Symptoms

Pain is insidious, sometimes described as a sharp pain or ache. Occasionally, there may be locking of the ankle joint and repetitive giving way.

Test

X-rays or MRI scans normally reveal the pathology. No orthopaedic tests have been shown to be reliable.

Treatment

Normally, OCD requires surgical intervention if conservative management fails. This may entail strength exercises and dynamic proprioception exercise in weight bearing.

Subluxation of the Peroneal Tendons

The peroneal tendon aids the calf muscle in plantarflexion of the foot and eversion. They are held in place by a small retinaculum, like a clasp, just posterior to the lateral malleoli. Sometimes, this retinaculum becomes loose, gets disrupted, or is strained, making the tendons sublux out of their groove (see Fig. 8.11). This is quite uncommon in children but normally is asymptomatic

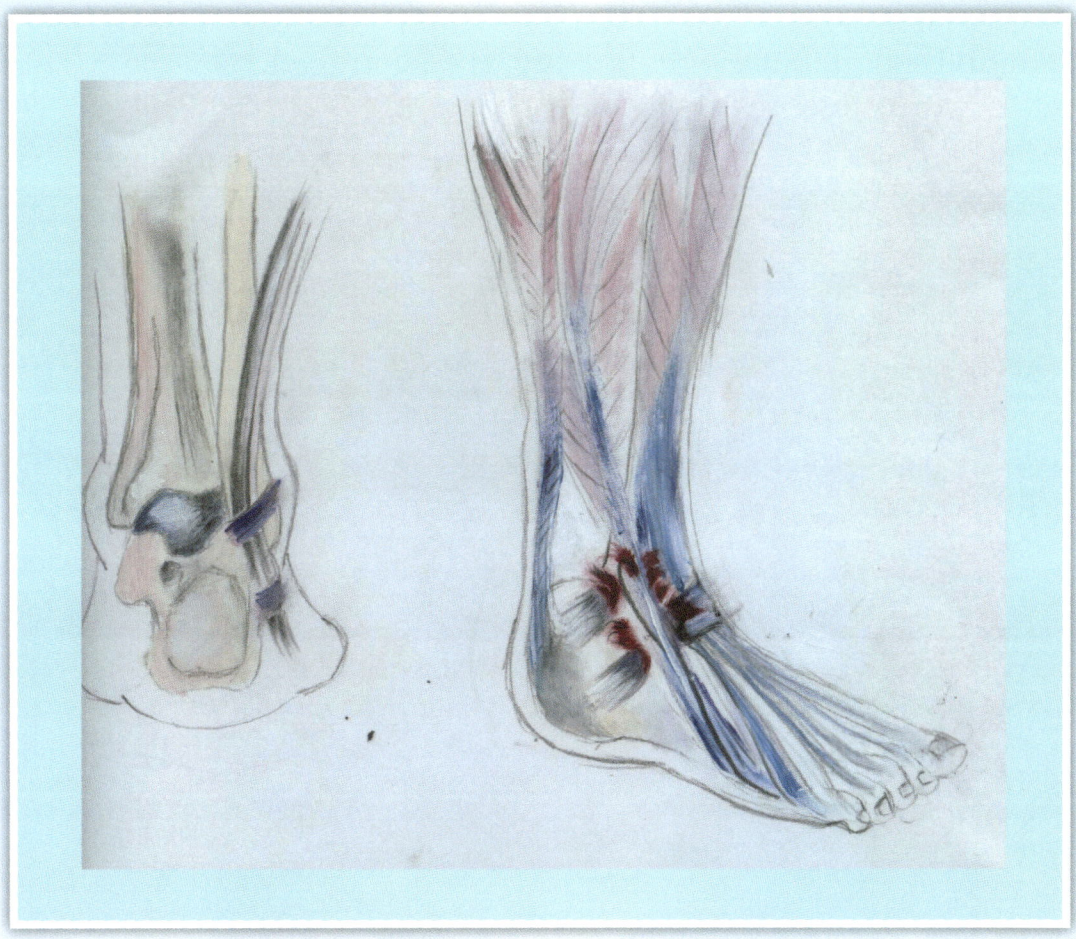

Fig. 8.11 Separation of the peroneal tendon from the trochlea

Signs and Symptoms

There is pain and clicking of the ankle at the posterior lateral portion of the lateral malleoli. Swelling is rare, and plantarflexion can exacerbate some symptoms.

Test

Plantarflexing the foot against manual resistance, can make the lateral ankle painful or a click is felt on palpation.

Treatment

If acute trauma is involved, rest, ice, and compression is indicated. In severe cases, immobilisation, but weight bearing, is encouraged.

Key Points

- Distal tibia plates (lateral) are common fracture sites due to late closure of plate.

- Sever's disease is bilateral in 60% of the cases.

- >2 mm gap on X-rays of physeal plates may indicate instability.

- Fibula fractures are common at physes.

References

Birrer, R., Griesemer, B., & Cataletto, M. (2002). *Pediatric sports medicine in primary care* (2nd ed.). Philadelphia, PA: Lippincott, Williams and Wilkins.

Cassas, K., & Cassettari-Wayhs, A. (2006). Childhood and adolescent sports-related overuse injuries. *American Family Physician, 73*(6), 1014–1022.

Frush, T., & Lindenfeld, T. (2009). Peri-epiphyseal and overuse injuries in adolescent athletes. *Sports Health, 1*(3), 201–211.

Hendrix, C. (2005). Calcaneal apophysitis (Sever disease). *Clinics in Podiatric Medicine and Surgery, 22*(1), 55–62.

Hosgören, B., Köktener, A., & Dilmen, G. (2004). Ultrasonography of the calcaneus in Sever's disease. *Indian Pediatrics, 42*(1), 801–803.

Hunt, G., Stowell, T., Alnwick, G., & Evans, S. (2007). Arch taping as a symptomatic treatment in patients with Sever's disease: A multiple case series. *Foot, 17*(1), 178–183.

James, A., Williams, C., & Haines, T. (2010). Heel raises versus prefabricated orthoses in the treatment of posterior heel pain associated with calcaneal apophysitis (Sever's disease): Study protocol for a randomised controlled trial. *Journal of Foot and Ankle Research, 3*(1), 1–7.

Patel, D., Greydanus, D., & Baker, R. (2009) *Pediatric practice sports medicine* (2nd ed.). New York, NY: McGraw Hill Medical Books.

Scharfbillig, R., Jones, R., & Scutter, S. (2008). Sever's disease: What does the literature really tell us? *Journal of the American Podiatric Medical Association, 98*(3), 212–223.

Sitati, F., & Kingori, J. (2009). Chronic bilateral heel pain in a child with Sever disease: Case report and review of literature. *Cases Journal, 2*(9365), 1–3.

Soprano, J. (2005). Musculoskeletal injuries in the pediatric and adolescent athlete. *Current Sports Medicine Reports, 4*(1), 329–334.

CHAPTER 9

Foot Pathologies in Children and Adolescent Sport

Christian Schafer and Solomon Abrahams

Juvenile Hallux (Abducto) Valgus (HAV)

It is a condition where the hallux is both abducted and valgus rotated in relation to the first metatarsal.

Aetiology

Given that most children have excessively pronated feet, we know that it is more than just rearfoot hyperpronation involved. Poor alignment and posture of the metatarso-phalanageal joint as well as the metatarso-cuniform joint result in a mobile plantarflexed first ray and hypermobile midtarsal joint. These tend to be major influencing factors, as well as a long or short first metatarsal. Different studies have demonstrated a positive family history in 68–80% of cases. The child in this case has inherited the specific poor lower limb mechanics that will predispose them to developing HAV.

Footwear, although significant as an exacerbating factor, will not cause HAV singularly, as the above 2 factors will usually need to exist.

Prevalence

The literature is varied with the incidence higher in shod populations. Piggot reported that 57% of adults with HAV recall problems starting in their teenage years. Cole reported that 36% of children aged 6–18, with girls making up approximately 75% of these, have this problem.

Signs and Symptoms

Pain is often not associated with juvenile HAV, with studies reflecting only 21% cases being painful. The complaints tend to be more around deformation and difficulty in getting shoes, and cosmesis. (Typically juvenile cases present between ages 11 and 14, where the child is becoming more self-aware of their appearance. In the author's experience, this is also when there tends to be a significant growth spurt in height, creating a temporary ankle equinus. This, in turn, compounds the deformity.) Parental concern of the younger patient between ages 6 and 10 years may be the driver.

Tests

The clinical diagnosis should be made with a digital goniometer or a dorso-plantar weight-bearing X-ray, with greater than 15 degrees first MTP joint angle noted. Further angular measurement may be calculated from X-rays, but these would be reserved for severe surgical cases due to the avoidance of unnecessary exposure to X-rays.

To summarise, there are 4 criteria that the author recommends when considering the severity of juvenile HAV:

1. Extent of pain: this may be from dorso-medial irritation of the first Metatarsal Phalangeal Joint (MTPJ) or dorsal compression of the first Metatarsal phalangeal (MTP) joint.

2. Footwear: difficulty in wearing footwear, both in terms of accommodation space at medial forefoot and the extent of deformation of this area.

3. Function of the first ray and first MTPJ: as long as sufficient stability of the first ray and functional ROM of the first MTPJ coexist, the foot is theoretically still able to operate through forefoot loading and propulsion.

4. Consideration of how the deformity will progress: a good indicator being looking at family history and the impact that it has had.

Management is based around empowering the patient to minimise progression as much as possible, along with maintaining a reduction in symptoms. This is best achieved through ensuring that footwear is accommodative enough at the toe box and the midfoot, stretching out tight hamstrings and triceps surae, wearing night splints, and improving poor foot mechanics with orthotics.

Turf Toe

Otherwise known as first MTP joint sprain, this is a common hyperextension injury to the first metatarso-phalangeal joint, resulting in partial or complete disruption of the fibrocartilage plantar plate ligament. In patients playing substantially on hard Astro Turf, this may advance to cause tearing of the joint capsule and eventual osteoarthritic change and a hallux rigidus. Very flexible unsupportive football boots have also been implicated in the cause.

Diagnosis is made by noting the history of joint tenderness and swelling and looking for instability and a varus and valgus stress test combined with a dorso-plantar drawer test of the first MTP joint. The clinician should aim to identify collateral ligament damage or a plantar plate tear. Management in acute cases consists of ice, anti-inflammatory modalities, and pressure redistributive padding and strapping. For long-term management, in-shoe deflective padding or orthotics to reduce excessive pronation can be considered.

Osteochondroses (Avascular Necrosis)

It is described as a disease of the growth plate or ossification centres in children, often due to trauma. Initially, there is necrosis of the bone, followed by re-calcification and remodelling. The following are diseases that occur in the foot.

Freiberg's Disease

The head of the second metatarsal is the most common site for this osteochondrosis caused by avascular necrosis. The end result is a flattened reorganisation of the metatarsal head with consequent arthritis of the second MTPJ. One study showed a 68% incidence at the second metatarsal head, 27% at the third, and most rarely, 5% at the fifth (Gauthier & Elbaz, 1979). Old Freiberg injuries are often identified years on when the foot is being investigated for something else.

Signs and Symptoms

While there is usually a history of a trauma, mechanical and anatomical causes should be ruled out. The joint ROM at the second metatarsal is limited, and dorso-plantar X-rays would help confirm a flattened reorganised shape to the head of the metatarsal in late stages only. (See Fig. 9.1.)

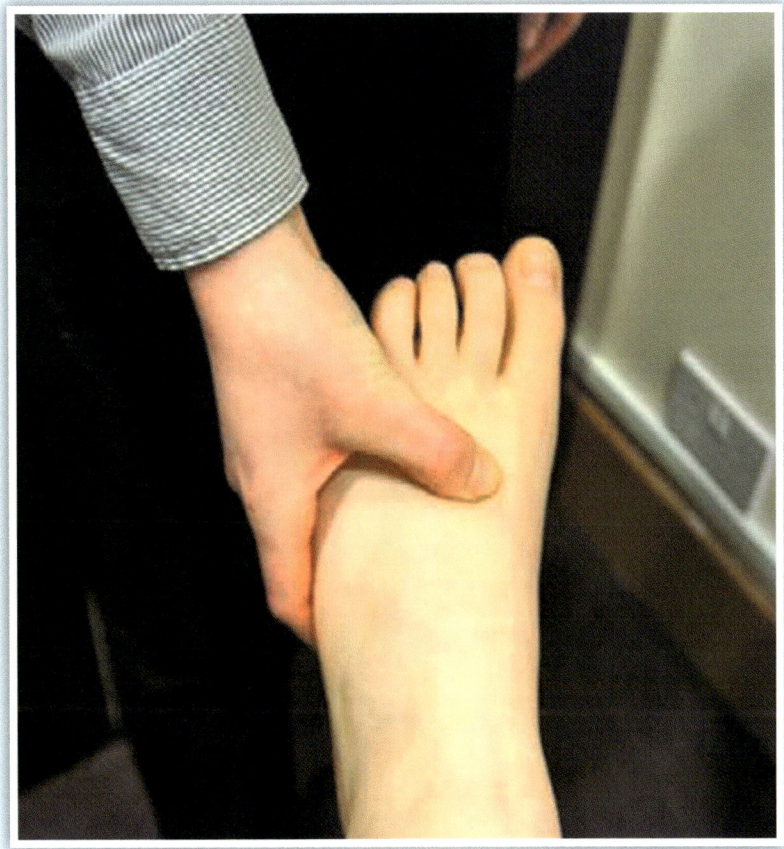

Fig. 9.1 Palpation of Freiberg's disease

Incidence

This is hard to ascertain as there are probably a large number of undiagnosed cases that spontaneously resolve. It is most prevalent in the 13–15 years age range with a 1:4 male:female ratio.

Management

Supportive footwear with pressure redistributive padding and reduced activity for 4–6 weeks is advisable. In an extreme case, a below-the-knee-cast for 4–6 weeks is indicated, while surgery is rarely indicated. But in cases of poor foot mechanics, orthotics will be needed for long-term management in order to reduce progressive osteoarthritic changes.

Köhler's Disease

Affecting the navicular bone, this disease is found in children between the ages 3 and 9 years, with peak incidence around 4–5 years. It is rare, and normally presents with a limping child often supinating to avoid pressure over the Navicular area.

X-rays normally reveal a dense sclerotic irregular shape to the navicular. It does, however, return to regular size, shape, and density.

Management should be through offloading the navicular by valgus support of the longitudinal arch, combined with supportive footwear.

Fractures

Metatarsal Stress Fractures

These are described as spontaneous fractures due to an accumulation of stresses and account for 3.7% of all sports injuries, with the second and third metatarsals accounting for 80–90% of these. With the deep transverse metatarsal ligaments and interosseous muscles acting as anchors between the second to fourth metatarsal heads, there is reduced displacement from the ground reaction force. 95% of second metatarsal fractures are on the shaft and distal neck. Although much rarer, proximal fractures are both harder to diagnose and have less favourable prognosis in terms of rehabilitation. They are found in ballerinas from standing on pointe. According to a study of 320 children with stress fractures, 34% were confirmed to have the fractures in the tarsal and metatarsal region of the foot (Shanmugam & Maffulli, 2008).

Signs and Symptoms

Pain is noted on activity; it resolves with rest, with the patient needing to limp. Eventual tenderness and swelling will ensue. X-rays may be unhelpful as it can take 2–3 weeks for changes to show. Where diagnosis cannot be confirmed by history and X-rays, bone scans and MRIs are used.

Management

This requires 4–8 weeks of rest, with pressure redistributive padding and supportive footwear or surgical boots and crutches designed to offload the forefoot. In cases of a short first metatarsal and/ or a hyperpronating foot, any predisposing biomechanical features should be addressed with orthotics.

Fifth Metatarsal Fractures

Three types have been noted with varying prognosis. The fifth metatarsal base avulsion fracture, where the peroneus brevis pulls a chip off the bone from the tuberosity at the lateral base of the shaft, often seen with inversion injuries. The head, neck, or shaft fracture to the fifth metatarsal may be seen in dancers who are balancing laterally on the forefoot and lose their balance, spiralling into inversion on the fifth metatarsal. Least favourable is the Jones fracture, which may often require prolonged non-weight-bearing and fixation due to a likelihood of non-union.

Signs and Symptoms

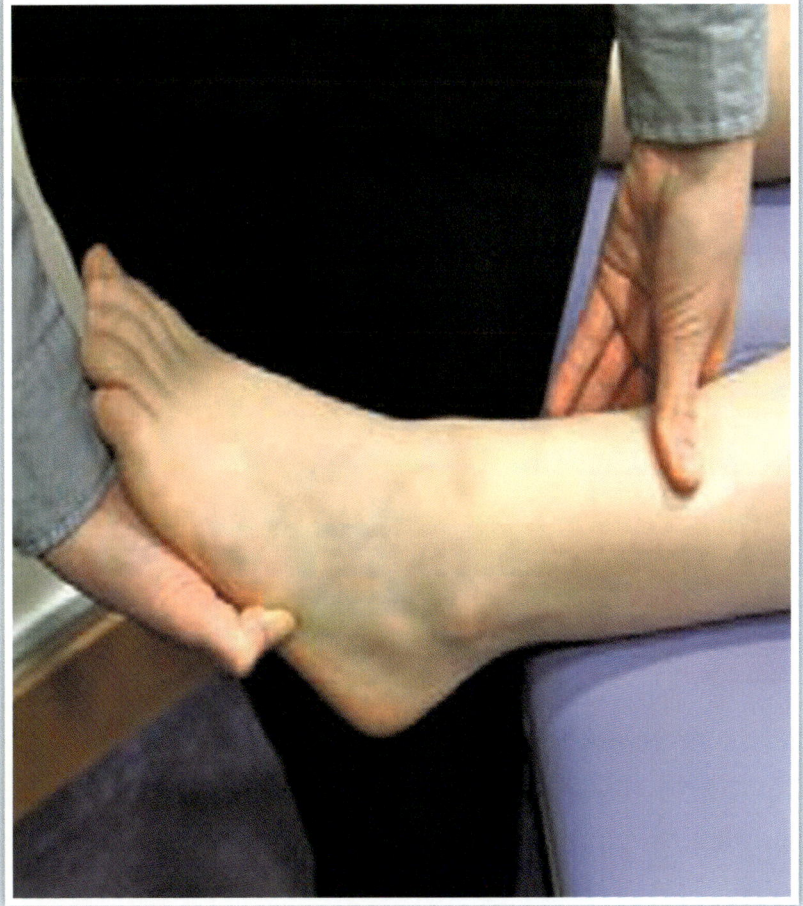

The patient will limp, trying to offload the lateral forefoot by pronating excessively to load the foot medially. X-rays are vital to distinguish between the different types as management varies significantly. An avulsion displays an oblique fracture line through the tubersosity. Palpation of the base of the 5th is normally very painful. (See Fig 9.2.)

Fig. 9.2 Palpation of base of fifth

Management

The fifth metatarsal avulsion fracture fairs best within 4 weeks without immobilisation but reduced weight-bearing activity, which can be achieved with an adapted orthotic or insole to offload the base of the fifth metatarsal and reduce load on the peroneals. The shaft, neck, and head (non-proximal) fractures are best managed in a weight-bearing cast, if tolerated, and the fractures heal between 4 and 6 weeks. However, the Jones fracture requires a prolonged healing time with 8 weeks completely non-weight bearing, and then weight bearing in a cast as tolerated. One study (Clapper, O'Brien, & Lyons, 1995) found that Jones fractures took between 21.2 and 25 weeks to heal with 28% requiring fixation.

Iselins Disease

Differentiation from this overuse osteochondritis at the base of the fifth metatarsal, and Jones fracture is key. The main difference is that Iselin's disease is self-limiting and will spontaneously resolve with closure of the growth plate.

Incidence

This is unknown as there is little data but it is speculated that there are many undiagnosed cases, so it may not be as rare as first thought. Like Sever's heel, it is typically more often seen in boys between the ages of 8 and 13 and is associated with impact-activity sports.

Signs, Symptoms, and Management

An X-ray will confirm diagnosis, and management is through anti-inflammatory modalities as well as offloading through padding, supportive footwear, stretching of triceps surae, and orthotics to correct any underlying biomechanical problems.

Navicular Stress Fracture

These are among the most common stress fractures in young athletes, notably sprinters, jumpers, and hurdlers, and involve the middle third of the body of the navicular in mostly young males. Symptoms may persist from weeks to years as diagnosis is often delayed. Causative factors that have been reported are excessive pronation, limited ankle dorsiflexion, and tarsal coalition.

Signs and Symptoms

Diagnosis is based largely on suspicion as pain is often insidious, poorly localised around the dorsum of the foot and midway along the longitudinal arch. However, suspicion should be raised if there is tenderness over the proximal dorsal aspect of the navicular combined with pain that is notably worse on activity, and better on rest. X-rays are of little use, and either MRIs or bone scans are needed to confirm the diagnosis.

Management

This requires immobilisation and strict non-weight bearing in a cast for 6 weeks. This should be repeated if there is still tenderness on the dorsal proximal aspect of the navicular for a further 6 weeks. On return to activity, mobilisation of the ankle, subtalar joint, and midtarsals and calf strengthening and gradual exercises are required before impact activities are resumed. For prevention of recurrence, flexibility of the triceps surae and hamstrings should be maintained, and orthotics should be used to reduce excessive eversion or pronatory forces acting on the navicular.

Midtarsal Dislocations

The midtarsal joint (Chopart's joint or transverse tarsal joint) is a 'gliding joint' and consists of the combined articulations of calcaneocuboid and the talonavicular joints, allowing the rear foot and midfoot to articulate. Trauma to the midtarsal (Chopart's) joint is believed to be relatively common and is often overlooked; therefore, diagnosis may be easily delayed due to insufficient X-rays – 30 of 73 cases in one study (Main and Jowett).

Signs and Symptoms

It differs from subtalar dislocations because the talocalcaneal relationship remains preserved. (Both midtarsal and subtalar dislocations can, however, result in talonavicular dislocation.) Symptoms involve local tenderness and pain on isolating the midtarsal joint and putting it through its full range of motion.

Midtarsal injury has been described in a number of ways:

i)   medial force (sprain, subluxation),

ii)   longitudinal force associated with a fractured navicular,

iii) lateral force (sprains, flake fractures, and dislocations, 'cuboid crush injury', 'swivel injury'), having the most long-term implications and often resulting in a loss of lateral stability,

iv)   plantar force (impaction fracture, bifurcate ligament avulsion fracture), and

v)   crush injury.

A careful history is vital to ascertain which of the above forces has resulted in the injury. X-rays and MRI scans are indicated to ascertain the extent of the injury, and then management can be best planned.

Management

This will vary according to the injury. For a sprain, anti-inflammatory modalities, padding and strapping with compression to limit excessive movement, and rest will be required. For a medial fracture sprain, the above precautions will be needed, but then a weight-bearing cast will be required. A calcaneocuboid fusion may be required in a persistently problematic lateral-force injury. In the long term, orthotics may be indicated for correcting any predisposing biomechanical problems. Where joint inflammation is persistent, a cortisone injection into one of the two joints may be beneficial.

Tarsal Coalition

This is the congenital or aquired condition of bridges between the tarsal bones that restrict or prevent movement. The bridge may be fibrous (syndesmosis), cartilaginous synchondrosis, or synostosis (osseus).

Incidence

According to studies on large military sample sizes, the incidence in the general population varied between 0.04% and 1.4%, with calcaneonavicular being the most common, followed by talocalcaneal, and then the rarest being talonavicular and calcanecuboid coalitions.

Signs and Symptoms

In children and adolescents, it may present with a painful pes planus foot-type with peroneal spasticity from overuse with the rearfoot kept in valgus position. There may be a history of an adolescent beginning a sport and complaining of intense pain. On testing the ROM of the subtalar and midtarsal joint, there is a noticeable lack of independent movement combined with pain at the end of the range.

Management

Management of the secondary effects of the coalition, that is peroneal spasticity or pes planus, may be more important than the coalition itself as in operated cases, symptoms have still been reported. Orthotics are indicated to help manage these secondary effects by limiting end-of-range excessive pronation and supination.

Lisfranc's Joint Fracture-Dislocation

Lisfranc's joint, or the tarsometatarsal joints, are a collective arc-shaped series of midfoot joints joining the metatarsals to the cuneiforms and the cuboid.

Signs and Symptoms

History of the injury will often reveal a load having been applied along the axis of Lisfranc's joint when the foot was plantarflexed. It is seen most frequently in industrial injuries, road traffic accidents, and equestrian injuries where the foot remains in the stirrup during a fall from the horse.

A fracture-dislocation may be obvious both clinically and on X-ray in all planes as oedema in the midfoot, and there may be difficulty in walking and pain on gentle supination. However, an *occult reduced fracture-dislocation* is possible, requiring a high index of suspicion. The patient may recall an audible 'snap' or 'pop'. On examination in this case, there may be a noticeably more abducted or adducted forefoot, often with a dorsally and plantarly mobile second metatarsal base or even excessive mobility right across Lisfranc's joint.

Management

This will vary according to the severity, with anatomical reduction being the main goal. Mild cases require 6 weeks of non-weight bearing in a cast, with severe cases requiring internal fixation.

Tibialis Posterior Tendinopthy

Most commonly seen in the excessively pronated foot, this tendon's function is to supinate the foot and is most vital for maintaining the structural integrity of the medial-longitudinal arch.

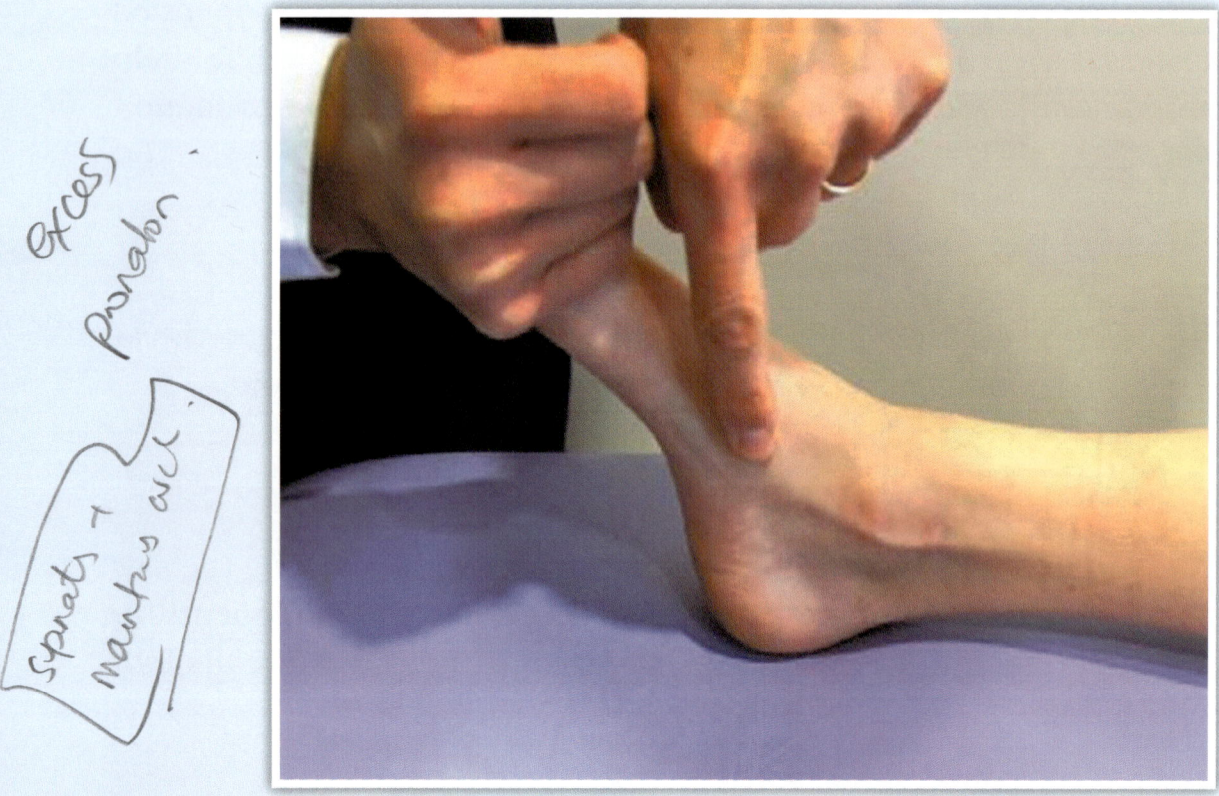

Fig. 9.3 Palpation of tibialis posterior tendon

By virtue of its anatomical placement, in excessively pronated-foot-types, there is increased potential to overuse the tendon, leading to either strain or inflammation. In cases of excessive repetitive stresses or a single large pronatory stress, the tendon may increase in length due to strain, rendering the foot's arch profile more 'collapsed'. This tendon, which has a synovial sheath, is the most likely to develop a stenosing tenosynovitis at the posterior medial malleolus, and navicular tuberosity.

Signs and Symptoms

Tenderness and oedema around the course of the muscle posterior to the medial malleolus (see Fig. 9.3), or inferior around the navicular which it uses for traction, may be present.Clinically, the patient would classically be unable to perform an inverted heel raise adequately or comfortably. It is often seen in hypermobile feet, where there is a more prominent plantar displaced navicular tuberosity. In chronic cases, ultrasound and MRI scans are required to see the extent of any changes in the tendon, and X-rays/ MRIs can check the presence of an accessory ossicle os navicularis, which can cause irriation and may require excision.

Management

Anti-inflammatory modalities as well as strengthening the muscle/tendon with single leg inverted heel raises are important for long-term management, along with orthotics and supportive footwear in most cases. Stretching the triceps surae in addition will reduce the pronatory forces during gait.

Peroneal Tendons

These refer mostly to the peroneus brevis and longus muscles and tendons which are commonly affected at sites where they change direction, in this case posterior to the lateral malleolus. They are evertors of the subtalar joint and may be overused after bad inversion injuries, where the lateral ankle ligaments have become weaker and the lateral ankle is more unstable. As these tendons have synovial sheaths, there may be tenosynovitis, where the sheath diameter narrows through inflammation and the tendon adheres to the sheath. If this process is chronic, over time, it may progress to stenosing tenosynovitis, where fibrous scar tissue build up in the sheath, which restricts movement of the tendon further.

Signs and Symptoms

Tenderness and swelling would be noted posterior to the lateral malleolus, plantar lateral aspect of the cuboid, and between the cuboid and the base of the first metatarsal, where the Peroneal Longus inserts. Symptoms would normally be felt when everting the foot against resistance from a maximally inverted position, and maximally everted position.

Management

In acute injuries, RICE, physiotherapy, and anti-inflammatory modalities are suggested. For the more chronic cases and to avoid recurence, supportive footwear is required to minimise midfoot/ forefoot instability, and orthotics should be used to reduce the end range of inversion at the midtarsal and subtalar joints.

Osteochondral Defects (OCDs) of the Talus

Also known as talar dome injuries, these lesions were described (Berndt & Harty) in 1959 as a transchondral fracture through articular cartilage and into the subchondral cancellous bone of the talus. In most studies, trauma was the aetiology, often with an inversion injury. Non-traumatic cases have been reported and are rare, but they are likely to be due to repetitive microtrauma and poor foot and ankle mechanics. The osteochondral fragment itself may remain in situ and become partially/totally detached or even displaced within the defect.

Incidence

One study reported talar dome injuries as representing 0.9% of all fractures and 0.1% of all talar fractures. However, the true incidence is likely to be higher due to the frequency of missed diagnoses. Footballers who suffer inversion ankle injuries may be particulary prone.

Signs and Symptoms

As mild cases can be asymptomatic, the clinician would need a high index of suspicion after an inversion injury, as X-rays and clinical tests will yield little. Repeat X-rays may be indicated following an inversion injury if there are symptoms of swelling, exercise-related pain, or clicking or catching of the ankle. If X-rays are negative but suspicions are still high, then an MRI may be warranted, even as long as 5 months after the injury. In the worst cases, there may be avascular necrosis and contralateral ligament injury.

Management

Immobilisation is vital in most cases to allow the union of the fracture fragment. Physiotherapy modalities would be needed for post-injury rehabilitation with orthotics to limit both excessive rearfoot pronation and midfoot and ankle supination (determined by whether the lesion is medial or lateral) to limit shearing forces to the talar dome.

Excessively Pronated Feet

There has been much debate about the significance of pronation in the child and adolescent, especially with sport. Certainly there are milestones in the child's development where excessive pronation would be regarded as perfectly normal, and any early intervention through orthotics are not deemed necessary until the ages of 6–12 years, when the hips have rotated. Beyond age 6, there may be a good reason to prescribe orthotics when there is a history of knee pain and balance and coordination difficulties with or without hypermobility in the feet. In older adolescents, conditions such as Achilles tendonopathy or shin splints may develop through having excessively pronated feet.

Signs and Symptoms

In terms of the foot position, the extent of pronation can be gauged by checking how many toes are visible laterally as the patient walks away from you. In addition, looking at the relative positions of the talus, navicular, and vertical displacement of the bisection of the calcaneum during gait will help.

A careful detailed history of symptoms and sporting activity is helpful to determine if the patient is actually being held back by his feet. They may present with Achilles tendinopathy or shin splints or, in the case with teenage girls who play a lot of sport, medial knee pain. Reference to footwear and seeing the patient walking in them will reveal the extent to which they may be deforming or excessively wearing the shoe.

Management

In cases where there are symptoms obviously relating to a patient's foot mechanics, intervention is truly justified. However, before orthotics is considered, it is essential to consider the whole lower limb mechanics. There are numerous cases where the feet 'have to be able to pronate excessively' to accommodate for insufficiencies elsewhere. For example, where there are tight hamstrings and/or tight triceps surae muscles, or where there is a genu varum, orthotic intervention may reduce the foot's ability to offload the knee, so the patient may develop knee pain as a result.

It is, therefore, always vital to reduce any soft-tissue influence around the hips, knees, and feet that could be having a significantly bad effect.

Orthotics is indicated, however, to help with the management of many lower limb and foot conditions in the sporting child and adolescent, many of which have been mentioned in this chapter. Conditions such as accessory navicular or *os navicularis,* which may coexist with tibialis posterior overuse in an excessively pronated adolescent, may need orthotics in the long term according to the degree. In cases like these, casts should be taken and the orthotics made bespoke to ensure they are truly fit for the purpose and fit the exact bony contours of the feet. There is no real substitute for casted orthotics, because despite the advent of pressure plates and laser scanners to map the contours of the feet, the image created from pressure plates and laser scanners is 2-dimensional, just like a photograph, so creating a 3-dimensional shape from this is debatable.

Key Points

- Most common cause of chronic ankle pain remains osteochondral lesion.

- Freiberg's disease affects the second Metatarsal in 68% of cases, 27% being the third Met.

- 70% of hallux valgus in children is genetic. Hallux valgus is common in children with flat feet.

References

Agosta, J. (2001). Foot pain. In *Clinical sports medicine* (2nd ed., pp. 584–600). Sydney: McGraw-Hill.

Bia, F. J., Crawford, J., & Thompson, R. (1981). In John P. Friel (Ed.). *Dorland's illustrated medical dictionary* (26th ed., p. 942). Philadelphia, PA: W. B. Saunders.

Shanmugam, C., & Maffulli, N. (2008). Sports injury in children. *British Medical Bulletin, 86,* 33–57.

CHAPTER 10:

Shoulder Pathologies in Children and Adolescent Sport

Solomon Abrahams

The adolescent shoulder is one of the biggest and most complex joints within the human body, comprising of the humeral head, clavicle, and scapular (see Fig. 10.1 and 10.2). It is not too dissimilar from that of an adult. The joint and ligaments are the same as that of a fully grown adult; however, they are not as strong or stable, as they are still very much immature. They remain one of the most unstable and injured joints in adolescents, more so than in adults (Ciullo, 1996).

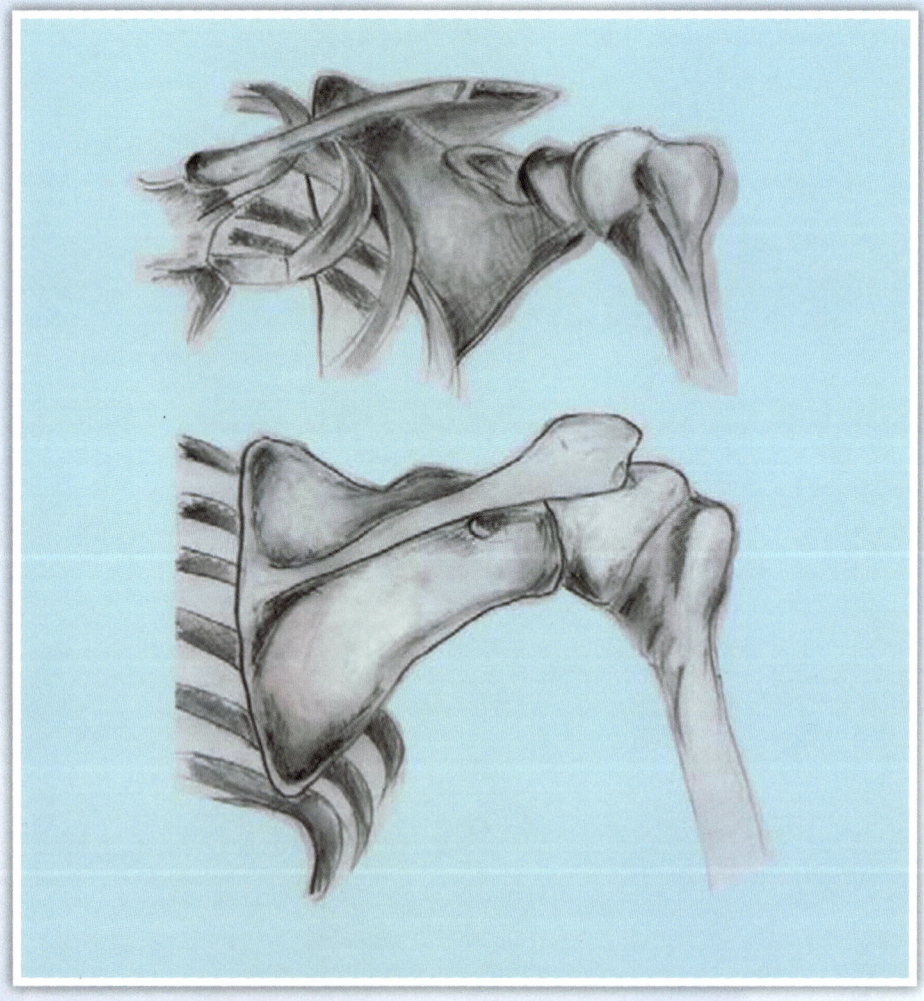

Fig. 10.1 The bony congruencies of the shoulder

The clavicle is a slightly 's-shaped' long bone; the superior surface of the clavicle is smooth and rounded, where the inferior surface is flat and rough because of the strong ligaments that bind it to the first rib near the sternal end. It also has grooves and ridges for muscle attachments. The medial or 'sternal' end is enlarged and rounded with a hammer-like head for articulation with the manubrium creating the sternoclavicular joint. The lateral or 'acromial' end is concave anteriorly and is flat where it articulates with the acromion, creating the acromioclavicular joint. It also has a roughened tuberosity called the conoid tubercle for the attachment of the conoid ligament (Saladin, 2012).

The clavicle supports the shoulder by keeping the upper limb away from the midline of the body and also transfers weight from the upper limb to the axial skeleton and vice versa. The clavicle is the most fractured bone within the adolescent body as a result of a child who falls with their arm out to try and cushion a fall (Moore, Dalley, & Agur, 2010).

The adolescent scapula is a triangular flat bone that lies on the posterolateral aspect of the thorax covering the second to seventh ribs; its only direct attachment to the body is by way of muscles. Rarely is this injured in a child or an adolescent. The convex posterior surfaces are divided into the infraspinous fossa, the smaller supraspinous fossa, and the larger subscapular fossa – the concave costal surface. The three bony fossas provide attachment for muscles. The body of the scapular is thin and translucent superiorly and inferiorly to the scapular spine. As the spine continues laterally, it forms the flat acromion that articulates with the clavicle.

Superolaterally, the lateral surface of the scapula has a glenoid cavity; this receives and articulates with the head of the humerus, creating the glenohumeral joint. The glenoid cavity is especially shallow in children; it is concave and an oval-shaped fossa (Saladin, 2012). It is considerably smaller than that of the humeral head, for which it serves as a socket, making it unstable. The coracoid process is superior to the glenoid fossa and projects anteriorolaterally. This provides the inferior attachment for the passively supporting coracoclavicular ligament (Moore et al., 2010).

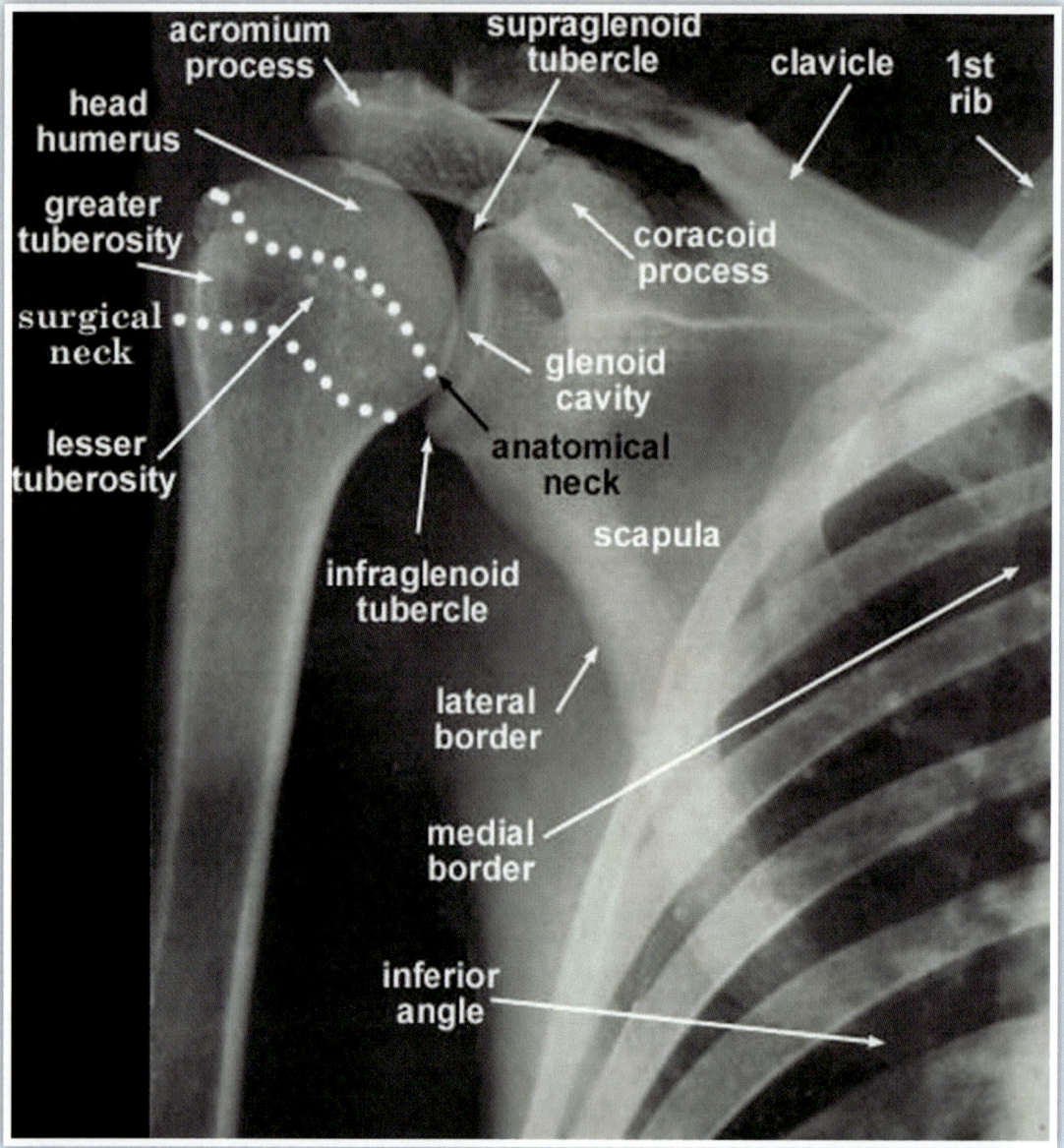

Fig. 10.2 Normal shoulder X-ray

The humeral head is spherical in shape and articulates with the glenoid cavity of the scapula. The anatomical neck is formed by a groove circumscribing the head and separating it from greater and lesser tubercles. This also indicates the line of attachment for the glenohumeral joint capsule. The greater tubercle is at the lateral margin of the humerus, whereas the lesser tubercle projects anteriorly from the bone. The intertubercular groove separates the greater and lesser tubercles and allows for passage of the long head of the bicep tendon (Moore et al., 2010).

The immature humerus is a long bone and grows and elongates from the epiphyseal growth plates at either end.

Clavicular Fractures

The clavicular fracture is arguably the most common fracture seen in children and accounts for between 5% and 15% of all fractures (Calder et al., 2002). The most common site of a clavicle fracture is the middle third, with the medial and lateral aspects rarely fractured. This is simply because its anatomical 'S' shape is more accentuated and is remarkably thin at this particular area in the growing child (Birrer, Greisemer, & Cataletto, 2002).

The most common type of fracture seen in children is a greenstick fracture (Drake, Vogl, & Mitchell, 2005). A greenstick fracture occurs when the bones are still soft and immature, and rather than breaking, the bones bend under the stress. The bone will tend to buckle on the opposite side to the force. Greenstick fractures do heal quickly; however, they normally take a few weeks and still need to be placed in a cast or a sling to ensure union of deformity or slippage (Marcovitch, 2010). Any fracture of the clavicle is normally visible (see Fig. 10.3), and the child will be very reluctant to move their shoulder.

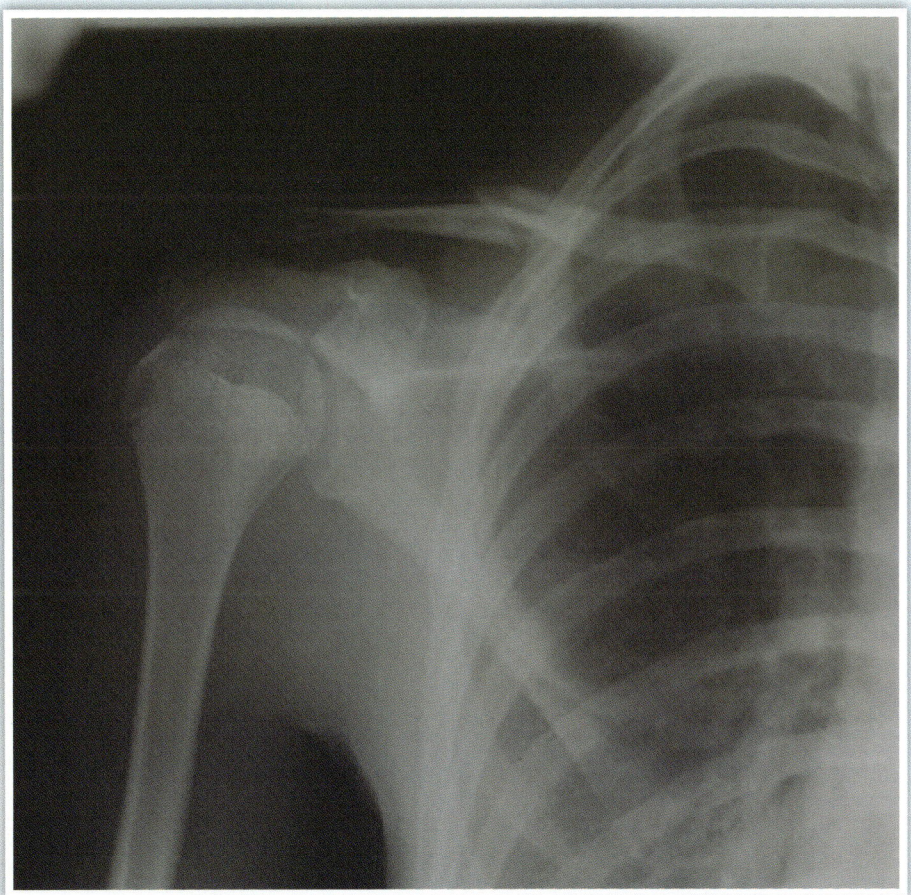

Fig. 10.3 Mid-clavicular fracture in a 15-year-old male

In children, the most common cause of a clavicle fracture is falling on an outstretched arm, accounting for 52% of cases; sports related fractures account for 24%, a car collision causes 15%, and 9% are caused by a fall down the stairs (Calder et al., 2002).

Diagnostically, a fractured clavicle has a number of components that are commonly seen; the outer portion of the clavicle tends to be pulled down because of the weight of the arm, and the arm may look 'limp' and present with local tenderness and swelling. The child will hold their arm to their side, as they feel they are unable to support it. They will be extremely reluctant to move the arm, and any palpation can cause apprehension.

To truly identify a fracture, an X-ray is needed.

Treatment and management of the fracture would be immobilisation with a sling for 4–6 weeks. Surgery may also have to be used if the child has an open fracture.

Once the sling has been removed, the next stage is gentle movements (Baker, Flandry, & Henderson, 1995). It has been suggested that the child or young athlete should proceed with light arm and shoulder exercises within the areas of pain to try reduce the chance of atrophy of the muscles.

Acromial Fractures

A fracture of the acromion is extremely rare, but when it does occur, it normally is the result of a direct superior blow or overloading the axial. The most common place of fracture is usually lateral to the acromioclavicular joint, resulting in minimal displacement. Children under the age of 13 years are more likely to sustain this kind of fracture due to the strength of the acromioclavicular ligamentous complex, which normally stays intact (Birrer et al., 2002).

Children presenting with an acromion fracture may experience pain on attempted abduction of the arm, a flattened shoulder, localised pain, swelling, and tenderness. Sometimes, this may be mistaken for a subluxation of the acromioclavicular joint. Normally, the fracture site is enormously sore and tender on palpation.

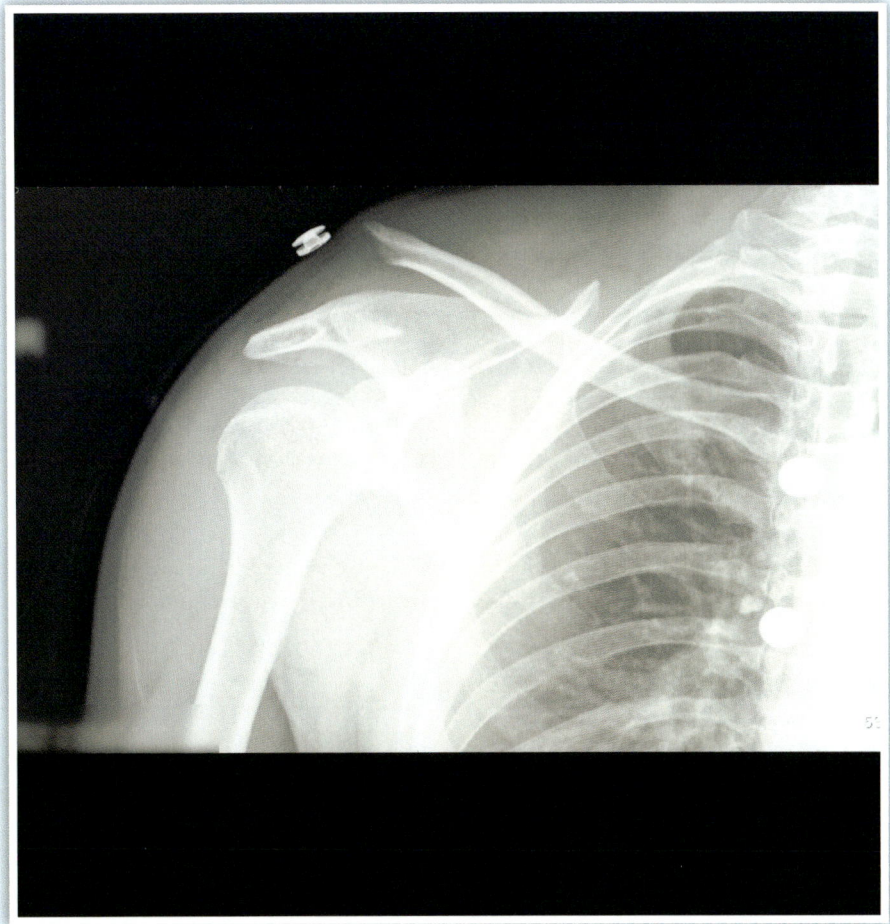

Fig. 10.4 Fracture to acromion end of the clavicle

Diagnostically, an anterior–posterior X-ray (see Fig. 10.4) and/or lateral views of the shoulder are used. In young athletes, it is vital not to confuse acromial epiphysis with a fracture. To ensure that this doesn't happen, a 30 degrees caudal tilt and a supraspinatus outlet view may be used. A non-displaced acromion fracture responds well to conservative treatment and immobilisation in a sling; for displaced fractures, a tension wire band can be used for fixation.

Rehabilitation can begin immediately after an isolated acromion fracture. It can include passive range of motion exercises, progressing to isometric exercises, and after full healing, active resistance exercises can be done (Baker et al., 1995).

Humeral Fracture

Proximal humeral fractures comprise fractures of the greater and lesser tubercles, neck, shaft, metaphysis, and the epiphysis. These fractures are usually caused when the child or the young athlete is in a state of abduction, extension, and external rotation at the time of a fall or physical trauma (Donatelli, 2004). This position is also a common dislocation position in children. Fractures of the humeral head in children tend to be more common than dislocations of the shoulder (Birrer et al., 2002).

Sometimes, just going down on a stretched arm can cause a fracture, where the humeral head shunts against the acromion. The child or young athlete may incur some moderate pain due the fall, with bruising and swelling.

For a fracture at the lesser tubercle, there can be some associated posterior dislocation of the glenohumeral joint; however, this type of fracture is tremendously rare. Treatment for this would involve closed reduction if found within 2–3 weeks and if there is minimal articular involvement (Donatelli, 2004).

Greater tubercle fractures are generally retracted posteriorly and superiorly, making reduction very difficult. They can also be linked to an anterior dislocation in which a closed reduction of the glenohumeral dislocation may reduce the fracture of the greater tuberosity. Also, a displacement superiorly or medially may result in a longitudinal tear of the rotator cuff. For non-displacement fractures, splinting or casting should be avoided so as to allow for active exercises as soon as possible. However, if a displacement is present, surgery and fixation via a screw would limit the likelihood of impingement of the acromion or coracoacromial ligaments (Donatelli, 2004).

Rehabilitation for all proximal humeral fractures will include similar points. Rehabilitation of a non-displacement fracture can begin after 7 days of the injury occurring, starting with heat packs and/ or warm showers and applying light stretches while at home. The next stage should be closely monitored as it includes elbow flexion and extension and supine/pronation movements. As strength is regained, full abduction, external rotation, and internal rotation are added. Exercise should be performed 3–4 times a day with isometric exercises starting at 3 weeks (Baker et al., 1995).

For a scapular fracture, the adolescent or child must have endured significant force as the scapular is well covered by muscles. Because of this, they are usually associated with other injuries such as rib fractures and are caused by high falls or high-energy sports such as motocross racing and snowmobiling.

A fracture can also occur though acromial growth plates, an avulsion of the coracoid tip or superior aspect of the scapular spine. The most common aetiology is subluxation or dislocation of the humeral head. The presentation for a scapular fracture would consist of extreme pain on movement, if movement is possible, with swelling and tenderness.

Injuries of the scapular are classified as follows: Type A involves scapular spine or acromion, Type B includes the body of the scapular, Type C involves the coracoid, and Type D involves injuries to the scapular neck or glenoid fossa.

Diagnosis would include a radiographic evaluation using an anterioposterior view of the shoulder, a tangential oblique view of the scapular, and an axillary view. Tangential and anterioposterior radiographs may be used to identify fractures of the scapular body or neck.

Diagnosis of a scapular fracture may be delayed by surrounding injuries and also during treatment for life-threating injuries. For comfort, the shoulder may be placed in a sling to immobilise the arm; only if there is a significant amount of damage will a surgical intervention be necessary. Management depends on the extent of the injury. For a scapular fracture, a rest period of 3–4 weeks is suggested followed by a gradual return to strength; after 6–12 weeks, the child or young athlete should be aiming to return to sport (Ciullo, 1996).

Nerve Injuries

The suprascapular nerve branches from the upper trunk of the brachial plexus at Erb's point and typically carries the fifth and sixth cervical nerve roots. It supplies the supraspinatus and the infraspinatus and is unique because it travels through the suprascapular notch of the scapular, which is bridged by the transverse scapular ligament (Ciullo, 1996).

The suprascapular nerve can be compressed or injured in many ways such as traction due to weight training, repetitive throwing, or a contusion by continuous use of a heavy backpack or sports such as rugby, football, and gymnastics. Depending on the level of entrapment, both the supraspinatus and infraspinatus may be involved, and there will be loss of strength of the short external rotators in abduction and external rotation (Porterfeild & DeRosa, 2004).

The child or athlete may complain of radiating pain, tingling, or numbness down the neck into the arm, into the medial aspect of the forearm and into the ring finger. Treatment would be rest, anti-inflammatory medication, sports massage, muscle strengthening and stretching exercises (Tyldesley & Grieve, 1989).

The long thoracic nerve originates from C5, C6, and C7 ventral rami at the level of the intervertebral foramen. It is also one of the few nerves that travel on the external surface of the muscle; it lies on the superficial surface of the serratus anterior muscle and is solely responsible for its complete nerve supply (Ciullo, 1996).

The common mechanism of injury is compression by a direct blow of the scapula against the second rib or a distracting stretch. Initially, no pain may be felt but scapular winging may be seen, and also the child or the young athlete may notice that they are throwing unevenly or the action is more one-sided (Porterfeild & DeRosa, 2004). It can also be the result of sustained trauma and as a result of sleeping in a funny position or carrying a heavy backpack (Tyldesley & Grieve, 1989).

Shoulder Instability or Dislocation

The glenohumeral joint is a very unstable joint in children and adolescents, more so than in adults, due to the articulations between the humeral head and the glenoid fossa as the glenoid fossa only accepts 1/3 of the humeral head at any one time. But more importantly, the ligaments at this age also remain quite loose compared with those of an adult.

There are 3 angles in which the adolescent shoulder can dislocate or sublux: anteriorly, posteriorly, and inferiorly. Dislocation is defined by the displacement from the normal position of bones meeting at a joint such that there is a complete loss of contact of the joint surfaces. A subluxation is defined as a partial dislocation of the joint so that the ends of the bones are misaligned but still in contact (Oxford Concise Colour Medical Dictionary, 2010).

Anterior Dislocation

The anterior dislocation occurs most frequently and is commonly caused by a sports-related injury (Bahr, Maehulm, & Bolic, 2004). Forced movements involving lateral rotation and abduction are regularly seen as mechanisms of injury such as falling on to an outstretched arm (Norris, 2004).

Signs and Symptoms

The common signs and symptoms of an anterior dislocation are as follows: The child or young athlete may position or hold the arm into a slight external rotation and abduction. Active or passive range of motion will be extremely restricted with the contours of the shoulder looking altered. Upon closer inspection, it can be seen that the acromion process is more prominent and a hollow is clearly visible as to where the humeral head should be located. The humeral head will also be readily palpated on the anterior aspect of the shoulder. The child will also be in extreme pain and will be reluctant to allow persons to touch or feel the entire shoulder and arm area (Patel, Greydanus, & Baker, 2009).

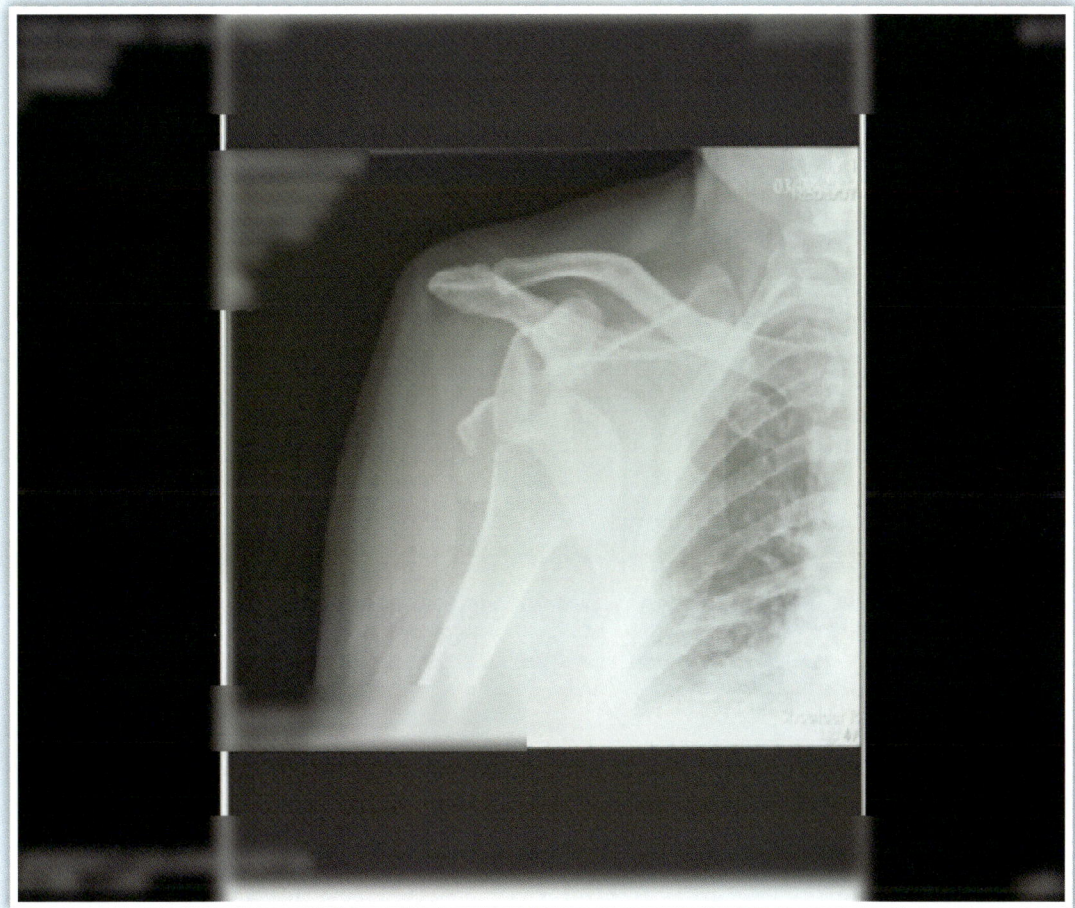

Fig. 10.5 Anterior inferior dislocation of the shoulder joint

Tests

An apprehension test (for shoulder instability) can be performed (see Fig. 10.6) with the child lying in the supine position and the arm passively taken into abduction 90 degrees and lateral rotation 90 degrees. Apprehension can be felt as lateral rotation is added. This could be a sign of apprehension.

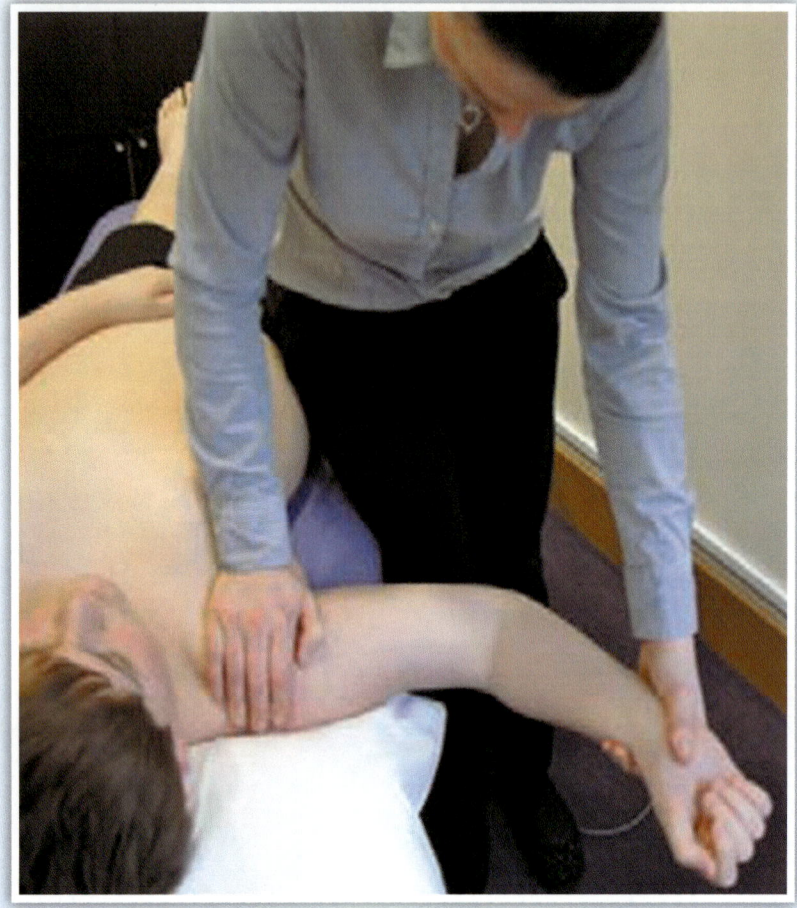

Fig. 10.6 Apprehension test

Diagnosis should be confirmed with an X-ray (see Fig. 10.5); this will be highly uncomfortable as the radiographer must take images from both the frontal and lateral angles. This is to rule out any fractures that may have been sustained from the mechanism of injury as 5–13% of all adolescent anterior dislocation involve a greater tubercle fracture.

Treatment and Management

The treatment, as with most injuries, depends on the severity of the injury and whether this is a first-time dislocation. The earlier the diagnosis, the more quickly treatment can begin. Similarly, the longer the humerus is out of the glenoid fossa, the higher is the risk of neurovascular damage, but there may be less muscle spasms, making it easier to relocate.

If the shoulder dislocation is a recurring injury, the child may be taken for surgery as the ligaments around the shoulder are lax and need to be tightened to reduce the chance of further dislocation (Bahr et al., 2004).

The initial treatment for an anterior dislocation is as follows: once the shoulder has been relocated, it is suggested that the area be rested and iced as to limit the inflammatory process. Also, the arm should be immobilised during the healing process to reduce the chance of re-dislocation for the first 3 weeks. Positions to avoid include extension, abduction, and lateral rotation for 3 weeks post injury.

Posterior Dislocation

The posterior dislocation represents less than 5% of shoulder dislocations. The injury is regularly seen with the mechanism of falling on to an outstretched arm; it has also been seen in children suffering from epileptic seizures. The pain is great, with the child holding or resting their arm in a position of adduction with internal rotation. Any attempt to move the arm will result in muscle spasms, and on occasions, the coracoid process is more visible than normal. Also, the head of humerus is easily palpated towards the posterior aspect of the joint. Posterior dislocation requires referral and reduction under sedation. Once again, the child would need an X-ray for an accurate diagnosis.

.

Acromioclavicular Dislocation

Acromioclavicular dislocations are common especially when falling off a bike or in contact sports such as rugby.

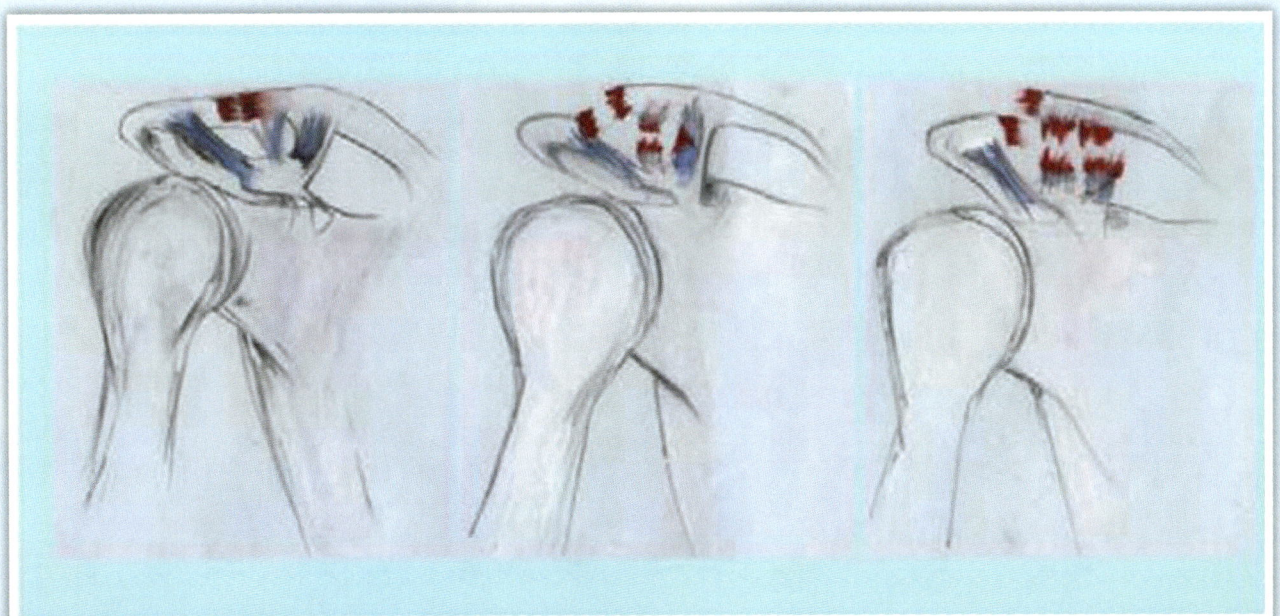

Fig. 10.7 AC joint separation of all the various ligaments

There are several ligaments that surround the joint, and depending on the severity of the dislocation, straining or rupture of these ligaments can occur (see Fig. 10.7). If this happens, there is a possibility of total separation between the acromion and the clavicle.

The mechanism of injury can be a result of direct or indirect force. The direct force involves the child falling on to their side with the arm slightly adducted, which can force the acromion inferiorly and medially.

The indirect force is that of the child falling on to an outstretched arm; this forces the humeral head into the acromion, disrupting the acromioclavicular ligament and stretching the corcacoclavicular.

Signs and Symptoms

The common signs and symptoms are localised pain and swelling over the acromioclavicular joint, shoulder deformities, and perhaps reduction of pain while holding the arm in a supinated position as it may feel directly supported (Bahr et al., 2004). A palpable lump may be felt at the AC joint, and compression of this is normally sore.

Tests

The joint is very sore on direct palpation (see Fig. 10.8) and normally is mobile. Sometimes a step may be felt. An X-ray will confirm diagnosis.

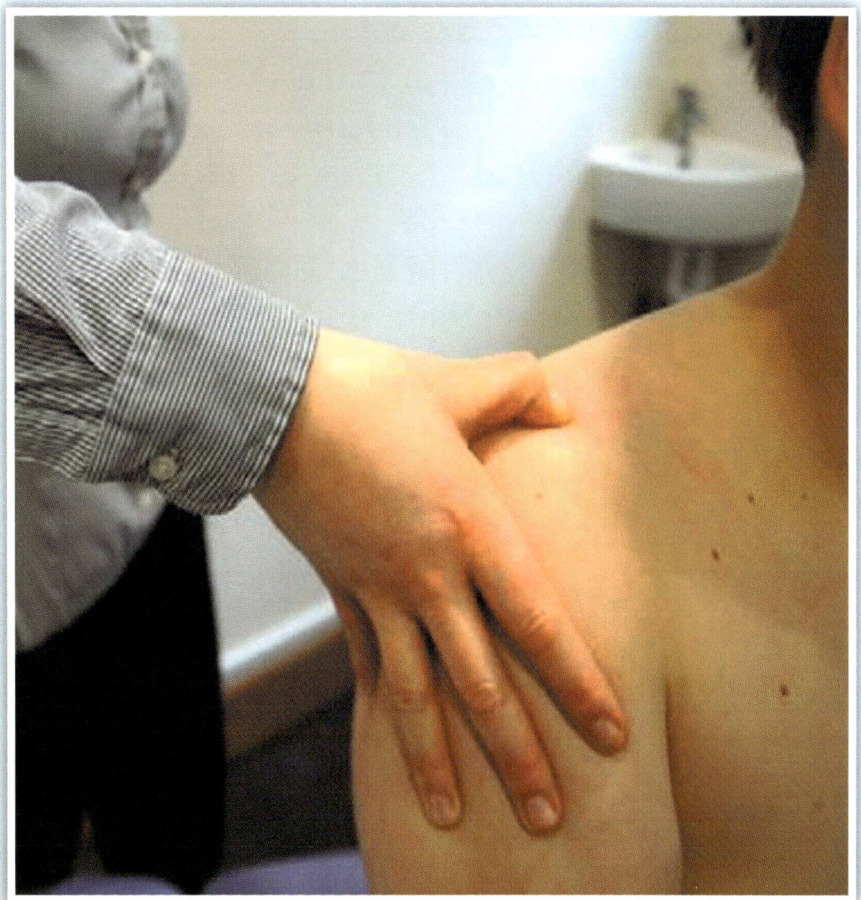

Fig. 10.8 Palpation of the acromioclavicular joint

Treatment and Management

Initial treatment should be ice, rest, and a sling to limit swelling; taking the weight off the arm; and immobilising the shoulder. Once the pain has reduced, it is important to try and return the child to as much active and passive range of motion as possible. After 2–4 weeks, the child should be returning to gentle activity.

Impingement

In children, nerve impingement in the shoulder is relatively rare. However; if it does occur, it usually involves the tendons of the rotator cuff muscles. These tendons include the supraspinatus tendon, the infraspinatus tendon, and the biceps tendon. (See Fig. 10.9.)

The supraspinatus tendon travels through the subacrominal space, which lies beneath the coracoacromial arch; this arch is covered by the deltoid and inferiorly is a continuation of the supraspinatus fascia. This arch prevents the upward dislocation of the humeral head.

During elevation and internal rotation, the supraspinatus that runs on the outside of the greater tuberosity may press against the anterior ridge of the underside of the acromion, causing the impingement pain (Bahr et al., 2004). This can also occur during flexion; however, the impingement is of the long head of the biceps (Norris, 2004). The impingement of the supraspinatus and the long head of the biceps compromises the integrity of the rotator cuff muscles.

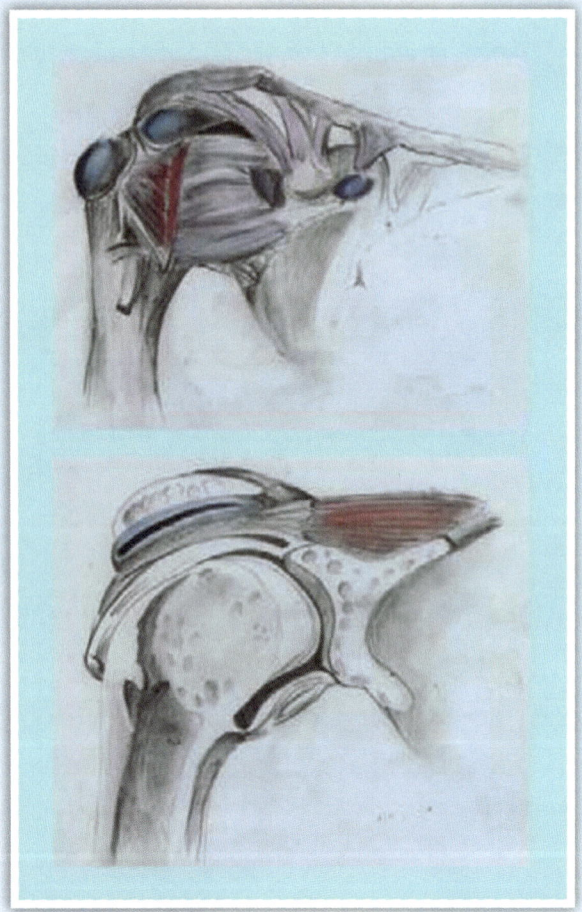

Fig. 10.9 Biceps tendon and supraspinatus tendon,
both commonly immplicated in impingement in children

Without the depressing action of the rotator cuff muscles on the humeral head, the deltoids pull the head of the humerus superiorly, progressively worsening the signs and symptoms of the impingement. With the shoulder impingement so rare in children and young athletes, if it is seen to be an impingement issue, they are usually diagnosed with multidirectional instability with secondary impingement. This can be common in adolescent swimmers and tennis players.

Signs and symptoms

The symptoms are usually related to a micro or repetitive trauma, with the pain starting as non-specific; as the impingement worsens, it becomes more localised to the anterolateral surface of the acromion. Impingement reduces shoulder function; without proper treatment and diagnosis, this can develop into tendinitis or tendinosis. Pain can be felt down the arm in acute stages, and it can even be sore at night. Elevation movements can be sore.

Tests

Tests used to help identify shoulder impingement include the Empty Can test, Hawkins sign, and active and passive ranges of motion with overpressure.

The Empty Can test is performed with the child lifting their arm into shoulder flexion and at 90 degrees, turning the arm medially so that their thumb is pointing downwards.

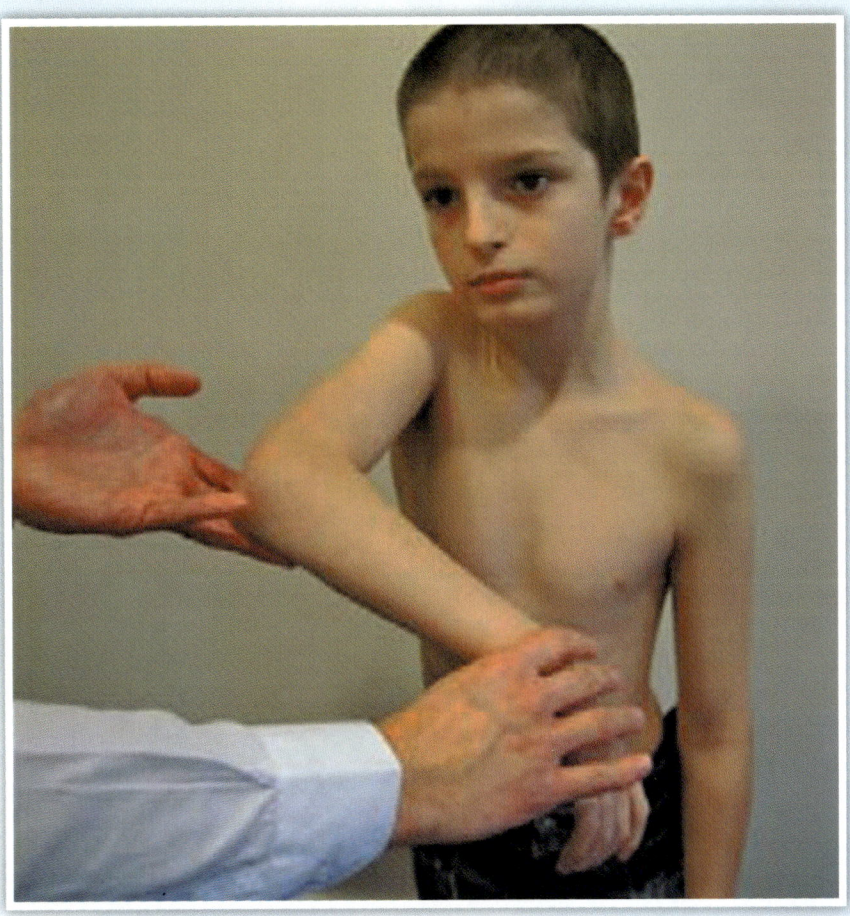

Fig. 10.10 Hawkins Kennedy test

Hawkins Kennedy test (see Fig. 10.10) is performed with the child in sitting position and passively taking their arm into horizontal flexion to 90 degrees, elbow flexion 90 degrees, and passively taking their forearm medially. This simply forces the greater tuberosity against the underside of the acromion.

Treatment

Conservative treatment is usually the first stage with children or young athletes. They are sometimes given anti-inflammatory drugs to help reduce the swelling and aggravation of the tissues. Strengthening programmes are also given to avoid muscle atrophy and to ensure that correct and full movements are still being performed. Management should be geared at prevention and modification of the cause (which sometimes can be wrong technique). Rotation exercises in varying degrees of abduction can help.

There are surgical treatments if symptoms persist; however, these are very rarely carried out on children as their bodies are still immature and surgery may cause more harm than good (Bahr et al., 2004).

Conclusion

The immaturity of a child's body, especially within the shoulder, accounts for the type and amount of injuries children sustain. However, as the shoulder is a relatively weak structure, throughout life, there will always be the injuries and pathologies associated with it.

It is, therefore, important that if a child should receive such an injury the right precautions and treatments are given to prevent lifelong effects.

Key Points

- The adolescent shoulder is more unstable than the adult shoulder.

- The clavicle is the most commonly fractured bone in children.

- Fractures of the humeral head are more common than dislocations.

References

Armstrong, N., Kirby, B., & Welsman, J. (1997). *Children and exercise XIX promoting health and well-being* (2nd ed.). E & FN Spon Pulishing house.

Bahr, R., Maehulm, S., & Bolic, T. (2004). *Clinical guide to sports injuries* (3rd ed.). Hammond.

Baker, C., Flandry, F., & Henderson, J. (1995). *Sports medicine book,* (2nd ed.). Baultimore: Williams and Wilkins.

Birrer, R., Greisemer, B., & Cataletto, M. (2002). *Pediatric sports medicine for primary care* (2nd ed.). Philadelphia, PA: Lippincott, Williams and Wilkins.

Calder, J., Solan, M., Gidwani, Y (2002). *Management of paediatric clavicle fractures – is follow up necessary.* Annuals Royal College Surgeons in England, 84: 5, 331–333

Ciullo, J. (1996). *Shoulder injuries in sport,* Evaluation, Treatment, and Rehabilitation. Human Kinetics, (2nd ed.). Human Kinetics, p206-218.

Donatelli, R. (2004). *Physical therapy of the shoulder* (4th ed.). New Harbinger Publications, St Louis.

Drake, R., Vogl, A., & Mitchell, A. (2005). *Greys anatomy for student* (2nd ed.).

Gallaspy, J., & May, J. (1996). *Signs and symptoms of athletic injuries* (2nd ed.). Mosby Publishing.

Huelke, D. (1998). An overview of the anatomical considerations of infants and children in the adult world of automobile safety design. *42nd Annual Proceedings Association for the Advancement of Automotive Medicine* (Vol. 97).

Marcovitch, H. (2010). *Blacks medical dictionary,* 42nd ed.

Moore, K., Dalley, A., & Agur, A. (2010). *Clinically oriented anatomy* (6th ed.). Baltimore: Lippincott Williams & Wilkins..

Norris, C. (2004). *Sports injuries diagnosis and management* (3rd ed.). London: Butterworth-Heinemann.

Patel, D., Greydanus, D., & Baker, R. (2009). *Pediatric practice sports medicine* (2nd ed.). New York, NY: McGraw-Hill Medical Books.

Porterfeild, J., & DeRosa, C. (2004). *Mechanical shoulder disorders* (3rd ed.). Willkins and Williams.

Saladin, K. (2012). *Anatomy and physiology the unity of form and function*(4th ed.). McGraw Hill Books.

Tyldesley, B., & Grieve, J. (1989). *Muscle, nerves and movement, Kinesiology in daily living* (3rd ed.). Oxford, UK: Blackwell Scientific.

CHAPTER 11

Elbow Pathologies in Children and Adolescent Sport

Solomon Abrahams and Georgia Parry

The child elbow is a typical synovial hinge joint, which allows uni-axial movements and is supported by collateral ligaments. The three articulating bones that make up the elbow joint are the distal end of humerus, the proximal ends of the ulna, and the biconcave superior aspect of the radius (Magee, 2002).

The ulna, radius, and humerus are all covered in hyaline cartilage, which helps to protect the bones from friction within the joint and, in turn, delays the onset of arthritis (Saraf and Khare, 2011).

There are three joints at the elbow: the ulnohumeral joint between the humerus and the ulna, radiohumeral joint between the humerus and the radius, and the radioulnar joint between the radius and the ulna – which is classified as a synovial pivot joint.

The fibrous capsule surrounding the joint attaches superiorly above the olecranon, radial, and coronoid fossae and inferiorly blends with the annular ligament, to the neck of the radius and margins of the coronoid process. Medially and laterally, the bone is thickest and reinforced by the radial and ulna ligaments. The synovial membrane lines the deep surface of the capsule (Hoppenfeld, 2009).

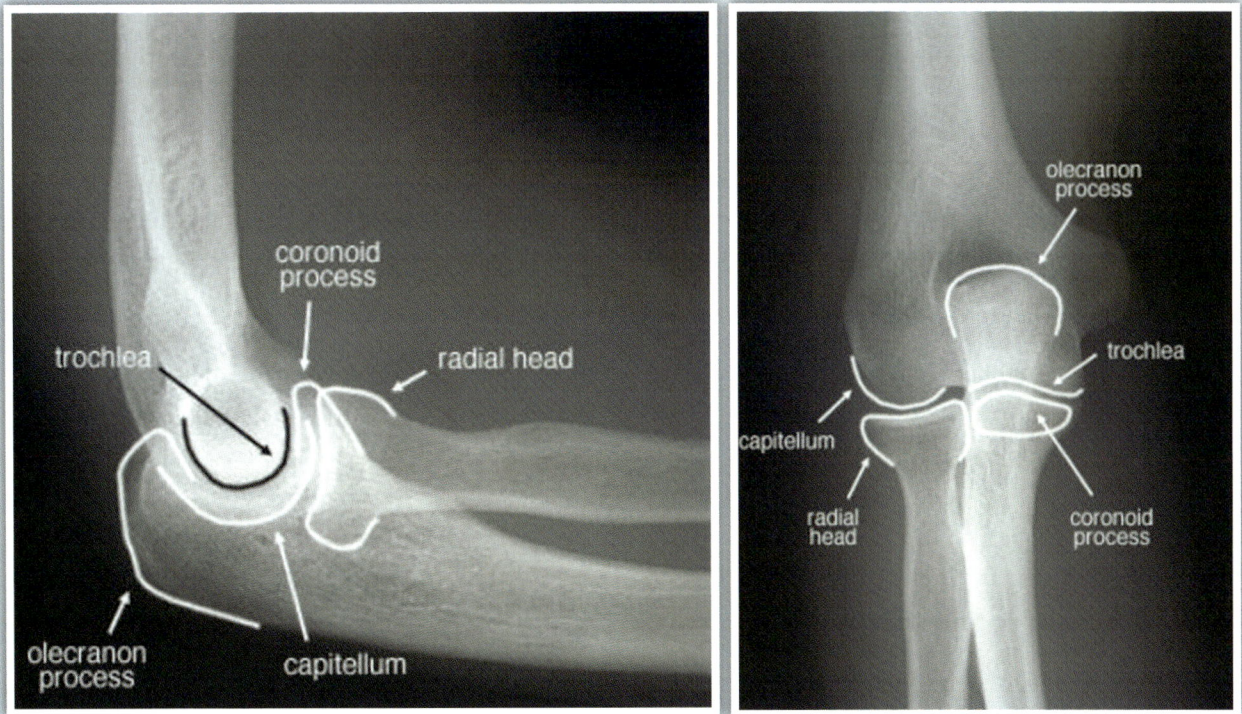

Fig. 11.1 Normal X-rays of the elbow

The capsule and joint are stabilised by ulnar and radial collateral ligaments. The lateral (radial) collateral ligament is the smaller of the two, and it goes from the lateral epicondyle to the annular ligament. Its function is to limit adduction and extension of the forearm. The ulnar collateral ligament is the stronger of the two and is typically made up of three bands: The anterior band attaches from the medial epicondyle to the medial coronoid process. The posterior band goes from the medial epicondyle to the medial olecranon. The transverse (oblique) band unites the distal attachments of the anterior and posterior bands. The annular ligament is also within the elbow joint; it circles the head of radius, and its function is to maintain contact between the radius and the humerus (Magee, 2002).

The joint is very stable due to three main factors: good congruency between the joint surfaces, the collateral ligaments, and the muscles surrounding the joint at certain angles.

The two movements allowed at the elbow joint are flexion and extension. Typically, 145 degrees of flexion is possible with muscular end feel being the main restrictor, and 0 degrees of extension is possible with a bony end feel. This may be increased in hypermobile individuals (Williams & Warwick, 1980).

The radioulnar joint allows pronation and supination, with normal ranges of movement being 70 degrees of pronation and 85 degrees of supination.

Saraf and Khare (2011) suggest that other than ligaments and the joint type (hinge or pivot) restricting the ranges of movement, the muscles across the elbow joint also control and restrict the movements allowed. These include biceps brachii, triceps brachii, brachialis, brachioradialis, pronator teres, and extensor carpi radialis brevis.

Ossification of the growth centres of the elbow occurs at the following times:

- Capitulum: 11 months
- Medial epicondyle: 4–6 years
- Radial head: 5–6 years
- Olecranon: 6–8 years
- Trochlea: 9–10 years
- Lateral epicondyle: 10–12 years (Moore & Dalley, 2001).

Common Fractures

Medial Epicondyle

The medial epicondyle is the bony bump on the inner side of the elbow. In children and adolescents who are actively growing, there is a growth plate at the medial epicondyle. The growth plate is made up of cartilage cells, which are softer and more vulnerable to injury than mature bone.

The forearm muscles that bend the wrist are anchored to the elbow at the medial epicondyle growth plate. A single, forceful contraction of these muscles can cause them to pull the growth plate away from the bone. This is called an avulsion fracture.

Medial epicondyle avulsion fractures most commonly affect adolescent baseball pitchers during periods of rapid growth, typically between 9 and 14 years of age. This is when the growth plate cartilage is most vulnerable to injury. It is the rapid contraction of the muscles that cause the avulsion fracture. Less commonly, it can affect athletes in other throwing or overhead sports such as football, water polo, and volleyball. The mechanism of injury can also come from falling on an outstretched arm.

Signs and Symptoms

Farsetti, Potenza, Caterini, & Ippolito (2004) suggest that the symptoms present themselves as a sudden onset of severe pain on the inside of the elbow following a forceful pitch or throw, or falling on an outstretched arm. Some athletes feel or hear a 'pop' at the time of the injury. There is usually swelling and some limitation of elbow motion. Occasionally, the ulnar nerve, which sits next to the medial epicondyle, becomes irritated after an avulsion fracture, causing numbness and tingling in the forearm and fourth and fifth fingers. There will be tenderness on the medial aspect of the elbow, and valgus instability.

Tests

A diagnosis can be confirmed by examining the child's elbow and arm for tenderness at the medial epicondyle. An X-ray will show the avulsion fracture as a separation of the growth plate from the humerus.

Management

Most avulsion fractures can be successfully treated with cast immobilisation for 4–6 weeks. During this time, ice can be placed on the elbow for 20–30 minutes every 3–4 hours while there is pain or swelling.

After 4–6 weeks of immobilisation, if X-rays show that the fracture is healing, a course of physiotherapy is prescribed. While most avulsion fractures heal well with this treatment, those with a very wide separation on X-rays may require surgery. Rosemont (2004–2010) found that the recovery time after surgery is similar to that for non-surgical treatment. The surgical treatment is an open reduction in internal fixation, where the fracture is screwed together again.

Complications with the treatment can be injury to the ulnar nerve, limited range of movement in the elbow, and a non-reunion of the bone fragments.

Treatment to an avulsion fracture includes regaining the full pain-free motion of the elbow and adequate strength in the arm, upper back, and core muscles. A gradual return to throwing programme can then begin. It typically takes 4–6 weeks in this programme before the athlete can pitch in games (Farsetti et al., 2004).

Lateral Epicondyle

Saraf and Khare (2011) suggest that lateral epicondyle fractures are rare. They usually occur between ages 6 and 7 years. They are believed to occur during sudden traction on the common extensor origin by the extensor musculature.

The cause of a lateral epicondyle fracture is related to the age of ossification in the bones, which is usually between ages 10 and 11 years.

Treatment depends on whether the bone has been displaced completely or minimally. In completely displaced fractures, rigid internal fixations are placed, which still allow movement.

Supracondylar

In children, supracondylar fractures typically remain extra-articular and involve thin bone fragments between coronoid fossa and olecranon fossa of distal humerus; the fracture line is typically from the anterior distal point to the posterior proximal site. (See Fig. 11.2.)

Fractures most often occur between the ages 6 and 7 years.

There are two types of fractures of the suprcondylar: extension (95%) and flexion.

Tests

Palpate the distal radius for a fracture; it occurs only in 5–6% of cases. Distinguishing between an extension or flexion injury is vital, as it will change your treatment method.

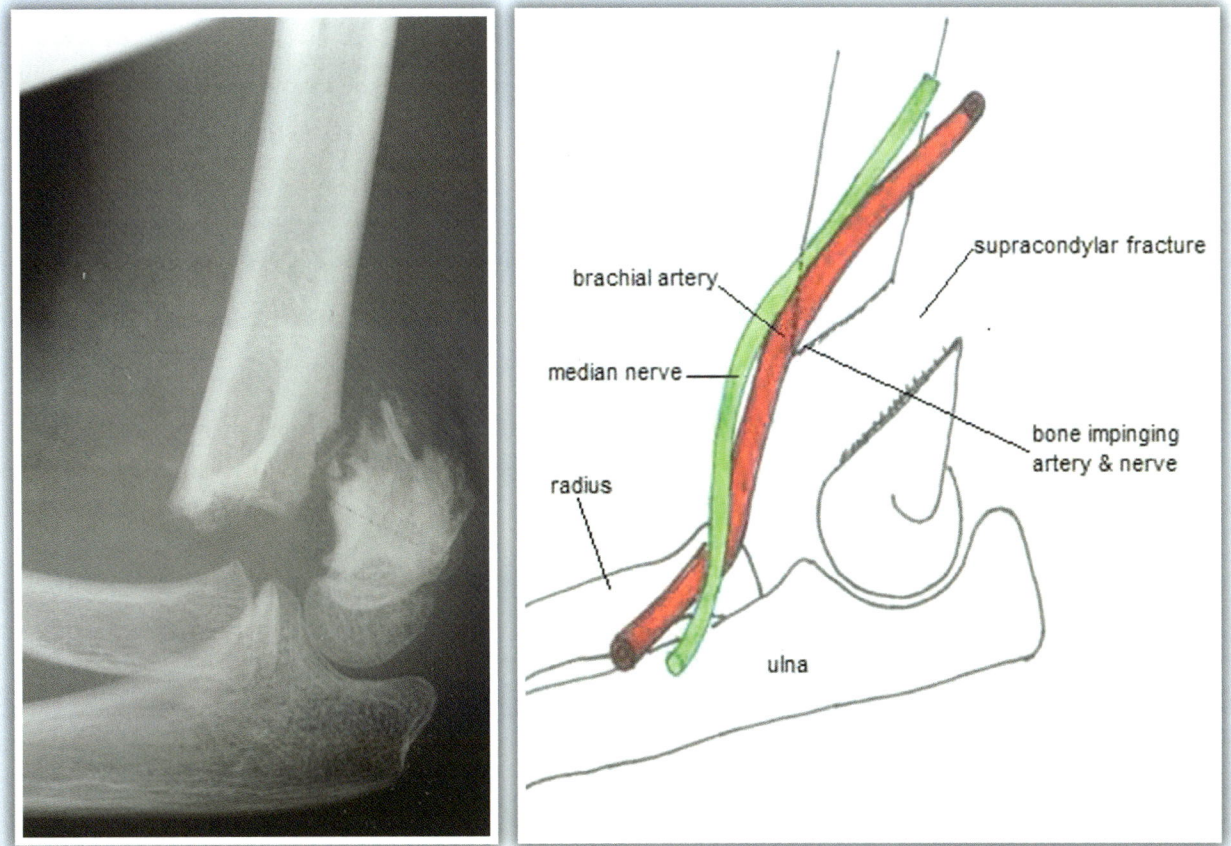

Fig. 11.2 X-ray to show severe supracondylar fracture and drawing to represent potential damage to nearby blood vessels

Treatment

For the treatment of an extension-type injury, the supracondylar fracture is splinted in 20 degrees of flexion to make the joint stable during recovery.

Mehlman et al. (2001) evaluated complications from early surgical treatment (<8 hours) and delayed treatment (>8 hours) of displaced supracondylar fractures; 52 patients had early surgical treatment, and 146 patients had delayed surgical treatment of a displaced supracondylar humeral fracture. Perioperative complication rates of the 2 groups were compared with the use of bivariate and multivariate statistical methods; no significant difference between the 2 groups were found. No compartment syndromes occurred in either group, and there were no significant differences with regard to preoperative complication rates between early and delayed treatment of displaced supracondylar fractions. Therefore, non-surgical methods should be attempted first as it is less invasive and the recovery times are the same.

Complications of this fracture include the disruption of nearby blood vessels and nerves. Any fracture of this region should have vascular tests performed (such as radial pulse) to ensure there has been no compression of the brachial artery, and if so, is treated as an emergency (see Fig. 11.2).

Radial Head Fractures

In children, the fractures of the proximal end of the radius typically involve the physis or radial neck. Most cases are Salter-Harris type II fractures with radial head involvement, rare. The most common age to get a radial head fracture is between ages 9 and 10 years which counts for 1–5% of all paediatric elbow fractures, and it is as common in boys as girls.

The mechanism of injury is most often associated with valgus loading. It is also linked to the age of ossification of the radial head, which appears between 3 and 5 years of age, yet the radial head doesn't fuse with the radial shaft until ages 16–18 years. (Magee, 2002).

Signs and Symptoms

A child with a radial head fracture will present symptoms of pain within the elbow and a very restricted range of movement, if any.

Test

To test for a diagnosis, start with observation. There will often be lateral swelling and pain with motion, especially with supination and pronation. Pain may be referred to the wrist. An X-ray will confirm a fracture, although non-displaced fractures may be difficult to visualise. However, an effusion of the fat pads will confirm the fracture, as these only become absent when a fracture is present (Hoppenfeld, 2009).

Treatment

To treat a radial head fracture non-operatively, reduce movement by immobilisation. However, do begin movement through the joint after 3–7 days, depending on severity, to avoid stiffness. Rosemont (2008) claims that for operative treatments, percutaneous reduction or open reduction operations can be carried out. Percutaneous reduction is better in children as it doesn't limit range of movement like the open reduction does.

There are complications linked to radial head fractures and the treatments for them. There is decreased range of motion, especially in pronation and supination. Radial head overgrowth occurs in 20–40% of fractures; however, it doesn't affect the function. Osteonecrosis and synostosis can also occur, synostosis being the most severe complication.

Lateral Condyle Fractures

Lateral condyle fractures most often occur in children between ages 6 and 10 years and account for 20% of elbow injuries in paediatrics. The mechanism of injury is usually from falling on an outstretched arm with the forearm in abduction and the elbow in extension. A fracture to the lateral condyle causes the humerus to become unstable, and it tends to become displaced, even once immobilised due to the pull from the forearm extensors. Lateral condyle fractures are prone to non-union as the fracture is intra-articular and is surrounded by synovial fluid (Kobayashi, Oka, Ikeda, & Munesada, et al., 2002).

Signs and Symptoms

The child will often present pain only on the lateral side of the elbow.

Ossification of the lateral condyle begins at the age of 18 months and continues up until 2 years; it doesn't then ossify until age 13 years, where it then fuses with the capitulum at age 16.

Test

X-rays can confirm the fracture.

There is a grading system for lateral condyle fractures to distinguish the severity of the fracture, namely the Salter-Harris classification system.

Milch type I fracture: This is a Salter-Harris IV fracture in which the fracture traverses the ossification centre of the capitellum so that the lateral wall of the trochlea remains attached to the main portion of the humerus; because the fracture line lies lateral to capitello-trochlear groove, the elbow is stable and the relationship between the forearm and the humerus remains intact. This is a less common variant than a type II fracture.

Milch type II fracture: This is the most common variant. It involves a fracture line beginning at the lateral side of distal metaphysis of humerus and extends obliquely downwards and medial to the capitellum (or in some cases through the trochlear groove), traverses the physis, and enters the joint in the lateral portion of trochlea. The fracture is described as being an SH type II physeal fracture; the distal fragment contains epiphysis of capitellum, lateral trochlea, and epicondyle, as well as part of metaphysis with radial collateral ligaments and forearm extensor tendons.

This fracture passes across the trochlear groove which, therefore, allows subluxation of the ulna (lateral wall of the trochlea remains attached to fractured condylar fragment). With non-displaced fractures, determine whether there is lateral elbow tenderness and whether lateral elbow tenderness increases with elbow flexion (Kobayashi et al., 2002).

Medial type II variant: Some type II fractures will not exit through the trochlea but will, instead, exit at the medial aspect of the physis; this is a Salter Harris type II fracture. It may be difficult to distinguish between a classic lateral type II fracture and a medial type II variant when trochlea and medial epicondyle remain un-ossified; while examining, look for medial tenderness and swelling (Birrer, Griesemer, & Cataletto, 2002; Netter & Craig, 2002).

When making a diagnosis, the fracture line may not appear for 7–10 days following the injury, and a correct diagnosis may be difficult as the capitellum will not ossify until 9–10 years of age.

An X-ray will show a fracture; if it is not visible on the first attempt, retry after 1 week (Birrer et al., 2002; Kobayashi et al., 2002; Netter & Craig, 2002).

Treatment

For non-opeative treatment of the lateral condyle, arthography can be used for non-displaced fractures. For completely displaced fractures, a cast is used to immobilise the joint, with the elbow left at 90 degrees of flexion and the forearm in poronation to minimise the pull from the extensor muscles. The cast is removed every 2 weeks to check for recovery and range of movement.

For operative treatment, closed reduction percutaneous pinning is often used and is very successful (Rosemont, 2002).

Medial Condyle Fracture

Medial condyle fractures are less common than lateral fractures. During adolescence, the distal humerus is the second-most common site of physeal injury (second only to the distal radius). It is most commonly injured between ages 8 and 12 years. The medial condyle fracture is most commonly caused by a fall on to an outstretched upper extremity or a fall on to a flexed elbow (Magee, 2002).

Signs and Symptoms

The symptoms present with this fracture would be pain and swelling on the medial side of the elbow. Unlike medial epicondyle fractures, a dislocation is rare with a condyle fracture.

Test

X-ray first.

When testing for a medial condylar fracture, test the radial, median, and ulna nerves. Palpation is also important; also test the child's range of motion.

Management

Treatment for a medial condyle fracture would include immobilization of the elbow joint, using a cast or sling for 4–6 weeks. It is important that the cast is removed every 2 weeks for the joint to be mobilised. Surgical treatment can be carried out through pinning the bone fragments together again (Magee, 2002).

The complication of experiencing a medial condyle fracture was reported by Farsetti et al. (2004), who performed a retrospective study of 21 medial condylar fractures. The study revealed that the complication rate for these rare fractures was 33%; most of the minimally displaced fractures healed uneventfully with immobilization.

The trochlea does not ossify until age 8 years; therefore fractures of the medial condyle may be mistaken for fractures of the medial epicondyle. This is especially true if there is significant pain, swelling, and instability (but no dislocation); a fracture into the metaphyseal bone helps with the diagnosis. If the diagnosis is in question, an MRI will confirm a diagnosis.

Elbow Dislocation

Elbow dislocation is rare, but it happens to be the second-most common dislocation in teens in the upper limb apart from the shoulder (Birrer et al., 2002). It is caused by a fall on an extended hand or with the elbow in flexion.

Most dislocations are anterior (see Fig. 11.3), and therefore, care must be taken to ensure that the brachial artery is not compressed. A check of the radial pulse should be done.

Signs and Symptoms

Pain is normally immediate, and the elbow cannot be moved actively or passively. Reduction should be avoided in the event for fracture dislocation.

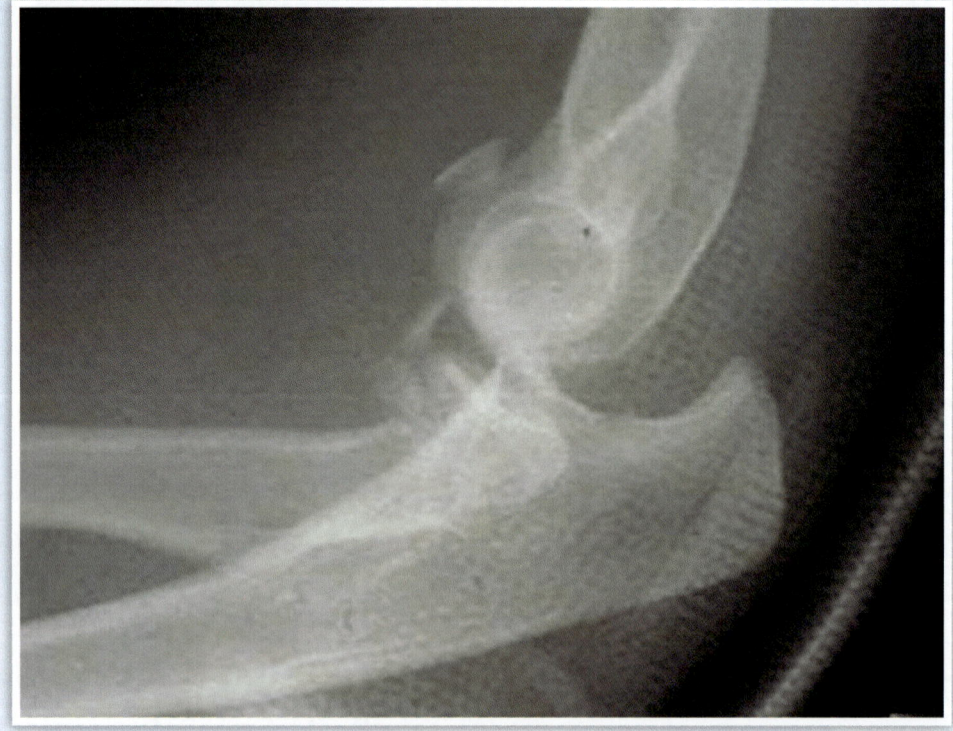

Fig. 11.3 X-ray revealing anterior dislocation of the elbow

Test

X-ray, especially if they are unable to flex or extend. Treat as an emergency if the brachial artery is compressed.

Management

Once the artery is checked to ensure non-compression and once X-rays confirm there is no fracture, then reduction can occur. The patient is placed in the prone position with the elbow off the end of the bed in flexion, and a traction is added to the hand to pull the radius and ulnar away from the elbow – which should slip the joint back (Birrer et al., 2002).

Immobilisation is then insitu for 3 weeks, and thereafter, a repeat X-ray is recommended to ensure that there is no avascular necrosis.

Avascular Necrosis (Panner's Disease)

Numerous studies carried out on Panner's disease have found that this affects mainly boys in their childhood between 5 and 10 years of age. For unknown reasons, normal growth in the outer edge of the elbow is disrupted, which causes a small area of bone to flatten.

The child will feel pain within their elbow during activity, and the pain will ease during rest. There is usually an account of trauma to the elbow to explain the injury. After injury, the bone calcifies for the next 2 years, reducing the symptoms of pain; however, the child's arm may never fully straighten again. It is especially common in baseball players and gymnasts.

Panner's disease affects the developing bone within the capitellum of the humerus, where the growth plate within the capitellum is disrupted. It is not yet known why these growth plates are disrupted. It is thought that it may be hereditary or may be caused by repetitive movements through the capitellum. Another thought is that it is the poor blood supply during chilhood that causes the Panner's disease.

Once there is the onset of Panner's disease, the cells within the growth plate of the capitellum begin to die. This death of the cells is caused by avascular necrosis (loss of blood supply). When necrosis begins, the bone of the capitellum begins to flatten out due to newly forming bone being absorbed by the body. Gradually, over a period of 1 or 2 years, new blood vessels enter the area and new cells begin to form within the growth plate. Eventually, the original shape of the capitellum is created, but limited range of motion is often a long-lasting symptom of Panner's disease (Birrer et al., 2002; Hoppenfeld, 2009; Magee, 2002; Netter & Craig, 2002).

Signs and Symptoms

On palpation, the injured elbow will be tender, and the movement possible on the injured side will be significantly reduced.

Test

Verbal questioning will be taken of the child's account of the initial injury, the symptoms, and their age and activity level. An X-ray is needed to confirm the diagnosis.

Treatment

Non-surgical treatments available for Panner's disease can be as simple as rest. This allows the inflammation and tenderness of the joint to calm down, and the joint may become pain-free. Anti-inflammatory pills may be prescribed. In severe cases, a cast may be recommended for 3–4 weeks to prevent movement. Surgery is not generally an option as the symptoms do go gradually (Netter & Craig, 2002).

Golfer's Elbow (Medial Epicondylitis)

Golfer's elbow is most common in males aged between 10 and 14 years. It is an overuse tendinopathy linked with racquet sports (Plancher Halbrecht, Lourie, 1996).

It only accounts for 10–20% of all epicondylitis diagnoses. The medial epicondyle is the common origin of the forearm flexors, and it is the region between the pronator teres and flexor carpi radialis that is most commonly injured (Plancher et al., 1996).

Signs and Symptoms

The symptom present with golfer's elbow is an aching pain over the medial elbow (see Fig. 11.4), and in severe cases, there is pain whilst gripping, which was supported by Vicenzino, Brooksbank, Minto, Offord, and Paungmali. (2003). The child may experience pain during throwing, especially in the acceleration phase. The ulnar nerve can cause some discomfort in up to 20% of individuals with golfer's elbow.

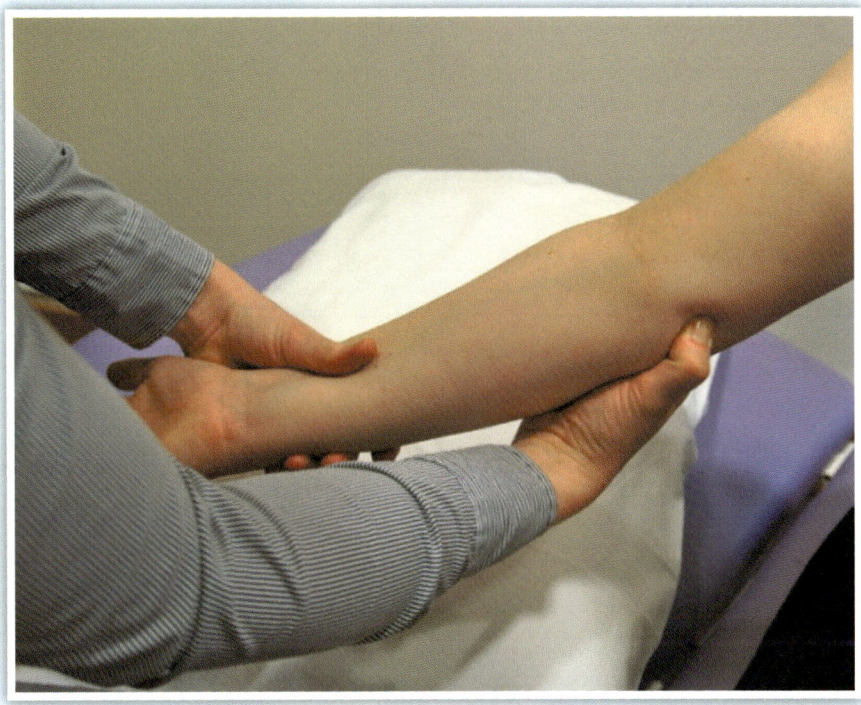

Fig. 11.4 Palpation of the medial epicondyle

Test

When examining the individual for golfer's elbow, palpation is essential. The child may feel discomfort during resisted wrist flexion, and the medial epicondyle will be tender when palpated. Pronation when resisted is also often painful. In more chronic cases, there may be pain with resisted flexion of the elbow. The Tinel's sign should be checked to rule out ulnar neuropathy.

Treatment

Localised treatment helps, such as ice, compression, and rest. Addressing the cause is important (Birrer et al., 2002).

The causes of golfer's elbow is hugely down to poor technique, where tennis players and other racquet sports players use poor serving technique and forehand strokes. Individuals may cause risk to themselves if they are not physically fit for the activity – if they have poor endurance, poor flexibility, or weakness. The size of the racquet handle and tightness of the strings on the racquet head can all have a bearing.

The equipment is also an important factor. If it is not the correct size or weight or if generally the equipment is not used for the individual, this can predispose them to sustaining golfer's elbow (Plancher et al., 1996).

Tennis Elbow (Lateral Epicondylitis)

Tennis elbow is a tendinopathy to the lateral epicondyle of the elbow. It is sustained from excessive wrist extension. It most commonly affects the extensor carpi radialis brevis (Hoppenfeld, 2009). It is less likely to be seen in children and more so in an older adolescent.

The individual will experience one of two types of onset: A sudden onset where the individual can recall a single instance where the wrist went in to full extension and the wrist became strained. Or, a late onset, where pain is not usually felt for 24–72 hours after severe wrist extension.

Signs and Symptoms

The individual may complain of pain around 1–2 cm distal of the lateral epicondyle (see Fig. 11.5). Some everyday tasks will become difficult, like opening a door handle. When the elbow is in extension along with the wrist and resistance is given, the individual may complain of pain on the lateral element of the elbow. The pain can also continue if the individual extends their fingers. On palpation, the lateral elbow will be tender.

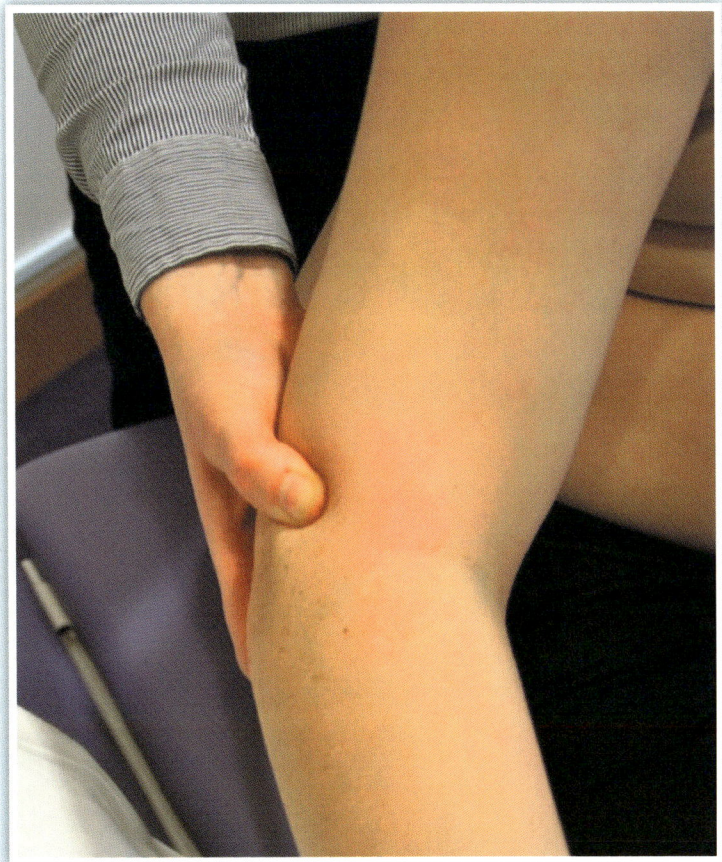

Fig. 11.5 Palpation of the lateral epicondyle

Test

When diagnosing tennis elbow, and after palpation, resisted wrist extension and resisted middle finger extension should be carried out. Both may be painful, but if limited range of motion is possible, then tennis elbow is likely. A diagnostic ultrasound will confirm a diagnosis (Magee, 2002).

Treatment

There are a number of possible causes of tennis elbow such as overuse or repetitive strain caused by extension of the wrist against resistance; poor technique of backhand in racquet sports; the wrong grip size, handle size, or racquet size; and if the individual uses wet or heavy balls.

Treatments for tennis elbow are yet to be conclusively effective; however, a combination of techniques can dramatically decrease the symptoms. Ice and rest are recommended to control inflammation, reduce plain, and minimise further damage. In severe cases, a brace or a support can be worn to help immobilise the joint. Some doctors may prescribe anti-inflammatory drugs. Ultrasound by a physiotherapist and soft-tissue massage can also help to promote the healing process and reduce pain and swelling (Birrer et al., 2002).

Addressing the cause is essential to prevent recurrence of pathology.

Key Points

- There are 6 different growth plates around the elbow.

- Closure of growth plates range from 11 months to 12 years.

- Supracondylar fractures can compress on brachial artery in children.

- Avascular necrosis (Panner's) affects the capitullem bone.

References

Birrer, R., Griesemer, B., & Cataletto, M. (2002). *Pediatric sports medicine in primary care* (2nd ed.). Philadelphia, PA: Lippincott, Williams and Wilkins,.

Biyani, A., Gupta, S. P,. & Sharma, J. C. (1989). Ipsilateral supracondylar fracture of humerus and forearm bones in children. Journal of Bone & Joint Surgery; 83: 27, 253–258.

Chapman, V. M., Grottkau, B. E., Albright, M. (1995). Multidetector computed tomography of pediatric lateral condylar fractures. *Journal of Computer Assisted Tomography*, 12, 1, 45-49.

Eilert, R. E., & Erickson, M. A. (2006). Fractures of the proximal radius and ulna (6th ed.). In J. H. Beaty & J. R. Kasser (Eds.). *Rockwood and Wilkins.*

Farsetti, P., Potenza, V., Caterini, R., & Ippolito, E. (2004). Long-term results of treatment of fractures of the medial humeral epicondyle in children. Journal of Bone & Joint Surgery, 53;83-A:1299-305.

Fischgrund, J. S. (2008). *Orthopaedic knowledge update 9.* Rosemont, IL: American Academy of Orthopaedic Surgeons.

Hoppenfeld, S. P. (2009). *Surgical exposures in orthopaedics: The anatomic approach.* Philadelphia, PA: Lippincott Williams & Wilkins.

James, P., & Heinrich, S. D. (1991). Orthopidics. Supracondylar elbow fractures with impaction of the medial condyle in children (3rd ed.). Fractures in Children, Rockwood and Wilkins

Kobayashi, Y., Oka, Y., Ikeda, M., & Munesada, S. (2002). Avulsion fracture of the medial and lateral epicondyles of the humerus. *Journal of Shoulder and Elbow Surgery.* 5, 67, 200-205.

Kraushaar, B. S., & Nirsch, 1 R. P. (1999). Tendinosis of the elbow (tennis elbow). Clinical features and findings of histological, immunohistochemical, and electron microscopy studies. *Journal of Bone and Joint Surgery-American* , 75A(11): 1585–1592.

Ljung, B. O., Forsgren, S., & Fridén, J. (1999). Substance P and calcitonin gene-related peptide expression at the extensor carpi radialis brevis muscle origin: implications for the etiology of tennis elbow. *Journal of Orthopaedic Research.* 28(3): 186-189.

Magee, D. (2002). *Orthopedic physical assessment* (4th ed.). Philadelphia, PA: Saunders.

Malinzak, R. A., Albritton, M. J., & Pickering, T. R. (2009). *First Aid for the Orthopaedic Boards*, McGraw Hill Medical, New York.

Miller, M. D. (2008). *Review of orthopaedics* (5th ed.). Philadelphia, PA: Saunders, an imprint of Elsevier.

Netter, F. H., & Craig, J. A. (2002). *Netter's concise atlas of orthopaedic anatomy.* Teterboro, NJ: Icon Learning Systems.

Nirshal, R. P. (1993). Muscle and tendon trauma: tennis elbow. *The elbow and its disorders.* Philadelphia, PA: W. B. Saunders.

Plancher, K. D., Halbrecht, J., & Lourie, G. M. (1996). Medial and lateral epicondylitis in the athlete. *Clinics in Sports Medicine.* 15 (2), 283–305.

Rosemont, IL. 2004–2010. *OITE questions.* American Academy of Orthopaedic Surgeons.

Rosemont, IL. 2008. *Orthopaedic knowledge update 9.* American Academy of Orthopaedic Surgeons.

Saraf, S. K., & Khare, G. N. (2011). Late presentation of fractures of the lateral condyle of the humerus in children. *Indian Journal of Orthopaedics.* 20;45:39-44

Sponseller, P. D. (Ed.) (2002). *Orthopaedic knowledge update: Pediatrics 2.* Rosemont, IL: American Academy of Orthopaedic Surgeons.

Stanitski, C. L., Michel, C., & Derech, K. (1980). Simultaneous ipsilateral fractures of the arm and forearm in children. Clinics in Orthopedics. 153: 218-222. 233.

Vicenzino, B., Brooksbank, J., Minto, J., Offord, S., & Paungmali, A. (2003). Initial effects of elbow taping on pain-free grip strength and pressure pain threshold. *Journal of Orthopaedic & Sports Physical Therapy.* 33(7): 400–7.

Waters, P. M. (2006). Injuries of the shoulder, elbow, and forearm. In: M. F. Abel (Ed.). *Orthopaedic knowledge update: Pediatrics 3.* Rosemont, IL: American Academy of Orthopaedic Surgeons.

CHAPTER 12

Hand and Wrist Pathologies in Children and Adolescent Sport

Solomon Abrahams

Introduction

Hand and wrist injuries are common in children and adolescents. Actually, both children and teens suffer more wrist injuries than adults do (Kopjar & Wickizer, 1998).

Stoner et al. (2012) found in a Swedish study that in children between 0 and 18 years, upper extremity fractures make up 68% of all fractures, 26% being of the distal radius, and 17% to the wrist/hand.

Previously, injuries to the wrist and hand were acute as a result of a single microtrauma, such as dislocations and fractures. However, recently there has been an increase in the number of overuse injuries through repetitive microtrauma in sports such as tennis or gymnastics (Gill & Micheli, 1996; Klein & Micheli, 1991).

The adolescent wrist is a compound joint connecting the forearm to the hand.

Movements available are extension, flexion, radial and ulnar deviation, pronation, and supination. The distal ends of the radius and ulna and 8 carpal bones articulate to form the wrist joint. There are various complex ligaments in place to provide stability whilst allowing mobility, and the joints are all surrounded by a fibrous capsule (Moore & Dalley, 1999; Waters, 2001).

Pronation and supination are achieved through the distal radioulnar joint. This small J-shaped joint is between the ulnar head and the ulnar notch on the distal radius. Flexion and extension comes through the radiocarpal joint, formed by the distal radius, scaphoid, and lunate (Moore & Dalley, 1999).

The adolescent hand itself is formed by the 8 carpal bones, 5 metacarpals, and 14 phalanges. The carpal bones are divided into a proximal and a distal row, with the scaphoid connecting them to provide more stability. The other 7 carpals are lunate, triquetrum, pisiform, (proximal), capitate, trapezium, trapezoid, and hamate. (Moore & Dalley 1999).

There are three phalanges in each finger and two in the thumb. The distal interphalangeal joint is between the distal and middle phalanx and the proximal interphalangeal joint is between the middle and proximal phalanx. At the thumb, the one joint is known as the interphalangeal joint (Hoynak, 2010; Larsen, 2003).

Other joints at the hand include the intercarpal joint, between the two rows of carpal bones and the carpometacarpal joint, between the distal row and the proximal end of the metacarpals. Between the metacarpals and the fingers/thumb are the metacarpophalangeal joints.

Three nerves supply the hand: the ulna, radial, and median (Larsen, 2003).

Merkel and Molony (2012) state that bones of the immature hand generally have more collagen and cartilage as well as increased vascularity and a thickened periosteum than an adult hand. This simply means they should are able to heal faster. Similarly, during this healing process, most children do not face the complications that adults do, such as joint stiffness or non-union of fractures.

The other main anatomical difference seen between adults and children is of the physis (growth plates). They are located at the distal portion of long bones and are between the carpal bones. Schwab (1977) and Merkel and Molony (2012) suggest that the physis are made of cartilage, allowing the bones to expand and lengthen until they ossify at skeletal maturity(16–18 years), but in doing so, they remain vulnerable to injury in the upper limb.

The epiphyseal plates are much weaker than the surrounding tissues in adolescents, and therefore, an injury to the plates is the equivalent of a ligamentous tear in adults.

There are 2 mechanisms of injury in the wrist and hand of a growing athlete. The first results from a direct blow to the joint area and causes a separation across the plate. The second is traumatic epiphysitis which develops from a strong and repetitive muscular contraction, stressing the muscle attaching to the epiphysis.

Injury can be missed as pain and deformity are less obvious and radiographs may appear normal, so treatment can be delayed. The most common site for this injury to occur is at the distal radial epiphysis, similar to a Colle's fracture in adults (Schwab, 1977).

Research suggests males are more likely to get fractures, thought to be due to more high-risk and aggressive behaviours (Stoner et al., 2012; Wood et al., 2010).

Wrist Fracture

Gill and Micheli (1996) believe that the most common sport-related wrist injuries seen in the immature athletes are fractures. Rotational motions at the wrist or falling on to an outstretched hand with wrist extension can cause these fractures. Extension, whether repetitive (gymnastics) or traumatic, is responsible for 90% of wrist injuries (Gerbino, 1998).

Radius and Ulnar Fractures

A greenstick fracture is the most common type of upper limb fracture seen in children, where the bone is broken but the periosteum remains intact. These usually occur at the distal radius/ulna after falling on an outstretched arm. (See Fig. 12.1 and 12.2.)

Studies show that greenstick fractures are unstable and continue to displace after 2 weeks due to more complications (Randsborg & Sivertsen, 2009).

Merkel and Molony (2012) discovered that when a paediatric patient presents with a fracture, they will show certain signs and symptoms. These include pain on movement, which increases on palpation, and less ability to weight bear and swelling.

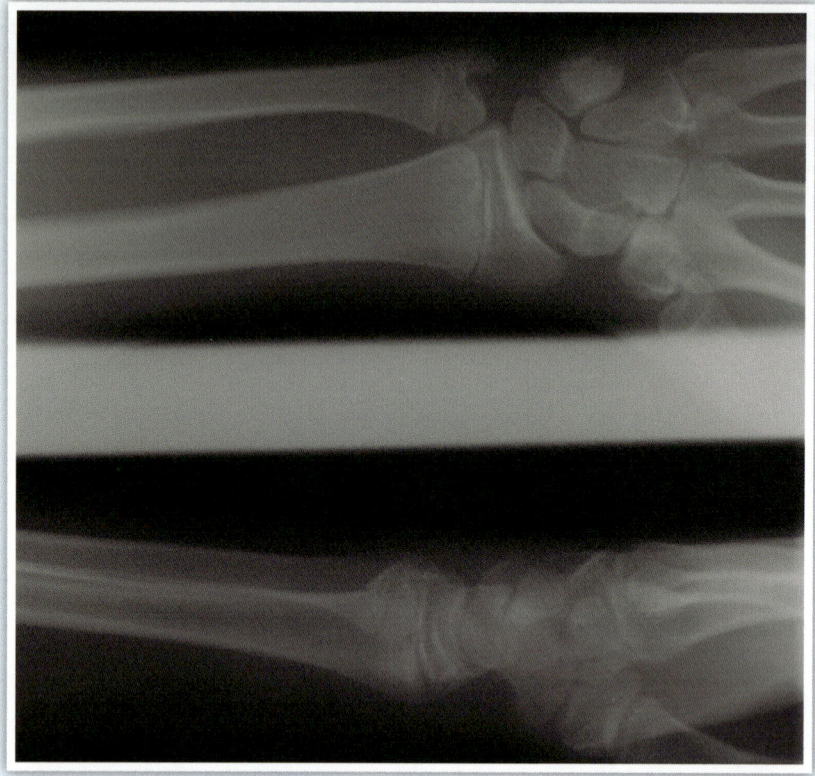

Fig. 12.1 Salter–Harris (type 2) fracture of styloid process of ulnar at distal radius ulnar joint

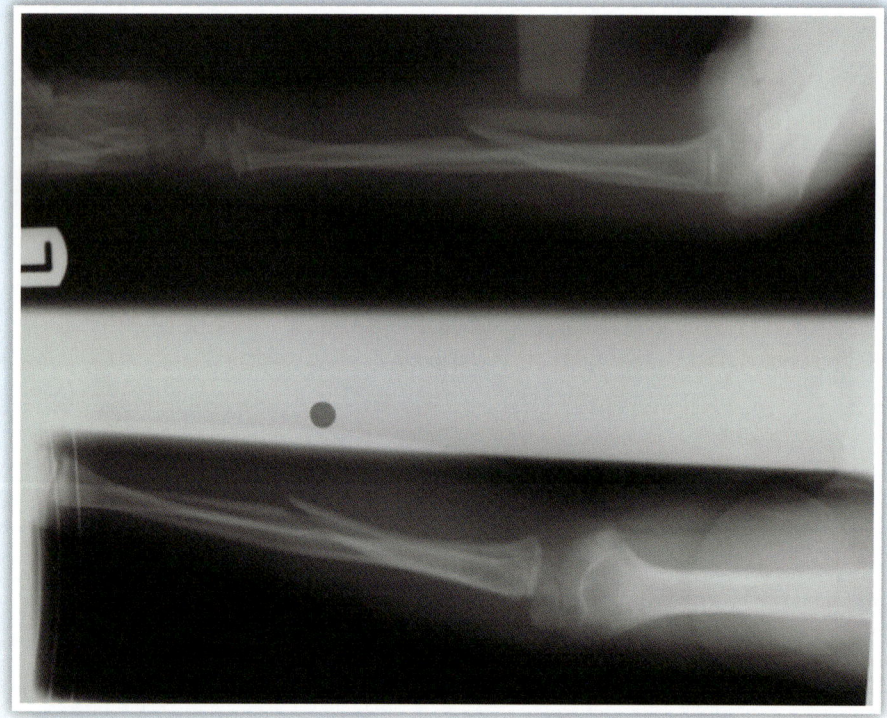

Fig. 12.1 Fracture of radius of 9-year-old girl

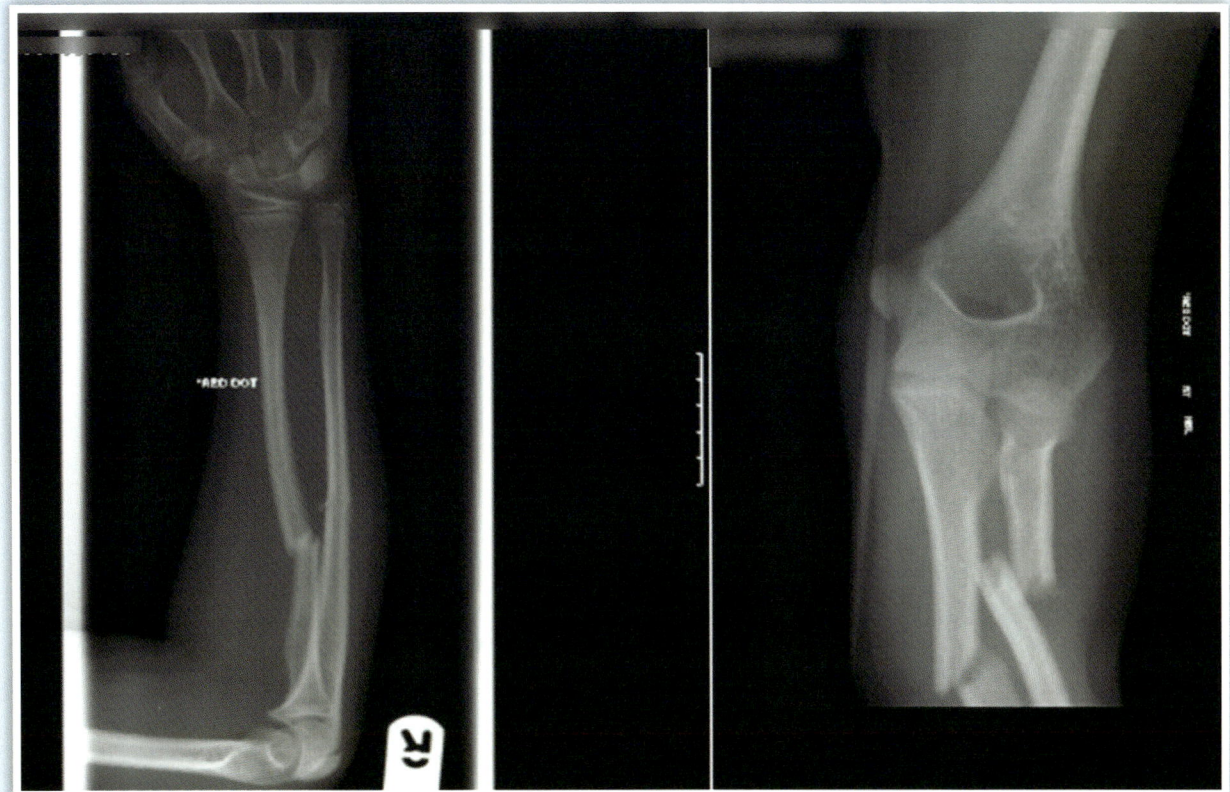

Fig. 12.2 Radial shaft fracture

Distal Radius and Ulnar Fractures

Randsborg and Sivertsen (2009) state that the most common fractures to occur in adolescents are the distal radius and ulnar fractures. Falling on an extended hand puts huge pressure through the wrist. Brudvik and Hove (2008) and Waters (2001) report that these fractures occur 3 times more often in boys than in girls. Deformities are usually a result of an indirect trauma from angular loading combined with rotational displacement.

Signs and Symptoms

Pain will present at the fracture site and in the distal forearm with limited range at the wrist. Sometimes, a visible deformity can be seen.

Test

An X-ray should be taken to confirm the diagnosis.

Management

Conservative management by immobilising the hand for 3 weeks is usually effective. Refer to orthopaedics.

Hand and Finger Fractures

In adolescencts, the hand is one of the most frequently injured body parts. The most commonly injured fingers are the little finger and the thumb. Young children are at risk of crush injuries, for example fingers getting caught in a closing door. As they get older, they are more likely to suffer injury through sporting activity. Due to risks with anaesthesia in children, surgery is not normally performed. Children can remodel fractures too, so non-operative techniques are usually preferred (Yeo, Sebastin, & Chong, 2010).

Volar Plate Injuries

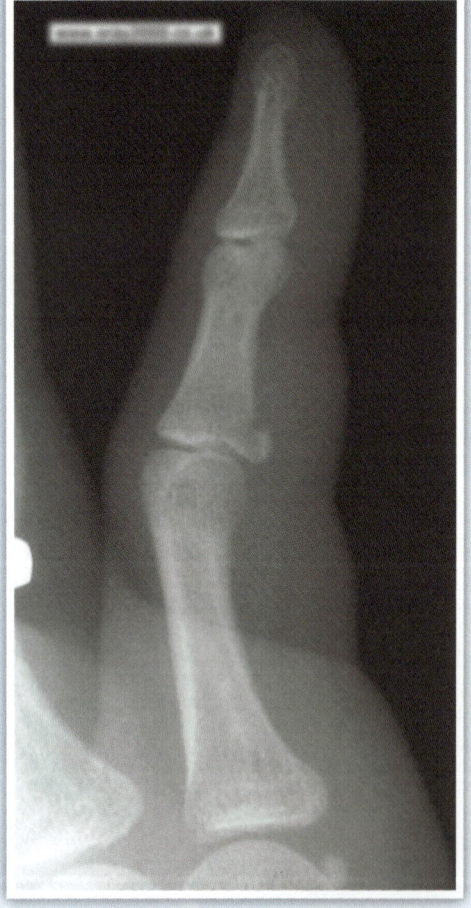

Volar plate injuries (see Fig. 12.3) occur at the distal interphalangeal (IP) joint and are normally caused by direct trauma. They normally involve a dislocation dorsally or laterally through a hyperextension injury. They are rare injuries and are normally seen in sports like cricket, baseball, and basketball (Merkel & Molony, 2012).

Fig. 12.3 Volar plate fracture

Signs and Symptoms

Localised pain, tenderness, swelling, visual deformity, and skin abrasions are some symptoms. Radiographs are a good indication of injury (Yeo et al., 2010).

Management

The joint is normally immobilised in extension for 2–3 weeks. After which, gentle mobilisations can resume.

Fracture to the Base of the Proximal Phalanx of the Thumb

Known as skier's thumb, this fracture causes instability at the first metacarpal-phalangeal joint. The mechanism is falling on to an outstretched thumb, which forces the thumb into hyperextension and abduction. Sometimes, the ulnar ligament of the thumb is sprained or ruptured, and sometimes there is even subluxation of the joint (see Fig. 12.4 and Fig. 12.6).

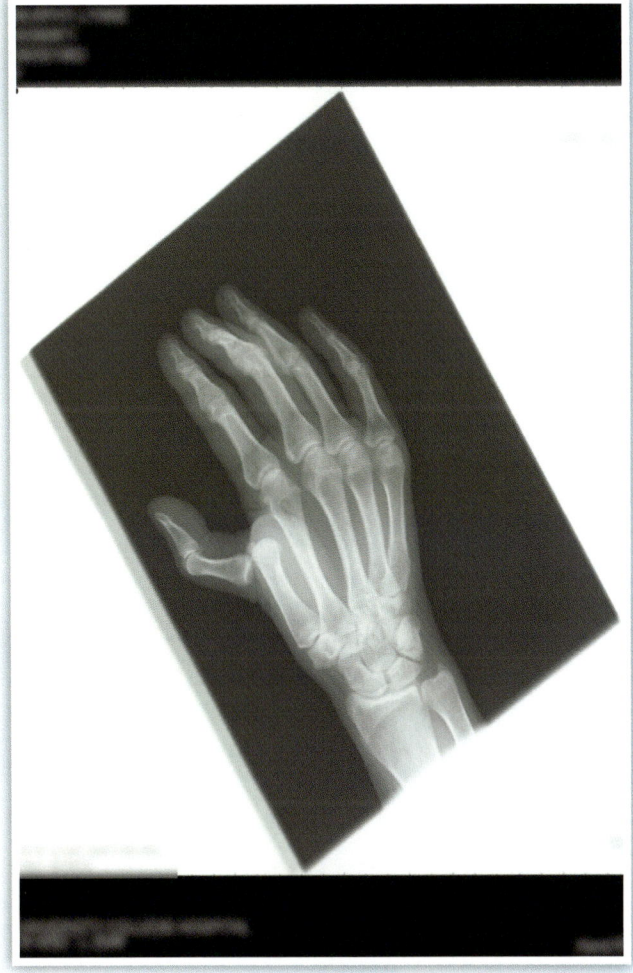

Fig. 12.4 Subluxation of the base of the first MCP

Signs and Symptoms

Localised pain, swelling and bruising, depending on the grade of sprain to the ligaments. Sometimes a physical deformity can be visible in cases of subluxation.

Test

A simple test is to add an adduction stress or valgus stress (see Fig. 12.5) to the base of the first metacarpophalangeal (MCP). Pain on the inner part may indicate damage to the ligament and capsule. Instability will present with excessive movement of this joint.

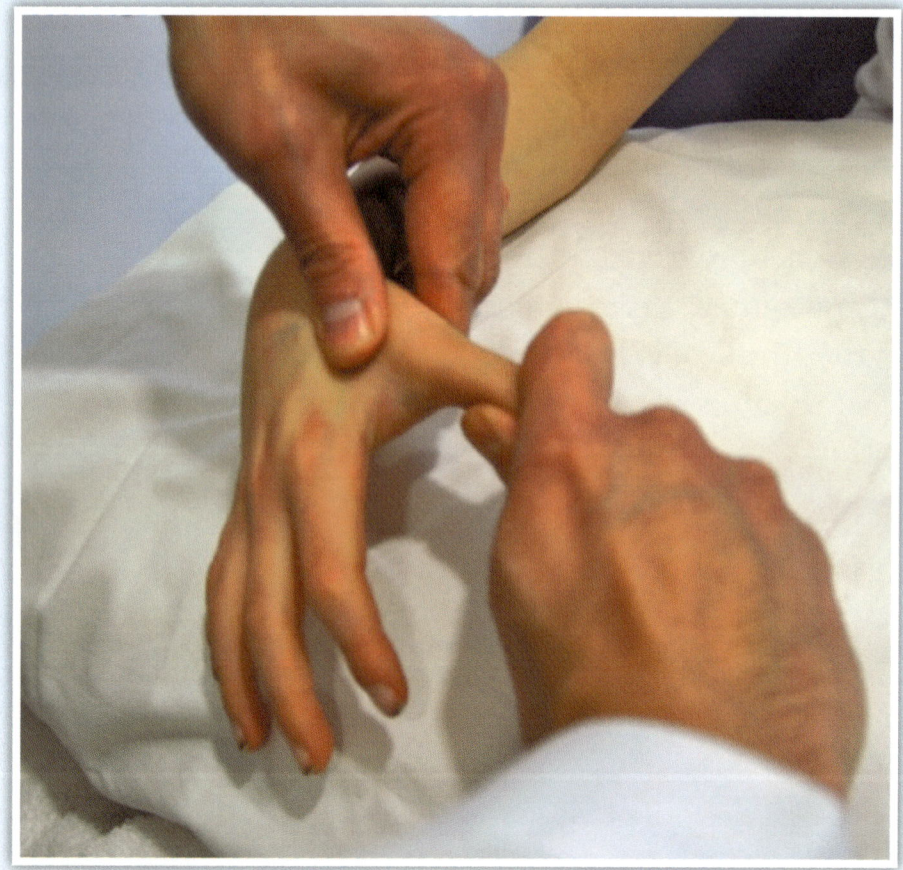

Fig. 12.5 Testing of ulnar collateral ligament of the thumb

X-ray should be done to exclude fracture/dislocation.

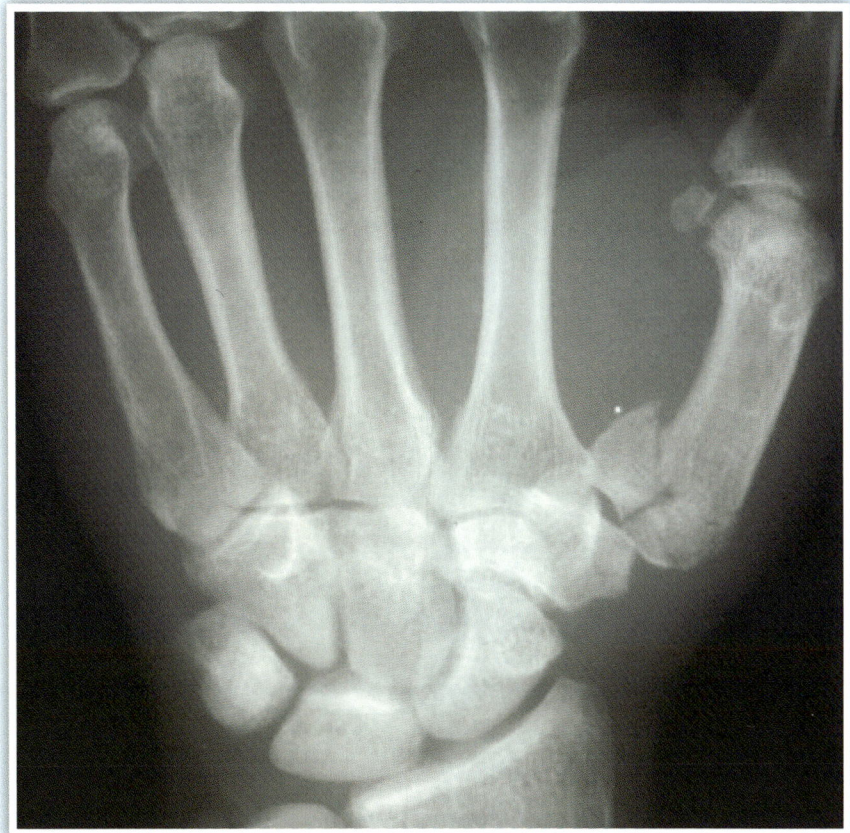

Fig. 12.6 Base of the first MCP fracture

Management

Management is mostly immobilisation between 2 and 4 weeks, depending on severity of injury. Slow mobilisation should be encouraged thereafter.

Scaphoid

In the carpal bones, the most common site of injury is the scaphoid, commonly seen in ages 12–15. These injuries make up 70% of all carpal fractures (Gerbino, 1998; Gill & Micheli, 1996; Moore, 2012; Stoner et al., 2012).

Normally, mechanism of injury is with direct impact, such as a fall onto an outstretched hand.

Signs and Symptoms

The fracture presents as pain on the radial side at the scaphoid tubercle (extend wrist and press on tuberosity), pain on range of motion, and tenderness over the 'snuff box' region (actively extend and abduct thumb, press between extensor pollicis longus and extensor pollicis brevis tendons) (Larsen, 2003; Manusov, 2002).

Test

Palpation directly over scaphoid or an X-ray reveals fracture.

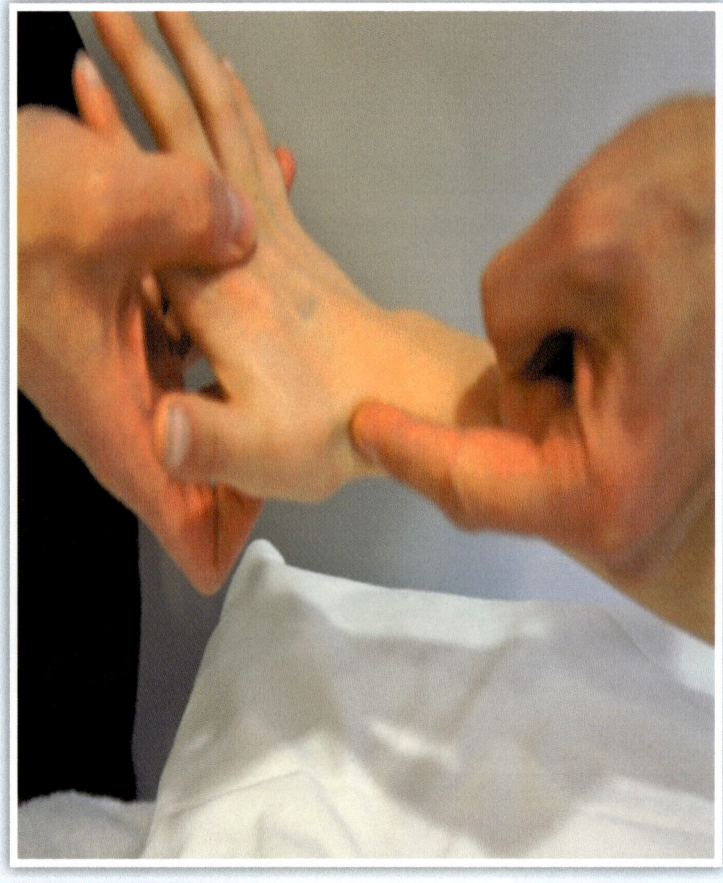

Fig. 12.7 Palpation of scaphoid bone

Management

Due to poor blood supply and difficulty immobilising a small structure, scaphoid fractures can take a long time to recover (Gerbino, 1998; Neumann, 2002).

Two to three weeks in a short cast is usually necessary, but in some cases, recovery can take 6–10 weeks. If displaced when presented to the clinician, internal fixation should be performed to prevent avascular necrosis or instability (Gill & Micheli, 1996). Gholson et al. (2011) have shown studies which quote surgery to be 96.5% effective of union; therefore surgery should be used when the injury is chronic.

Scaphoid fractures (see Fig. 12.8) in an adolescent typically occur to the distal half due to ossification. At bone maturation, there are more scaphoid wrist fractures seen in adults (Stoner et al., 2012). Scaphoid relies on an interosseous blood supply, and a fracture could result in avascular necrosis to the distal pole.

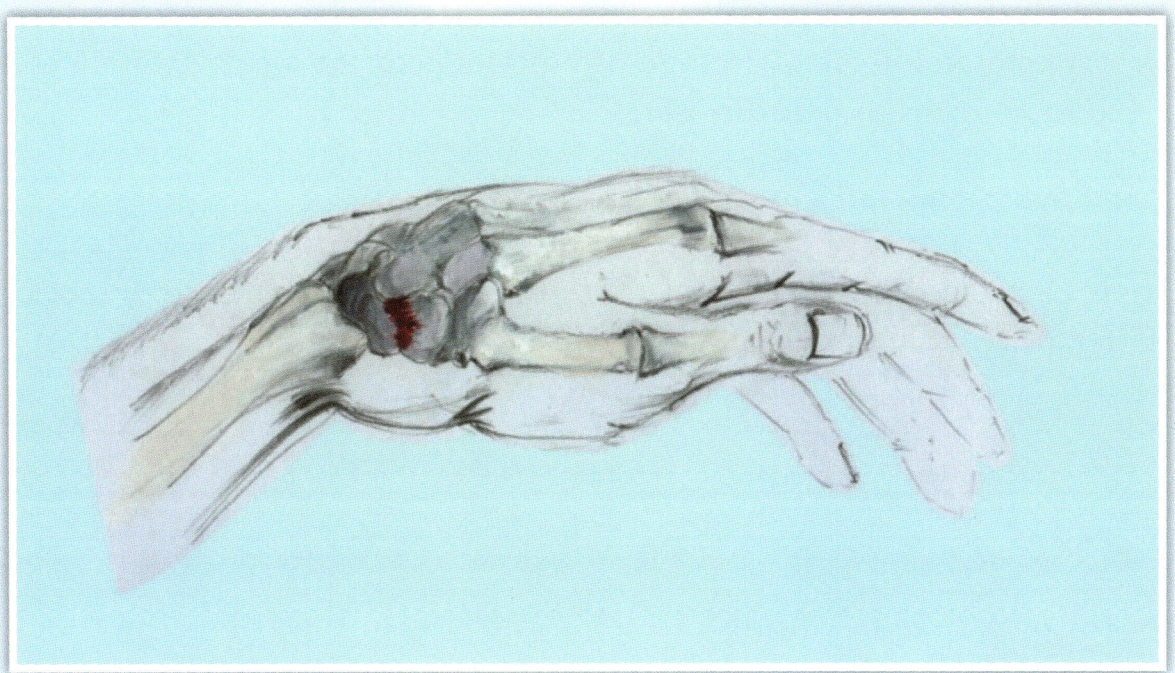

Fig. 12.8 Scaphoid fracture

Hamate

Fractures to the hook of the hamate bone, through repetitive microtrauma to the ulnar side, are frequently missed and require 6 weeks of immobilisation (Gill & Micheli, 1996). Another mechanism is falling on an outstretched arm, especially when holding an item which then gets trapped between the floor and the ulnar side of the palm.

Sign and Symptoms

Pain to the ulnar side is increased with gripping movements, and the clinician should test the ulnar nerve due to close proximity. An X-ray confirms fracture.

Management

Fracture of the hamate bone is treated conservatively with immobilisation for around 6 weeks, but if displaced, it requires internal fixation (Hoynak, 2010).

Lunate

Allan et al. (2001) describe that fractures to the lunate bone occur from either a direct blow or after chronic, recurrent trauma. If there is a fracture, the site is usually painful on palpation (just distal to radial tubercle). When recurrent, this can cause avascular necrosis of the lunate, known as Kienböck's disease. This occurs when the blood supply to the lunate is interrupted and causes weakness when gripping and decreased range of movement at the wrist. Eventually, this can lead to bone death or arthritis.

Sign and Symptoms and Test

There is pain directly over the lunate, centrally. Patient is unable to move the wrist, in particular in flexion and extension.

An X-ray confirms diagnosis.

Management

Refer for orthopaedic opinion to see if the pressure needs to be released off the bone to increase blood flow (revascularisation). Surgery is sometimes indicated.

Tendinitis

Tendinitis can occur in children, most commonly in gymnasts, from repetitive flexion and extension of the wrist (Gill & Micheli, 1996).

Signs and Symptoms

Pain increases when performing the activity or with a passive stretch of the tendon.

Test

Resist the tendon action (see Fig. 12.8b). More pain indicates tendinitis of a specific tendon.

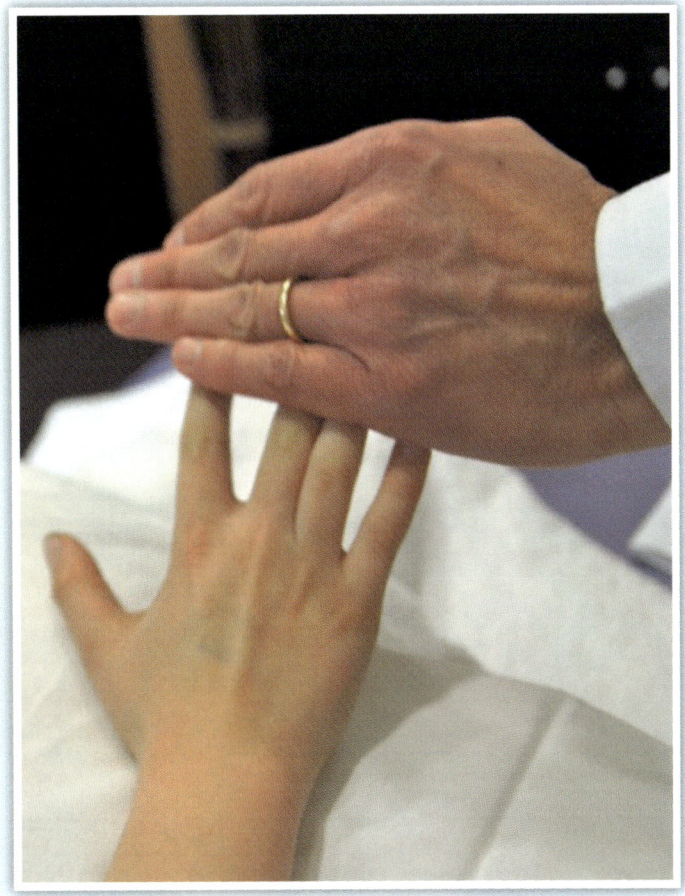

Fig. 12.8b Resisted extensors of the wrist

Management

Rest and anti-inflammatory drugs can help ease the pain, but biomechanics should be assessed in order to prevent reoccurrence.

Distal Radioulnar Ligament Strain

The radius and ulna articulate distally at the lower aspect of the forearm. The fibrous capsule of the distal radioulnar joint is strengthened by anterior and posterior ligaments (Moore, 2012). This structure allows the radius to fully rotate around the ulna during forearm rotation.

Due to this function, the rotational movement can lead to radioulnar joint injury in the form of ligament damage.

Repetitive movements such as pronantion and supination can result in gradual tears or strains from overuse (Miller, 2012). Children are at risk of suffering from these types of injury by falling on to an outstretched hand or a flexed wrist.

Signs and Symptoms

It is common to suffer pain/tenderness in the area. There may be swelling around the wrist, and hotness and redness may also present as symptoms. These ligament sprains are graded from 1 to 3 depending on severity, grade 1 being micro tears of the ligament and grade 3 being a severe or complete rupture.

Test

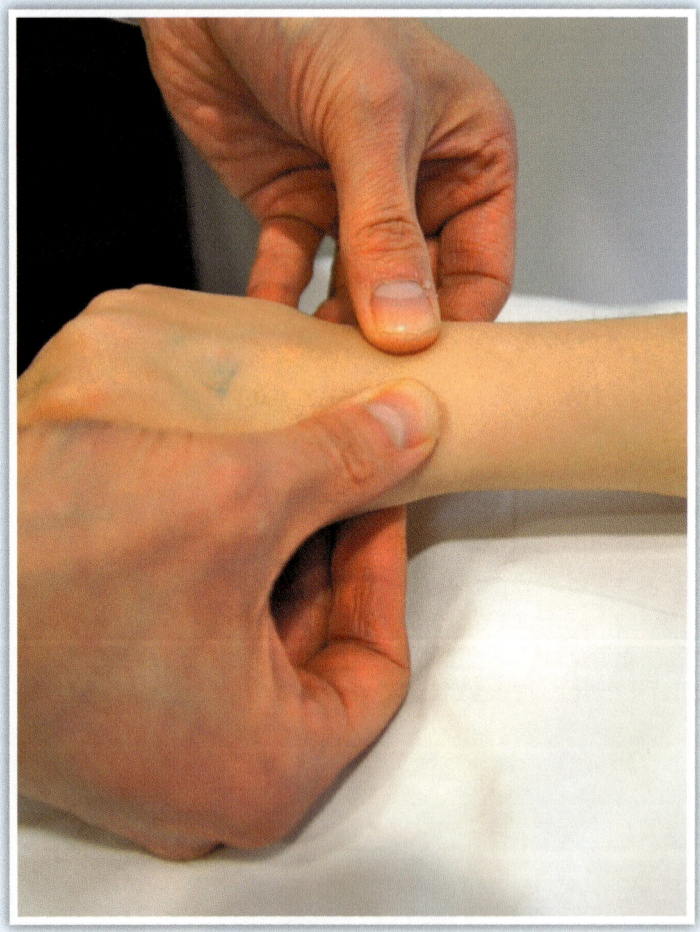

There is tenderness directly over the ligament (see Fig. 12.9) and soreness on accessory movements of the distal radius and ulnar in opposing directions. An MRI or diagnostic ultrasound scan should confirm.

Fig. 12.9 Palpation of inferior radioulnar joint

Management

The first line of treatment for this injury is to rest it and stop any forms of activity. Ice, compression, and elevation helps. An elastic compression bandage can also be used to control the swelling. It is also important to keep the hand elevated as much as possible above the heart so that the swelling is limited (Quinn, 2011).

Scapholunate Ligament Strain

The Scapholunate ligament is among the most commonly injured ligament in the wrist in children and teens. This ligament connects the scaphoid and the lunate bones and enables them to move together. A tear in this ligament forces a gap to appear between the two bones as the scaphoid flexes and the lunate extends and they move away from each other (Bissel & Bedi, 2011).

This injury is commonly a result of a fall on to an outstretched hand; however, a violent twisting motion of the hand can also be responsible for a tear.

Signs and Symptoms

Symptoms include pain in the wrist, stiffness, and swelling (Your Hands, 2012).

Test

A positive Watson test is a way of indicating a scapholunate ligament tear. The test will present a 'clunking' noise during ulnar/radial deviation (Moore, 2012).

Watson Test:

This test provokes dorsal subluxation of the proximal scaphoid over the dorsal rim of the radius, as the wrist is radially deviated;

- is performed by grasping the patient's hand from its ulnar aspect of the small metacarpal with the examiner's thumb on the palmar surface of the distal pole of the scaphoid;

- alternatively, the patient's hand is grasped by the examiner's hand from the radial aspect of the index metacarpal with the thumb and the palmar surface;

- it is critical for the examiner's thumb to apply pressure to the distal pole of the scaphoid, in order to prevent it from flexing;

- move wrist from ulnar to radial deviation with distal tuberosity compressed;

- as scaphoid flexes to more vertical orientation with radial deviation, tuberosity compression forces proximal pole subluxation dorsal to lip of radius;

- as the examiner's thumb pressure is removed, the subluxed scaphoid reduces, and may produce a palpable clunk and dorsal wrist pain (indicating instability of the scapholunate ligament). (Patel, Graydanus, & Baker, 2009).

Management

The injury is managed differently depending on whether it is a partial or complete tear. Partial tears are often managed conservatively using a splint and rest. Complete tears require surgery, where wires are inserted to hold the bones together whilst the ligament heals (Your Hands, 2012). Scapholunate ligament injuries are uncommon in the paediatric and adolescent population, with the treatment not being well explained (Earp, Waters, & Wyzykowski, 2006).

However, if this injury is left untreated, then it can progress to a severe joint instability, a condition known as a SLAC wrist. This is when the instability leads to arthritis in the radiocarpal and midcarpal joints (Vital, 2012).

Triangular Fibrocartilage Complex

Triangular Fibrocartilage Complex (TFCC) affects the ulnar side of the wrist, and it is commonly referred to as a wrist sprain. A TFCC injury can be a very serious condition that can leave the wrist joint with a considerable amount of instability. The soft tissues surrounding the wrist all work together to ensure joint stability, and as the name implies, they are very complex (eOrthopod, 2012).

Anatomically, the TFCC separates the distal radioulnar joint from the radiocarpal joint; it comprises the articular disc, the dorsal and palmar radioulnar ligaments, the meniscus homologue, and the extensor carpi ulnaris tendon sheath. The TFCC sits between the ulna and the two carpal bones, the lunate and the triquetrum, and helps stabilise the distal radioulnar joint while also improving wrist congruency and range of motion. A TFCC injury usually involves tearing of the articular disc and the meniscus homologue.

This injury is caused through direct trauma such as falling on to an outstretched hand that is in a pronated position (Chidgey, 1995). If there is sufficient force through the ulnar side of the hyperextended wrist, then an injury or a tear will occur. Athletes such as gymnasts and tennis players are likely to suffer from TFCC because of high stresses to the wrist joint. The injury is also very common in children and adolescents, although in children, it occurs more often after an ulnar styloid fracture doesn't heal properly. This is important to know because young children often take falls and bumps, so correct management of these forms of fractures can prevent TFCC injuries from developing.

Signs and Symptoms

Signs and symptoms include wrist pain; this pain is sometimes diffused so that it may feel as though the entire wrist is painful. This pain is then made worse by forearm rotation or by any movements in the ulnar direction such as opening a door handle. Other symptoms include swelling, cracking sounds, and a feeling of instability, as if the wrist is about to give way (eOrthopod, 2012).

Tests

There are tests that can be carried out to examine and diagnose TFCC injury.

There can be pain and clicking during ulnar deviation and extension of the wrist (see Fig. 12.9b) (Verheyden & Palmer, 2012).

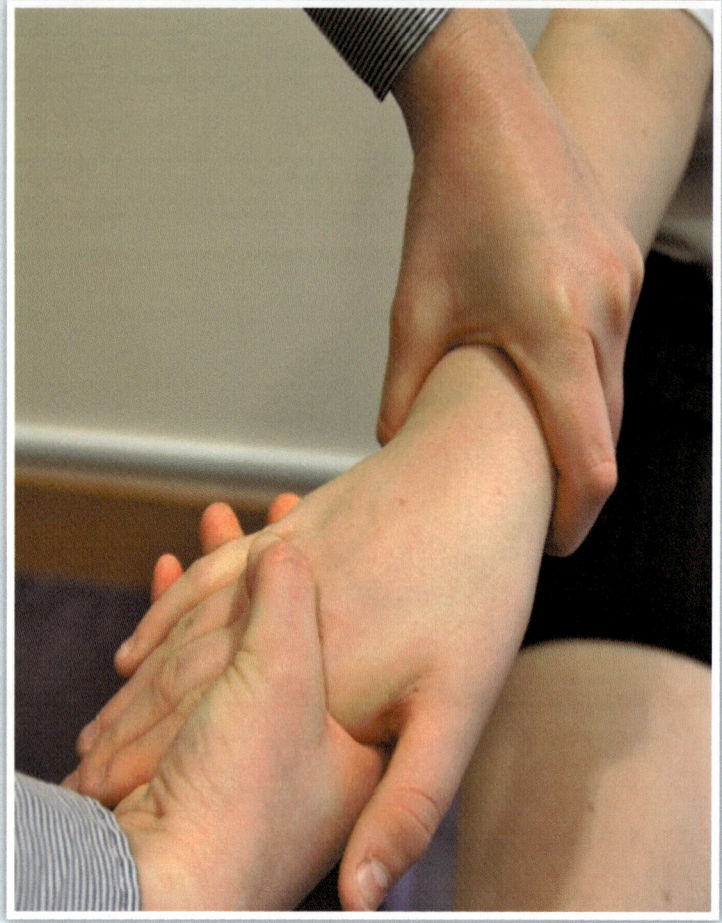

Fig. 12.9b Ulnar deviation

Shuck Test – The examiner takes the distal part of the ulna between index finger and thumb with the forearm in supination. Increased laxity or movement indicates TFFC instability (eOrif, 2012).

Fovea Sign – External pressure is applied to the ulnar fovea. This is the groove that separates the ulnar styloid from the ulnar head. If pain is reproduced, then it may be a sign of a split-tear injury (eOrthopod, 2012).

MRI scans can also be used to confirm ligament damage (eOrthopod, 2012).

Management

This injury can be managed surgically and non-surgically. If the wrist shows signs of stability, then it can be managed conservatively. This will involve wearing a splint for anything up to 6 weeks. However, if the wrist is unstable but if the patient doesn't want surgery, then a cast can sometimes be used instead of a splint. Patients are often able to return to pain-free movement and work following injury (eOrthopod, 2012).

If the wrist joint is unstable as a result of a complete rupture/avulsion fracture, then surgery is advised as soon as possible. The outer portion of the triangular fibrocartilage has a good blood supply and will therefore heal; however, the central portion is avascular, meaning that healing isn't possible. This is when an arthroscopic debridement is needed from surgery; this procedure works well for simple tears. Hard wires and screws are used for more complex tears, where the joint is needed to be fixed into position whilst it heals. Physiotherapy is required to regain full range of motion following surgery and the long period of immobilisation. Many patients return to pain-free activity 6 weeks post op, although a minority will require alterations to their activity as a result of restrictions or weakness (eOrthopod, 2012).

Jersey Finger Injuries

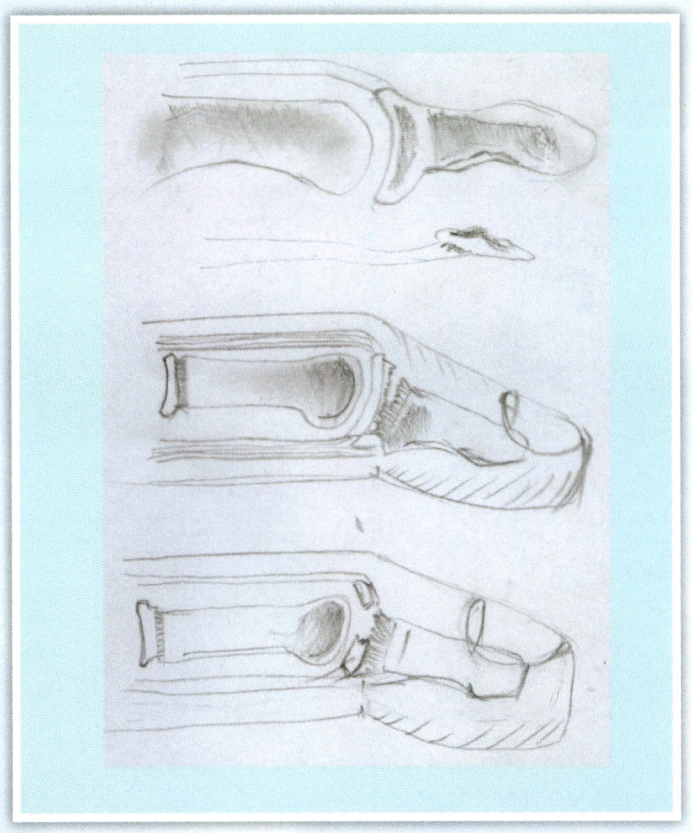

When the distal interphalangeal joint (DIPJ) is forced into extension during active flexion, it can cause trauma to the flexor digitorum profundus tendon; this injury is also known as jersey finger (Leggit & Meko, 2006). The tendon can either rupture or it can avulse and pull away part of the bone, meaning that a fracture is not that uncommon.

Fig. 12.10 Flexor profundus rupture

This type of injury occurs commonly in sports such as football and rugby, for example, where players try to grab on to other players' shirts. Jersey finger is an injury that isn't only isolated towards athletes; the injury is just as common in non-athletes of all age groups (eOrthopod, 2012). Although any finger can be affected, the ring finger, which is the weakest finger, is the most commonly injured, accounting for 75% of jersey finger injuries (Leggit & Meko, 2006; Yeo et al., 2010).

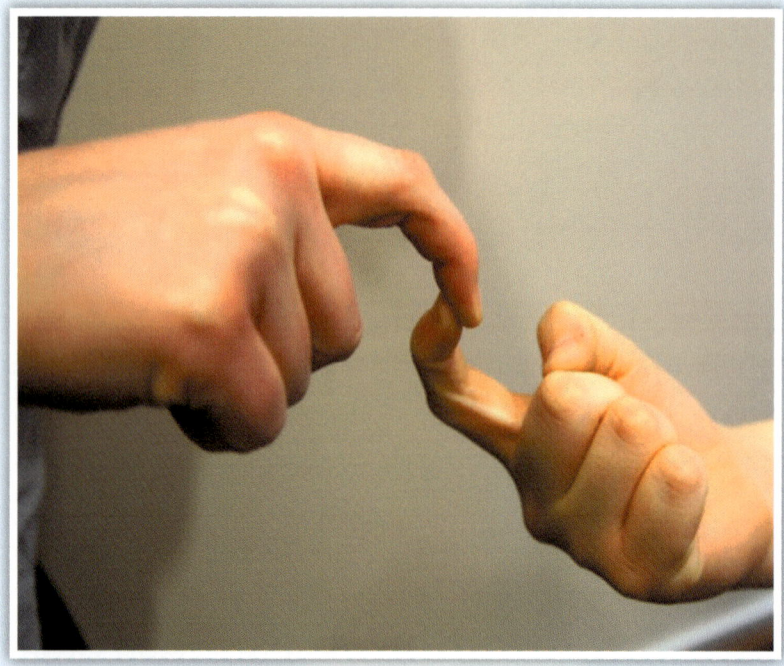

Fig. 12.11 Test of jersey finger

Signs and Symptoms

Signs and symptoms include pain and swelling, and the finger remains extended when the hand is at rest (Leggit & Meko, 2006). Immediately after suffering the injury, the patient will not be able to actively flex their DIPJ, and a lump may be visible and palpable over the proximal interphalangeal joint. This will be where the ruptured tendon has retracted (Yeo et al., 2010).

Test

In order to assess the flexor digitorum profundus tendon, the metacarpophalangeal (MCP) and proximal interphalangeal joint (PIPJ) must be held in extension as the patient attempts to flex their DIPJ (see Fig. 12.11). The other non-affected fingers should be flexed whilst doing so. If there is no movement, it is an indication of a rupture. The injury can be classified as type 1–5 depending on how far the tendon has retracted towards the palm of the hand.

Management

Treatment is dependent on the classification; the prognosis is worse if treatment is delayed as fibrosis and scar tissue can form. Patients should be referred to an orthopaedic or hand surgeon (Leggit & Meko, 2006).

Mallet Finger Injuries

When the Distal interphalangeal joint (DIPJ) is forced into sudden flexion during active extension, it can cause trauma to the extensor tendon; this is also known as mallet finger (see Fig. 12.12) (Leggit & Meko, 2006).

This injury is caused when an object such as a ball hits the tip of the finger, damaging the tendon and not allowing the finger to straighten. Sometimes, if the force is great enough, then a small piece of bone may be avulsed away from the distal phalanx (eOrthopod, 2012).

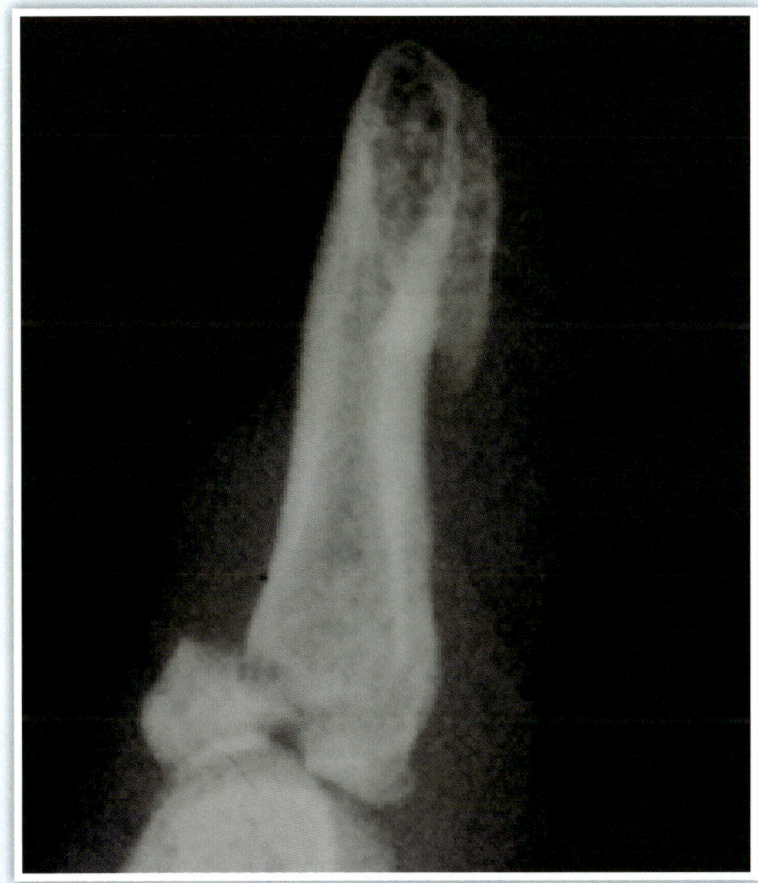

Fig. 12.12 Extensor tendon rupture

Signs and Symptoms

Signs and symptoms will include pain, swelling, and bruising. The fingertip will drop down, and it won't be able to straighten voluntarily. In some instances, blood can form beneath the nail (Orthoinfo, 2007). When evaluating the extensor tendon, it is important to isolate the DIP to ensure that passive extension comes from the tendon and not the central slip.

Test

If the finger cannot passively extend, then this indicates some form of bony entrapment that may require surgical intervention (Leggit & Meko, 2006).

Management

The majority of mallet finger injuries can be treated conservatively. Ice should be applied straight away, and the hand should be elevated above the level of the heart. Splinting can be used to hold the finger in extension or slight hyperextension for about 6 weeks, whilst the tendon heals. Injuries in children require special consideration when it comes to treatment. In children, mallet finger injuries may involve the cartilage that controls bone growth; this must be carefully evaluated so that the finger does not grow in a deformed or stunted fashion (Orthoinfo, 2007).

Trigger Finger

Trigger finger is a condition that affects the tendons of the fingers and the sheaths in which the tendons pass through. The movement of tendons through these sheaths allow the fingers to be pulled in towards the wrist when the forearm muscles are contracted. A disruption to this mechanism of movement causes trigger finger. It is a common problem that causes pain and snapping of the fingers and thumb.

The cause of trigger finger is unclear, and it seems to materialise out of nowhere. It is considered that an inflammation or swelling to the tendon results in a size discrepancy between the tendon and the sheath, resulting in resisted movement.

The condition can get to the stage where it requires force from other fingers to enable it to straighten, or it may not straighten properly at all (Cluett, 2011). This condition is mostly associated with adults, but occasionally, a child may be born with it and it often goes unnoticed by parents. This condition can be present at birth but it may be 4–6 months before the diagnosis is made.

In infants, the condition sometimes corrects itself, meaning no other treatment is needed. Around 30% of children who have the condition at birth cure themselves within 1 year. 12% of children who develop the condition between 6 and 30 months of age cure themselves within 6 months. However, if trigger finger develops in a child over the age of 3, then it rarely ever cures itself. Therefore, surgery is usually required to open up the sheaths to allow the tendons to pass through them freely (Trigger Finger and Thumb, 2012).

Signs and Symptoms

Pain and snapping of the finger during flexion and extension.

Test

An MRI scan should reveal a tenosynovitis, and calcification may be seen on more chronic cases

Management

Night splints and casts are normally indicated for a few weeks to avoid movement and allow inflammation to settle. Sometimes, surgery is indicated in more chronic cases, or where the pain does not settle.

Volkmann's Ischaemic Contracture

Volkmann's ischaemic contracture is the flexion deformity of the wrist flexors due to ischaemia of the flexor muscles because of an obstruction to the blood flow to the tendons. It is more commonly seen following a fracture of the radius, or supracondylar fracture of the humerus or any occlusion of the brachial artery. It is seen more in children.

Signs and Symptoms

Fingers are blue and cold. Radial pulse is limited or weak. Active movements of fingers are weak. Sometimes there is pain in the fingers, or there may be tingling and even numbness. Eventual flexion deformity occurs when the flexor tendons are contracted.

Test

Urgent diagnostic ultrasound scan or Doppler scan and MRI scan can confirm the injury.

Management

Immediate surgery is advised (Crawford & Hamblen, 1990).

Key Points

- Hand and wrist pathologies affect children more than adults.

- More repetition injuries are now being seen in this area.

- Distal radius and ulnar are common fracture sites in children.

- Scaphoid fractures remain the most common fractures of all carpal bones

- The scaphoid and the lunate have poor blood supplies in children.

References

Allan, C., Lichtman, D., Mack, G., & MacDonald, R. (2001). Kienbock's disease, diagnosis and treatment. *Journal of the American Academy of Orthopaedic Surgeons, 9*(2), 128–136.

Bissel, B., & Bedi, A. (2011). *Scapholunate ligament tear.* Retrieved from http://www.sportsmd.com/Articles/id/14/n/scapholunate_ligament_tear_.aspx. [accessed on 25/1/2013].

Brudvik, C., & Hove, L. (2008). Displaced Paediatirc fractures of the distal radius. *Archives of Orthopaedic and Trauma Surgery, 128*(1), 55–60.

Chidgey, L. (1995). The distal radioulnar joint: Problems and solutions. *Journal of the American Academy of Orthopaedic Surgeons, 3*(1), 95–96.

Cluett, J. (2011). *Trigger finger.* Retrieved from http://orthopedics.about.com/cs/handcondiitions/a/triggerfinger.htm [accessed 30/1/2013].

Crawford, A., & Hamblen, G. (1990). *Outline of orthopaedics* (11th ed.). Edinburgh: Churchill Livingstone.

Earp, B., Waters, P., & Wyzykowski, R. (2006). Arthroscopic treatment of partial scapholunate ligament tears in children with chronic wrist pain. *Journal of Bone and Joint Surgery–American Volume, 88*(1), 2448–2455.

eOrif (2012). *TFCC tear.* Retrieved from http://www.eorif.com/tfcc-tear-84209 [accessed on 27/1/2013].

eOrthopod (2012). *Triangular fibrocartilage complex (TFCC) injuries.* Retrieved from http://www.eorthopod.com/content/triangular-fibrocartilage-complex-tfcc-injuries [accessed on 26/1/2013].

eOrthopod (2012). *Treatment for jersey finger injury.* Retrieved from http://www.eorthopod.com/content/treatment-for-jersey-finger-injury [accessed on 29/1/2013].

Gerbino, P. (1998). Wrist disorders in the oung athlete. *Operative Techniques in Sports Medicine, 6*(4), 197–205.

Gholson, J., et al. (2011). Scaphoid fractures in children and adolescents: Contemporary injury patterns and factors influencing time to union. *Journal of Bone and Joint Surgery, 93*(13), 1210–1219.

Gill, T., & Micheli, L. (1996). The immature athlete: Common injuries and overuse syndromes of the elbow and wrist. *Clinical Sports Medicine, 15*(2), 401–423.

Hoynak, B. (2010). Carpal fractures and dislocations, *eMedicine.* http://emedicine.medscape.com/article/828746-differential.

Klein, J., & Micheli, L. (1991). Sports injuries in children and adolescents. *British Journal Sports Medicine, 25*(1), 6–9.

Kopjar, B., & Wickizer, T. (1998). Fractures among children: Incidence and impact on daily activities. *Injury Prevention,* 4(3), 194–197.

Larsen, D. (2003). Assessment and management of hand and wrist fractures. *Nursing Standard, 16*(36), 45–53.

Leggit, J., & Meko, C. (2006). Acute finger injuries: Part I. Tendons and ligaments. *American Family Physician, 73*(5), 810–816.

Manusov, E. (2002). *Pediatric sports medicine for primary care.* Philadelphia, PA: Lippincott Williams & Wilkins.

Merkel, D., & Molony, J. (2012). Recognition and management of traumatic sports injuries in the skeletally immature athlete. *International Journal of Sports Physical Therapy,* 7(6), 691–704.

Miller, S. (2012). *What are the symptoms of a radioulnar joint injury?* Retrieved from http://www.wisegeek.com/what-are-the-symptoms-of-a-radioulnar-joint-injury.htm [accessed on 24/1/2013].

Moore, D. (2012). *Scapholunate ligament injury & DISI.* Retrieved from http://www.orthobullets.com/hand/6041/scapholunate-ligament-injury-and-disi [accessed on 26/1/2013].

Moore, L., & Dalley, F. (1999). *Clinically oriented anatomy* (4th ed.). Philadelphia, PA: Lippincott Williams & Wilkins. pp. 803–804.

Neumann, D. (2002). *Kinesiology of the musculoskeletal system.* St. Louis, MO: Mosby.

Orthoinfo. (2007). *Mallet finger (baseball finger).* Retrieved from http://orthoinfo.aaos.org/topic.cfm?topic=A00018 [accessed on 29/1/2013].

Patel, D., Graydanus, D., & Baker, R. (2009). *Pediatric practice sports medicine* (2nd ed.). New York, NY: McGraw Hill Medical Book.

Quinn, E. (2011). *Sprained wrist – Treatment and prevention of wrist pain.* Retrieved from http://sportsmedicine.about.com/cs/wrist_hand/a/aa072503.htm [accessed on 24/1/2013].

Randsborg, P., & Sivertsen, E. (2009). Distal radius fractures in children: Substantial difference in stability between buckle and greenstick fractures. *Acta Orthopaedica, 80*(5), 585–589.

Schwab, S. (1977). Epiphyseal injuries in the growing athlete. *Canadian Medical Association Journal, 177*(6), 626–630.

Stoner, M., et al. (2012). Five key injuries of the pediatric wrist and hand. *Pediatric Emergency Medicine Reports, 17,* 53.

Trigger Finger and Thumb. (2012). *Trigger finger in children usually involves the thumb*. Retrieved from http://www.triggerfingersymptoms.com/trigger-finger-in-children [accessed on 30/1/2013].

Verheyden, J., & Palmer, A. (2012). *Triangular fibrocartilage complex injuries*. Retrieved from http://emedicine.medscape.com/article/1240789-overview#a0112 [accessed on 27/1/2013].

Vital, M. (2012). *SLAC (scaphoid lunate advanced collapse)*. Retrieved from http://www.orthobullets.com/hand/6043/slac-scaphoid-lunate-advanced-collapse [accessed on 26/1/2013].

Waters, P. (2001). *Distal radius and ulna fractures*. Philadelphia, PA: Lippincott Williams & Wilkins.William.

Wood, A., et al. (2010). The epidemiology of sports related fractures in adolescents. *Injury, 41*(8), 834–838.

Yeo, C., Sebastin, S., & Chong, A. (2010). Fingertip injuries. *Singapore Medical Journal, 51*(1), 78–86.

Your Hands. (2012). *Scapholunate ligament injury*. Retrieved from http://www.yourhands.co.uk/hand-wrist-surgery/hand-and-wrist-injuries/scapholunate-ligament-injury [accessed on 26/1/2013].

CHAPTER 13

Chest, Abdominal, Eyes, Nose, and Ear Pathologies

Solomon Abrahams

Chest Injuries

Chest injuries include bone injuries, pulmonary injuries, mediastinal injuries, and diaphragm injuries (Bliss & Silen, 2002). These can occur due to direct blows to the chest region. The number of chest injuries in adolescent sport is less than those in adult sport.

Bony Injuries

Bony injuries include fractures to the ribs and sternum. They are normally caused by direct blows to the ribs or sternum rather than overuse. A fracture to the rib cage could be caused by a direct blow (tackle) or a crushing of the chest. The function of the rib cage is to protect the internal organs such as the lungs and the heart. Damage to the ribs may allow damage to the organs. Signs of a fractured rib include bruising, tenderness on palpation (see Fig. 13.1) at the fracture site, an occasional dip on palpation of the bone, and pain on deep inspiration and when coughing (NYU Langone Medical Centre, 2012). Shortness of breath following trauma to the ribs could indicate a pneumothorax (punctured lung), and hence an X-ray should be considered.

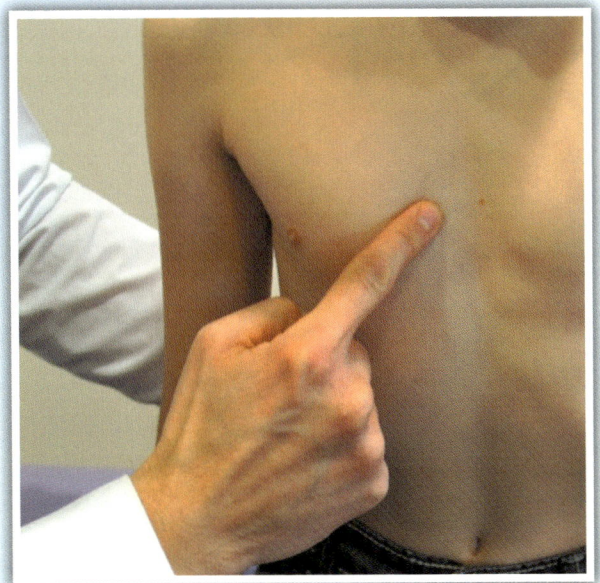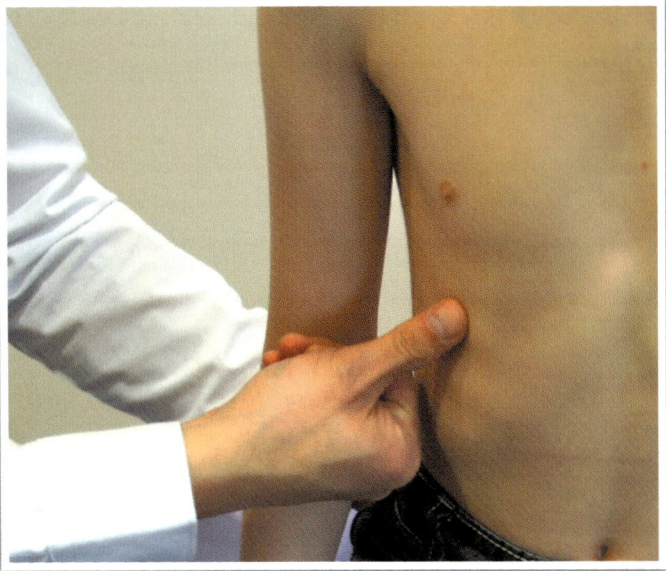

Fig. 13.1 Palpation of ribs

Sternal fractures are a cause of concern due to the proximity of the heart. Any potential chest pain in a child should be treated in an emergency department to determine the extent of injury.

Any fracture of the sternum will be acutely sore and very tender on palpation and should be X-rayed as a matter of urgency.

Stress fractures of the ribs can occur in adolescents predominantly in rowing and weightlifting. Pain is brought on by activity. Normally, rest is employed for at least 3–4 weeks. A bone scan will confirm diagnosis.

A rarer pathology of the joints at the ribs is costochondritis, normally affecting rib joints 2, 3, 4. Inflammation of the costal cartilage can occur in adolescents who have been doing excessive breathing such as seen in a viral infection (Birrer et al., 2002). Pain is felt directly over the costal cartilage which can be sore on deep breathing.

Pulmonary Injuries

A pulmonary contusion is a common injury to children in sport. They are prone to these injuries due to their lack of muscle mass which acts as a protector along with the rib cage. This is a bruising of the lung, usually due to a direct blow to the chest. The blow damages the capillaries, resulting in blood and other fluids accumulating in the lung tissue. This excess fluid interferes with the gas exchange, which is the function of the lungs (Bliss & Silen, 2002).

More of this will be discussed in later chapters.

These injuries are rarely life-threatening, but care must be taken to ensure that the internal organs have not been damaged. Direct trauma to the anterior rib cage can cause problems to the heart; even bruising of the heart, called cardiac contusion, can cause irregular heartbeats.

X-rays should always be considered in sternal and rib pain, if it causes breathing difficulties in the child or is very painful.

Mediastinal Injuries

Mediastinal injuries are rare in sport as the force of the blow must be high; they are usually seen in car accidents. With a mediastinal injury, fluid accumulates in the right pleural space. A thoracentesis reveals the presence of chylous fluid in the pleural space, indicating a rupture of the thoracic duct (Bliss & Silen, 2002).

Diaphragm

The diaphragm is a dome-shaped musculofibrous septum that splits the abdominal cavity from the thoracic cavity. There are 3 different parts of the diaphragm. The sternal fibres originate from the back of the xiphoid process. The costal fibres originate from the inner surfaces of the cartilages and adjacent portions of the lower 6 ribs on both sides. The lumbar fibres arise from the aponeurotic arches and the lumbar crura. All fibres then connect to a form a central membranous tendon (Shehata, Basma, & Shabann, 2006). Damage to the diaphragm occurs from a direct blow to the abdominal region. This is not often seen as high force is needed. Traumatic diaphragmatic rupture (TDR) only accounts for 4–8% of organ injuries due to a blunt trauma to the abdominal region. Traumatic diaphragmatic injuries include ruptures, tears, avulsions, and eventually, late necrosis (Shehata et al., 2006).

Lower Abdominal Trauma

The most common internal organ injured in adolescent sport is the spleen, caused by direct trauma to the left lower quadrant under the ribs. Pain would be progressive sometimes followed by fever. Unrelenting pain should be further investigated. Sometimes, pain in the left shoulder is seen with spleen injuries (Birrer et al., 2002).

Another injury common in children is injury to the kidneys, arguably more than the spleen (Lyle, 1984); it is normally sustained from direct or a blunt trauma. Some of these children may have a pre-existing problem with the renal system, but usually, most traumas cause a contusion. If, however, following a renal trauma, blood is passed in the urine, further investigation should be considered (Lyle, 1984).

Male external genitalia can also be damaged by direct trauma. Rarely does this give any long-term problems, and most settle down with conservative rather than surgical procedures. Most of the traumas in this region are contusions or haematoma-related, which can be treated with rest and ice packs. In more severe cases, trauma can cause a testicular rupture, which would produce a hematocele and require surgery (Lyle, 1984).

Eyes

Eye injuries in sports are common, and baseball is the leading cause of injuries in children up to 14 years of age. Basketball is the leading cause in teens between ages 15 and 24 years. Other sports such as squash, lacrosse, paintball, ice hockey, handball, tennis, badminton, and boxing are all high in eye injuries. Injuries to the eyes usually result from a direct blow to the eye either with a ball or an object (NEI, 2012).

Common eye injuries in sports include abrasions, contusions, eye socket fractures, detached retinas, corneal lacerations, haemorrhages, cataracts, and loss of an eye (Rivera, 2012). Most sports are now using protective eyewear such as goggles and eye guards to help reduce injury risk. These could prevent 90% of sports-related injuries (NEI, 2012).

Nose

'Nasal trauma is defined as any injury to the nose or related structure that may result in bleeding, a physical deformity, a decreased ability to breathe normally because of obstruction, or an impaired sense of smell. The injury may be either internal or external.' Fractures to the nasal bone are common as it only takes a force of 30 g to break it, whereas the jaw needs 70 g of force.

It is the third-most commonly broken bone, following the wrist and the clavicle. The most common mechanism of injury is a direct blow to the nose in sport using equipment (hockey stick) or bodies of other players (boxing). Protective measures such as a head guard are used in some sports such as amateur boxing. In young children (under 5 years old), this fracture is uncommon as the activities they partake in have a lower risk of exposure. It occurs most commonly during the ages 16–20 (Tursz & Crost, 1986).

Ears

A direct blow to the ear may result in a tear in the eardrum, dislocation of the ossicles, or damage to the inner ear. Sports such as wrestling and martial arts are common for this as there are repetitive hits to the head and the ears. Otitis externa or swimmer's ear is a common injury in children. This is an inflammation to the outer ear and the ear canal. This occurs when swimming in a polluted pool or from trapped water in the ear (E medicine health, 2012).

Conclusion

This section is a brief overview of injuries to the chest, abdomen, eyes, nose, and ear in children while participating in sport. Evidence shows that injuries suffered by children in sport are sometimes serious and affect their future life. Protective gear is being used in a lot of sports now to prevent the injuries. There have been few studies done on injuries in children as they are not as common as injuries in adults due to undeveloped anatomy, intensity of the sports, and the protective gear.

Key Points

- Spleen is the most commonly damaged internal organ in children.
- Stress fractures of the ribs are common in adolescent rowers.
- The nose is the third most common fracture site in adolescents.

References

Birrer, R., Griesemer, B., & Cataletto, M. (2002) Pediatric Sports Medicine for Primary Care (2nd ed.). Lippincott Williams and Wilkins.

Bliss, D., & Silen, M. (2002). Pediatric thoracic trauma. *Critical Care Medicine*, 30 (11), 409–415.

E medicine health (2012).

Grisogono, V. (1991). *Children and sport fitness, injuries and diet* (pp. 144–148). London: John Murry Ltd.

Karger D (2005). *Epidemiology of pediatric sports industries* (Vol. 1, p. 59). Switzerland: Reinhardt Druck.

Lyle, J. (1984) Pediatric and adolescent sports medicine (1st ed.). Boston, MA: Little Brown and Company.

Medscape General Medicine. (2000). *Common sports injuries in children and adolescents*. Retrieved from http://www.medscape.com/viewarticle/408524_4 [accessed on 25/1/2013].

NEI (2012). Retrieved from http://www.nei.nih.gov/sports/pdf/SpeakersGuide.pdf.

NYU Langone Medical Center. (2012). *Rib fracture*. Retrieved from http://pediatrics.med.nyu.edu/conditions-we-treat/conditions/rib-fracture [accessed on 25/1/2013].

Rivera, E. (2012). *11 Sports related eye injury facts*. Retrieved from http://visianinfo.com/11-sport-related-eye-injury-facts/ [accessed on 25/1/2013].

Shehata, S., Basma, S., & Shabann, S. (2006). Diaphragmatic injuries in children after blunt abdominal trauma. *Journal of Pediatric Surgery, 41*(1), 1727–1731.

Tursz, A., & Crost, M. (1986). Sports-related injuries in children: A study of their characteristics, frequency, and severity, with comparison to other types of accidental injuries. *American Journal of Sports Medicine, 14*(1), 294–299.

CHAPTER 14

Head, Brain, and Spinal Cord Pathologies in Children and Adolescent Sport

Nelson Lopes and Solomon Abrahams

Introduction

Head and spinal injuries are rare in adolescents; however, they remain an important problem in the paediatric population. International epidemiological surveys have shown that trauma is the leading cause of death among children aged 5–15 years in industrialised and some developing countries (Haller, 1983).

Traumatic injuries in adolescents are more often than not presented to be sports-related or following a road traffic accident or fall from height; this is a common feature found throughout the literature.

There are slight disparities between the mechanisms of injury and age. More adolescents will suffer brain or spinal injury from sports activity and road traffic accident (RTA) rather than infants who are injured through physical abuse and falls. The above injury events are more often than not the leading cause of paediatric head and spinal injuries.

Injuries of adolescents present in a different way from those of adults due to the differences in anatomical and physiological properties of the skull, brain, spine, spinal cord, and other relevant structures.

Spinal Injuries in Adolescents

As discussed already in earlier chapters, spines of children during growth are still immature; their intervertebral discs will have a higher water content, allowing for increased flexibility. This means it would require an incident of higher energy to cause injury in an adolescent compared with an adult. The paediatric population anatomically present with horizontal facet joints, underdeveloped and incompletely ossified spinous process, growth plates and ligamentous laxity, placing the spine at a higher risk of spinal cord injury due to the increased spinal mobility. The stages of skeletal growth differ in individuals, and there are discrepancies between genders.

There are different types of injuries stemming from excess spinal mobility in children such as compression fractures, burst fractures, seat-belt fractures (chance fractures), spondylolysis/spondylolisthesis, spinal cord injury, and spinal cord injury without radiological abnormalities.

Fractures

Paediatric spinal fractures represent between 2 and 5% of all acute spinal injuries (Clark & Letts, 2001). The low incidence is due not only to the plasticity and resilience of the paediatric spine but also to the difficulty of diagnosis and the severe, if not fatal, associated injuries.

Many recent studies have shown that younger children tend to have higher cervical spine lesions. To support this, Mathison et al. (2008) suggest that hypermobility combined with a large head-to-body ratio and poorly developed cervical musculature predisposes younger children (0–9 years old) to high torque forces at the upper cervical region.

C1–C2 fractures, despite being uncommon and rare, can occur through direct axial loading, but atlas-axis instability is more frequently presented in children. Baker et al. (1999) suggest that this instability is generally attributed to the higher fulcrum of flexion and greater ligamentous laxity present in young patients. Dislocation in the upper cervical region, in the atlanto-occipital articulation, can occur and is extremely dangerous, considering nearby structures such as the lower cranial nerves and the upper spinal cord. Kenter et al. (2001) state that a paediatric atlanto-occipital articulation is particularly vulnerable to hyperextension forces because of the horizontal orientation of the facet joints.

Thoracic and lumbar vertebral fractures are not as common as cervical fractures, although they are present in the paediatric population. Klassen (1994) identifies that the majority of thoracolumbar spine fractures in the paediatric population occur in children aged 14–16 years.

Lumbar compression fractures occur most frequently due to intervertebral disc herniation. This is more prevalent in adolescents rather than in children. Roaf, in (1960), demonstrated that the cartilaginous end plate often fails first, allowing herniation of the nucleus into the vertebral body instead of the spinal canal, as often seen in adult patients. As a result of the compression force, a burst fracture occurs to the vertebral body. The intervertebral discs of a paediatric patient are more elastic causing a wave of multiple compression fractures, unlike a single compression fracture in adults.

Adolescents who participate regularly in sports such as gymnastics, weightlifting, and/or football, where hyperextension is a constant stress, may suffer from an acute fracture of the pars interarticularis (spondylolysis). Consequently, the vertebral body can then be displaced forwards (spondylolisthesis). This is most commonly seen at the L5 to S1 level (97%) and should not be misinterpreted as an acute fracture–dislocation (Renshaw, 1994).

Spinal Cord Injury (SCI)

Traumatic spinal cord injury (SCI) is uncommon in the paediatric population, with approximately 1000 new cases occurring each year in children 0–15 years of age (Hamilton & Myles, 1992).

The effects can be devastating in terms of neurological disability. Spinal cord injury can be classified as either a complete or incomplete lesion. A complete lesion is where no motor and/or sensory function exists from more than three levels below the neurological level of injury.

One recent case review carried out by Singh et al. (2011) managed to analyse 122 patient cases of paediatric spinal injuries over a 2-year period. All the children were less than 20 years old and were allocated into three groups, depending on their age. All cases were from the All India Institute of Medical Sciences (AIIMS) Trauma Centre, suggesting the difficulty to generalise their findings to more developed countries. Their aim was to study the epidemiology, in-hospital outcome, and influence of various prognostic factors on the pattern of spinal injury in the paediatric population. 31% sustained a complete spinal cord lesion, 50% had an incomplete lesion, and 19% were neurologically intact. They also found that 54% suffered from autonomic dysfunctions such as hypotension and bladder/bowel problems. Cervical involvement was illustrated with 78% of cases in the 0–10 years age group, 63% in the 11–14 years age group, and 55% in 15–20 years age group.

This helps support the notion that the cervical region is more prone to injury as the development of growth progresses. This is also evident as '52 cases in which there was fracture along with subluxation/dislocation, 42 cases involved the cervical spine.' Alternatively, Singh et al. (2011) managed to concludethat there was no association between the level of injury and the mechanism of injury and gender.

Spinal Cord Injury Without Radiological Abnormalities (SCIWORA)

As discussed previously, a traumatic fracture can cause spinal cord damage along with many other mechanisms of injuries, such as excessive hyperflexion/ hyperextension without any fractures sustained to the vertebrae and arterial damage, leaving a haematoma and/or a thrombosis. Pang and Wilberger (1982) used the term SCIWORA for the first time to describe 28 clinical cases that were radiographically normal but neurologically abnormal.

SCIWORA is almost unique to the paediatric population and occurs as a consequence of a stretch or distraction injury to the relatively flexible spinal column (Pang & Wilberger, 1982). This occurs mainly following trauma with high energy, which dissipates in an adolescent's elastic musculoskeletal system but impacts the spinal cord and surrounding ligamentous structures. 90% of SCIWORA cases occur in the paediatric population with an average age of 7–8 years (Launay et al., 2005), with ¾ of SCIWORA injuries occurring in the cervical spine.

Examples of SCIWORA are hyperflexion injuries, causing distraction of the posterior ligamentous complex leading to potential ruptures. The hyperflexion forces may result in anterior subluxation, wedge-compression fractures, or facet dislocations (Mathison et al., 2008). These injuries are most commonly found in the cervical vertebrae; however, lumbar flexion-distraction injuries occur, as previously discussed, in seat belt fractures.

Hyperextension forces are most commonly seen as whiplash-associated disorders in road traffic accidents, they but can also be seen in sports-related activity.

Hyperextension injuries include avulsion fractures of the atlas, traumatic spondylolisthesis, and both laminar and pillar fractures (Mathison et al., 2008). These hyperextension/hyperflexion injuries may give rise to further complications when treating the patient.

Diagnosis

It is important to understand the anatomical and physiological differences in a paediatric spine in order to interpret radiographic studies and treat spinal injuries in adolescents. Kreykes et al. (2010) examined the literature regarding differences in cervical injuries between children and adult populations. They suggested that there is a common perception that the physical examination in infants and children, especially in those below the age of 3, is unreliable. This can also be even more difficult in infants where communication is difficult.

Associated injuries in children may be difficult to diagnose, secondary to an inability to communicate due to various factors such as age, non-compliance, or unconsciousness (Silber et al., 2001). Pain and crying can be misinterpreted, and neurological examinations can be challenging. However, with the scope of research out there and the low incidence of spinal cord injury in the paediatric population, a thorough subjective and physical examination is still considered.

In this age group, if radiographs are negative but there is still concern for injury, a dynamic flexion–extension radiography or an MRI is to be obtained. The literature suggests that in SCIWORA, neither plain radiographs nor CT scans of the neck reveal any injury; a magnetic resonance imaging (MRI) scan of the neck is likely the only way to define neural deficit (Kreykes et al., 2010).

Despite the low incidence of spinal cord injury in adolescents and infants, it is vital that clinical guidelines are met to ensure that nothing is missed as this could present with severe consequences down the line. Research illustrates the need for frequent imaging; however, this may have implications in terms of radiation risk. Children's organs are more sensitive to radiation, and their longer lifespan allows time for the deleterious effects to manifest (Mazrani et al., 2007). Kreykes et al. (2010) conclude that selective imaging is required but should be based on an adaptation of history and clinical findings employed in adult trauma management.

Management/Rehabilitation

Establishment of an airway, adequate ventilation, and cardiovascular support are cardinal principles in the management of any trauma patient (Gore et al., 2009). Due to the high incidences of associated spinal cord injury following a spinal fracture, it is vital to follow strict guidelines and protocols for management and rehabilitation. The literature also states the importance of individualising the treatment and follow-up rehabilitation to the patient's age, severity of injury, neurological compromise, and level of injury (Sibler et al., 2001).

Following a trauma, it is imperative to immobilise the adolescent or the infant in order to prevent further damage. In paediatric patients, this may be challenging as, following a traumatic event and when pain is present, they are restless and uncooperative. In the case of cervical spine injury, a collar is necessary for immobilisation. With the use of a rigid collar, paediatric patients still allow 15 degrees of flexion and extension. Huerta et al. (1987) suggest that a rigid collar combined with supplemental devices that partially enclose the head and tape provides the best immobilisation.

Operative Treatment

Eleraky et al. (2000) state, 'Indications for surgical intervention include an unstable injury, irreducible fracture or dislocation, progressive neurologic deficit from compression, and progressive deformity.' With a smaller anatomy, surgical procedures are challenging and require greater precision.

Advances in surgical techniques have made a good impact on recovery, particularly in methods of internal fixation. The treatment protocol should consist of early mobilisation post surgery in order to restore function.

Early mobilisation of paediatric patients with a spinal cord injury likely reduces the risk of deep venous thrombosis, decubitus ulcers, and respiratory infections (Brockmeyer et al., 1995). In a review by Singh et al. (2011), they found that out of their 122 paediatric cases, patients who underwent surgery had a significantly lower mortality (1%) as compared with those managed conservatively (13%).

Non-operative Treatment/Rehabilitation

An increasing number of patients are being offered surgery because it leads to early mobilisation, thereby preventing various complications related to immobility (Singh et al., 2011). Alternatively, conservative management can also be used. As discussed previously, for a majority of cervical spine fractures, rigid collar protocols are put in place. In response to a spinal injury, many complications can occur in the paediatric population as seen in adults.

Nash (2005) suggests that one out of four young people with spinal cord injury does not have the level of fitness required to perform essential activities of daily living. Injuries in the thoracic region can have implications to a patient's cardiorespiratory status.

Vogel (1996) states that complications such as these arise because of injury to the thorax and abdomen, as well as compromised pulmonary function due to respiratory muscle weakness from the neurologic deficit. Similarly, injuries to the cervical spine may cause respiratory weakness as accessory muscles are innervated by specific cranial nerves. These issues give rise to the importance of respiratory physiotherapy. Early aggressive ventilator management, if needed, as well as pulmonary toilet, suctioning, chest percussion, postural drainage, assisted coughing, incentive spirometry, forced vital capacity monitoring, and early mobilisation help prevent pulmonary complications (Zidek & Srinivasan, 2003).

Pain may also limit recovery in the adolescent patient. Botterell et al. (1954) state that pain affects 30–65.5% of adults and 6% of children with spinal cord injury. Along with analgesics, a physiotherapeutic view can be taken. Physical modalities such as transcutaneous electrical nerve stimulation (TENS), massage, and exercise can help alleviate the symptoms of pain by stimulating different pain mechanisms.

Spasticity can be a major problem in the paediatric population suffering from spinal injuries. It is stated by Little et al. (1989) that spasticity tends to be more severe in patients with incomplete lesions. Children with spasticity may find it difficult to mobilise, and therefore, appropriate medication should be administered. Spasticity may interfere with comfort, sleep, catheterisation, positioning, skin integrity, dressing, hygiene, bathing, orthotic use, transfers, sexual activity, activities of daily living, and seating (Zidek & Srinivasan, 2003). Physiotherapy interventions are useful in reducing these problems; this can be achieved with range of motion exercises and a regime of stretching and massage.

Splints are also conservatively used in order to manage spasticity as well as muscle weakness. A splint supports the weight of the upper extremity such that weak proximal muscles can move the arm and position the hand for such functions as eating, painting, computer use, strengthening, and neuromuscular re-education (Mulcahey, 1986).

Orthotics helps with muscular weakness, spasticity, posture and mobilising. Kelly and Stokes (1986) suggest that ankle-foot orthotics should be used for positioning in children with high-level tetraplegia, positioning and support in standing equipment in children with tetraplegia and paraplegia, and ambulation in children with paraplegia with injury at L5 or below.

Advancements in the field of science have reduced the use of orthotics, and there is a greater focus on functional rehabilitation such as locomotor training.

Harkema et al. (2012) highlight that the objective of locomotor training is to provide the damaged nervous system with appropriate sensory inputs to stimulate the remaining spinal cord networks and facilitate their continued involvement.

A wealth of studies have shown the benefits of locomotor training with subsequent reports showing gains in walking speed and increases in distance, as well as improvements in balance, body weight support, electromyographic activity, and kinematics (Harkema et al., 2012).

Brain Injuries in Adolescents

Morrow & Pearson (2010) identify that brain injuries represent the most common cause of mortality and long-term morbidity in paediatric trauma. The mechanism of injuries most prevalent still correlate with spinal injuries in children; these are: road traffic accidents, sports-related injuries, and falls.

Another mechanism has been highlighted specifically for injuries to the brain by the NSPCC (2009) as physical abuse. It is rarely a single event with children suffering from several episodes before brain damage is observed.

Case (2007) found that 80% of deaths from head trauma in children younger than 2 years were from inflicted injuries. It is important to note that the literature suggests brain injuries differ from a paediatric patient in comparison to an adult patient. A child's developing brain will present with more water, open sutures, lower cerebral blood flow per gram of brain tissue and reacts differently to medication (Morrow & Pearson, 2010). These structural differences offer a reduction in protection and difficulty in managing secondary complications as well as the choice in treatment options. This explains the high mortality rate in the paediatric population suffering from head trauma.

There is a growing body of research regarding the epidemiology and clinical findings of brain injuries in children; however, the results are difficult to generalise and compare because there are many varying methodologies used. Therefore, the clinical implications and recommendations differ. A piece of research carried out by Dean et al. (2007) found that physicians followed paediatric brain injury treatment recommendations only 60% of the time.

Concussion

Kirkwood et al. (2006) define a concussion as a type of mild traumatic brain injury caused by an impact or jolt to the head. The vast majority of paediatric concussions occur as a result of a sports-related incident. Among the more commonly played sports, American football and ice hockey have the highest incidence of concussion, followed by soccer, wrestling, basketball, field hockey, baseball, softball, and volleyball (Powell & Barber-Foss, 1999).

The signs and symptoms of a concussion are similar in young children and adults despite the anatomical and physiological differences. These are fatigue, contusion, slowing or slurring of speech, memory disturbances, loss of consciousness, increased emotion, un-coordination, headaches, dizziness, and vomiting.

The impact of a concussion to the physiology and anatomy of the paediatric brain was initially perceived to be minimal. A key historical piece of research by Kennard (1936) first defined that plasticity of a young brain would allow better and speedier recovery after an insult. However, more recent studies have proven otherwise as there is a lack of rehabilitation potential in children suffering from brain injuries due to the lack of learned basic skills. Any child with concussion should be sent to hospital to confirm the extent of injury. Parents should always be present when examining and managing the child where possible.

Traumatic Brain Injury (TBI)

Kay et al. (1998) identified that the clinical definition for mild traumatic brain injury has existed for 10 years as loss of consciousness <10 minutes or amnesia, Glasgow Coma Scale (GCS) of 13–15, no skull fracture on physical examination and on a non-focal examination. Consequently, we can deduce from this clinical definition the components needed in identifying the severity of the brain injury.

Another definition states that a TBI encompasses brain concussion, skull fracture, brain damage with clear neurological deficits and clinically observable cognitive deficits, post-traumatic amnesia, neurological sequelae, and any evidence of intracerebral or intracranial haemorrhaging (Tsai et al., 2004). These two different definitions illustrate the varying severity of brain injuries from mild to moderate and moderate to severe. Along with this, there are two forms of traumatic brain injuries that can be present: primary brain injury and secondary brain injury.

Primary Brain Injury

A primary brain injury is the immediate damage that the brain receives; this could be a physical deformation as in a skull fracture or bruising or shearing of neurons at the brain. One example is a contrecoup injury, most commonly seen in road traffic accidents. This injury occurs as the rapid deceleration causes the cerebral cortex to impact against the skull, causing potential damage to the brain with chance internal bleeding depending on the severity of the impact.

Fractures are more prevalent in children than in adults as children have thinner skulls. This explains the fact that skull deformation and bruising can occur more readily in children as less force is required for insult. A discrepancy identified in literature is the nature of fracture patterns between children and adults. Children are subjected and more inclined to receive facial and skull fractures simultaneously whereas adults will only have facial fractures alone. A study carried out by Chan et al. (2004) illustrated that from their sample of 201 young children, 20.3% received both facial and skull fractures compared with 50.4% of 139 adults who received just the facial fracture with no skull damage. The research can help support the idea that there is a higher vulnerability for skull fractures in the young population.

Secondary Brain Injury

These injuries occur as a result of the primary brain injury. It is commonly due to inadequate delivery of oxygen and nutrients to the brain, thereby causing severe consequences such as brain cell necrosis. The lack of oxygen to the brain is termed hypoxia. Low blood pressure (hypotension) can also occur; this is another detrimental factor in paediatric brain injuries, causing cardiorespiratory compromise. This can be in the form of cardiac dysfunction, respiratory failure as well as low vasomotor tone. A study carried out by Zebrack et al. (2009) identified from a sample of paediatric patients that the odds of death or long-term disability were 3 times higher for children who did not have their hypotension addressed.

A common pattern of injury in the developing brain is a subdural haematoma resulting from ruptured blood vessels in the subdural compartment and accompanying white matter damage (Raghupathi & Margulies, 2002). Haemorrhaging can be very dangerous. Hamilton and Keller (2010) identified that 20% of children with mild traumatic brain injuries sustain intracranial haemorrhaging.

Diagnosis

The signs and symptoms of brain injuries in infants and children are unconsciousness, seizures, paralysis, extreme irritability, increased head circumference, poor feeding, and/or excessive crying.

CT scans are performed primarily to identify any skull and/or facial fractures. This can also be done with an X-ray for further detail. If neurological symptoms and/or signs of brain damage are present, an MRI is requested. An MRI scan is best used for further detailed information regarding the extent of damage inflicted on the brain and better suggest the patient's prognosis. All tests are carried out and analysed by neurological specialists.

A key historical study by Kraus et al. (1987) reviewed 680 children and demonstrated that 23% had suffered at least one facial or skull fracture and 70% had been diagnosed with a concussion. In the total sample of patients, 85% received a skull radiograph and 82% received a CT scan. This illustrates the need for efficient diagnosis by combining diagnostic methods.

Along with imaging, a thorough subjective and physical examination is taken in order to guide and support treatment pathways. This is crucial and a GCS score is assessed immediately as a clinician must rely on clinical examinations, not on intercranial pressure (ICP) measurement, to see whether secondary brain injuries such as intracranial hypertension are developing (Mansfield, 2007).

Mansfield (2007) also states that frequent reassessment of the neurological examinations are required. These aspects of diagnosis are key to directing the paediatric patients' treatment and to observe progression or regression.

Management/Rehabilitation

With a spinal injury, it is vital to manage airways, breathing, and circulation. In severe head trauma, GCS scores are low and intubation is likely. As facial fractures and skull fractures may be present in conjunction in children, it is important to immobilise the region. This can be done using a collar to stabilise the cervical spine; this is a precaution in order to protect the spinal cord from damage and prevent neurological compromise.

Research shows that children who sustained mild traumatic brain injury with secondary brain injuries such as intracranial haemorrhage performed significantly worse in the Minnesota Multiphasic Personality Inventory-2 (MMPI-2). This test identified that children without intracranial haemorrhage scored no differently than the normative mean for educational length and employment rate.

Prito et al. (2007) identified that those who scored significantly worse also recorded more chronic fatigue, somatic complaints, and health problems. As a result, treatment can extend from treating symptoms such as flexion contractures and low blood pressure with medication as well as physiotherapy and rehabilitation. Active and passive range of movement along with massage and exercise prescription, amongst many techniques, are key in encouraging patients to re-learn lost basic motor skills.

In addition, functional rehabilitation is constantly adopted to aid in increasing a patient's quality of life. For the management of paediatric patients suffering from brain injuries, it is essential that all members of the multidisciplinary team address both short-term and long-term effects.

References

Baker, C., Kadish, H., & Schunk, J. E. *(1999). Evaluation of pediatric cervical spine injuries.* American Journal of Emergency Medicine, 17(3), 230–234.

Bazarian, S., McClung, J., Shah, M. N., Cheng, Y. T., Flesher, W., & Kraus, J. *(2005). Mild traumatic brain injury in the United States, 1998–2000. Brain Injury, 19(2), 85–91.*

Botterell, E. H., Callaghan, J. C., & Jousse, A. T. (1954). *Pain in paraplegia: Clinical management and surgical treatment. Proceeding of the Royal Society of Medicine, 47, 281–288.*

Brockmeyer, D., Apfelbaum, R., & Tippets, R., et al. (1995). *Pediatric cervical spine instrumentation using screw fixation. Pediatric Neurosurgery, 22, 147–157.*

Brown, R. L., Brunn, M. A., & Garcia, V. F. *(2001). Cervical spine injuries in children: A review of 103 patients treated consecutively at a level 1 pediatric trauma center. Journal of Pediatric Surgery, 36(8), 1107–1114.*

Case, M. E. (2007). *Abusive head injuries in infants and young children. Legal Medicine, 9(2), 83–87.*

Chan, D., Van Lierde, M., & Monstrey, S. *(2004). The age dependent relationship between facial fractures and skull fractures. International Journal of Pediatric Otorhinolaryngology, 68(7), 877–881.*

Clark, P., & Letts, M. (2001). *Trauma to the thoracic and lumbar spine in the adolescent. Canadian Journal of Surgery, 44(5), 337–345.*

Dean, N. P., Boslaugh, S., Adelson, P. D., et al. (2007). *Physician agreement with evidence-based recommendations for the treatment of severe traumatic brain injury in children. Journal of Neurosurgery, 107, 387–391.*

Eleraky, M. A, Theodore, N., Adams, M., et al. (2000). *Pediatric cervical spine injuries: Report of 102 cases and review of the literature. Journal of Neurosurgery, 92, 12–17.*

Gore, P. A. et al. (2009). *Cervical spine injuries in children: Attention to radiographic differences and stability compared to those in the adult patient. Seminars in Pediatric Surgery, 16(1), 42–58.*

Hachen, H. J. (1978). *Spinal cord injury in children and adolescents: Diagnostic pitfalls and therapeutic considerations in the acute stage. Paraplegia, 15(1), 55–64.*

Haller, J. A. Pediatric trauma. The no. 1 killer of children (commentary). 1983. *Journal of American Medical Association, 249, 47.*

Hamilton, M., & Myles, S. (1992). *Pediatric spinal injury: Review of 174 admissions. Journal of Neurosurgery, 77, 700–704.*

Hamilton, N. A., & Keller, M. S. (2010). Mild traumatic brain injury in children. Seminars in Pediatric Surgery, 19(4), 271–278.

Harkema, S. J. (2012). Locomotor training: As a treatment of spinal cord injury and in the progression of neurologic rehabilitation. Archives of Physical Medicine and Rehabilitation, 93(1), 1588–1597.

Huerta, C., Griffith, R., & Joyce, S. M. (1987). Cervical spine stabilization in pediatric patients: Evaluation of current techniques. Annals of Emergency Medicine, 16, 1121–1126.

Kay, T., Harrington, D. E., & Adams, R., et al. (1998). Definition of mild traumatic brain injury. Journal of Head Trauma Rehabilitation, 8, 86–87.

Kelly, M. A., & Stokes, K. S. (1986). Standing and ambulation for the child with paraplegia or tetraplegia. In R. R. Betz & M. J Mulcahey (Eds.), The child with a spinal cord injury (pp. 519–532). Rosemont, IL: American Academy of Orthopaedic Surgeons.

Kennard, M. A. (1936). Age and other factors in motor recovery from precentral lesions in monkeys. American Journal of Physiology, 115, 138–146.

Kenter, K., Zuckerbraun, B. S., Morrison, K., & Gaines, B. (2001). Pediatric traumatic atlanto-occipital dislocation: Five cases and a review. Journal of Pediatric Orthopaedics, 21(5), 585–589.

Kirkwood, Carroll, L. J., Cassidy, J. D., Peloso, P. M., & Borg, J. (2006). pediatric sport-related concussion: A review of the clinical management of an oft-neglected population. Pediatrics, 117(4), 1359–1371.

Klassen, R. A. (1994). Fractures and dislocations of the thoracolumbar spine. In R. M. Letts (Ed.), Management of pPediatric fFractures (p. 853) New York, NY: Churchill Livingstone,.

Kraus, B., Fife, D., & Conroy, C. (1987). Pediatric brain injuries: The nature, clinical course, and early outcomes in a defined United States' population. Pediatrics, 79(4), 501–507.

Kreykes, N. S. et al. (2010). Current issues in the diagnosis of pediatric cervical spine injury. Seminars in Pediatric Surgery, 19(1), 257–264.

Launay, F., Leet, A. I., Sponseller, P. D. (2005). Pediatric spinal cord injury without radiographic abnormality: A meta-analysis. Clinical Orthopaedics Related Research, 4, 67, 166–170.

Leonard, M. et al. (2007). Paediatric spinal trauma and associated injuries. Injury, International Journal of the Care of the Injured, 38(1), 188–193.

Little, J. W., Mickleson, P., & Umlauf, R., et al. (1989). Lower extremity manifestations of spasticity in chronic spinal cord injury. American Journal of Physical Medicine & Rehabilitation, 68, 32–36.

Lopez Alvarez, et al. (2011). Severe pediatric head injuries (I). Epidemiology, clinical manifestations and course. Medicina Intensiva, 35(6), 331–336.

Mansfield, R. T. (2007). *Severe traumatic brain injuries in children.* Clinical Pediatric Emergency Medicine, 8(3), 156–164.

Mathison, D. J. et al. (2008). *Spinal cord injury in the pediatric patient.* Clinical Pediatric Emergency Medicine, 9(1), 106–123.

Mazrani, W., McHugh, K., & Marsden, P. J. (2007). *The radiation burden of radiological investigations.* Archives Disease in Childhood, 92, 1127–31.

Morrow, S. E., & Pearson, M. (2010). *Management strategies for severe closed head injuries in children.* Seminars in Pediatric Surgery, 19(4), 279–285.

Mulcahey, M. J. (1986). *Upper eExtremity oOrthoses and sSplints. In R. R. Betz & M. J. Mulcahey (Eds.),* The child with a spinal cord injury *(pp. 373–392). Rosemont, IL: American Academy of Orthopaedic Surgeons.*

Nash, M. S. (2005). *Exercise as a health-promoting activity following spinal cord injury.* Journal of Neurologic Physical Therapy, 29, 87–103, 106.

NSPCC., & Cardiff University. (2009). Head and spinal injuries in children *(pp. 01–06). London: NSPCC Publications.*

Pang, D., & Wilberger, J. E. (1982). *Spinal cord injury without radiographic abnormalities in children.* Journal of Neurosurgery, 57, 114–29.

Powell, J. W., Barber-Foss, K. D. (1999). *Traumatic brain injury in high school athletes.* The Journal of the American Medical Association, 282, 958–963.

Prito. A., Chen. J. K., & Johnston, K. M. (2007). *Contributions of functional magnetic resonance imaging (fMRI) to sport concussion evaluation.* NeuroRehabilitation, 22, 217–227.

Raghupathi, R., Margulies, S. S. (2002). *Traumatic axonal injury after closed head injury in the neonatal pig.* Journal of Neurotrauma, 19, 843–53.

Renshaw, T. S. (1994). *Traumatic spondylolysis and spondylolisthesis. In R. M Letts (Ed.),* Management of pediatric fractures *(pp. 1195–1212). New York, NY: Churchill Livingstone.*

Seal, C. et al. (2005). *The management of pediatric cervical spine injuries.* Seminars in Spine Surgery, 17(2), 95–99.

Silber, J. S., Flynn, J. M., & Koffler, K. M. (2001). *Analysis of the cause, classification, and associated injuries of 166 consecutive pediatric pelvic fractures.* Journal of Pediatric Orthopeadics, 21, 446–50.

Singh, A., et al. (2011). *An overview of spinal injuries in children: Series of 122 cases.* Indian Journal of Neurotrauma, 11(1), 25–32.

Tsai, et al. (2004). *Pediatric traumatic brain injuries in Taiwan: An 8-year study.* Journal of Clinical Neuroscience, 11(2), 126–129.

Vialle, L. R., & Vialle, E. (2005). *Pediatric spine injuries.* Pediatric Spine Injuries, 36(2), S104–S112.

Vogel, L. C. (1996). *Management of medical issues. In R. R Betz & M. J. Mulcahey (Eds.),* The child with a spinal cord injury *(pp. 201–202). Rosemont, IL: American Academy of Orthopaedic Surgeons.*

Yucesoy, K., & Yuksel, Z. K. (2008). *SCIWORA in MRI era.* Clinical Neurology and Neurosurgery, 110(5), 429–433.

Zebrack, M., Dandoy, C., & Hansen. K., et al. (2009). *Early resuscitation of children with moderate-to-severe traumatic brain injury.* Pediatrics, 124, 56–64.

Zidek, K., & Srinivasana, R. (2003). *Rehabilitation of a child with a spinal cord injury.* Seminars in Pediatric Neurology, 10(2), 140–150.

CHAPTER 15

Emergencies in Children and Adolescent Sport

Solomon Abrahams

Introduction

Unintentional injuries in children's sport account for a significant number of admissions to emergency departments. Present-day emphasis on children participating in physical activity has produced a vast increase in the number of injuries to adolescents (Simon et al., 2004).

Recent research has suggested the most common emergencies in children's sports are superficial injury (i.e. contusions), ligament sprain (severe), musculotendinous strain, concussion, head and brain injuries, spinal injury, cardiopulmonary pathology, sudden death, seizure, pneumothorax, fractures of the extremities and head and neck trauma/injuries (Rennie & Court-Brown, 2007).

Head and neck (spinal) injuries, brain injuries, spinal cord injuries, muscular strains, contusions and pneumothorax are dealt with in more depth in other sections. This section will, therefore, focus on the other emergencies.

These more serious injuries generally occur through traumatic incidents or via the influence of external factors (Shanmugam & Maffulli, 2008). It has been stated previously that these injuries are less common in professional clubs and their academies, meaning most will occur in school sport and lower-league activity (Habelt & Hasler, 2011).

Extremity Fractures

A bone fracture is a complete or incomplete discontinuity of bone caused by a direct or indirect force. It is one of the most common injuries recorded in the youth and the elderly due to the porous structure of the bone that causes weak points where fractures occur. Within children's sports, fractures are due to falls that impact on the bone affected. They can also be caused by trauma or impact from an external force (Hedstrom & Svensson, 2010).

The most common type of fracture in this instance is to the extremities of the children, usually in the distal forearm; yet research remains controversial as to where the most common fracture site is. This was supported by a recent retrospective study, which suggested that fractures are more common in the upper limb due to the reactive breaking force when falling on to a playing surface. In addition to the falling mechanism of fractures in the upper limb, children can sustain lower limb fractures.

Lower limb fractures are mainly caused by a mechanism involving twisting and weight bearing. The incidence of fractures in cycling is relatively high among youths due to the involvement of the bicycle and the falling mechanism. Reviews of previous research state that long bone fractures were caused by falling; however, fractures of the axial skeleton, hands, and feet were more often caused by collisions or blunt traumas in sport (Rennie & Court-Brown, 2007).

Fractures frequently show similar signs and symptoms in the acute phase of children's injury. The most common signs of fractures are by the mechanism of injury to the area, such as falling or twisting while the extremity is fixed. However, this injury can also produce deformity of the bone and a dramatic reduction in range of motion, along with associated swelling and possible contusion due to the damage of surrounding soft tissues and blood vessels.

Assessment of fractures is limited initially to a clinical examination of the area. The child would have restricted mobility of this limb, and movement would cause unanticipated pain.

Fractures can often be associated with these problems due to possible displacement of the bone and link to swelling of the surrounding soft tissue. Diagnosis is made using radiography. Several types of images can be used to diagnose the fracture, although the methods used can vary depending on the type of fracture sustained. Some types of fractures can be considerably harder to analyse using methods that are used on simple fractures (Kraus & Wessel, 2010). Therapeutic ultrasound is a less common method of testing fractures; however, an ultrasound scan over the fracture site can reproduce the pain.

Fractures are immediately immobilised in order to aid pain relief and possible swelling, although the main reasoning is to aid alignment of bone displacement. Various conservative treatments, as well as surgical intervention, are available. The treatment option will depend on the damage to the bone, the location of the fracture, and the age of the child. Surgical intervention aims to stabilise the bone and reduce any risk of re-displacement. Conservative methods aim to manipulate the site to re-establish the structure of the bone, excluding the chance of re-displacement.

When this is achieved, rehabilitation will aim to re-establish the range of motion and stability around the area. This should be achieved after the fracture is stable enough to complete simple motion. In later stages of rehabilitation, full range of motion and strength of the bone and associated muscles will be further developed in order to weight bear and progress into movement and return to sport.

Concussion

Concussion is a mild form of trauma injury of the brain that is commonly caused due an impact injury to the head. This injury can also be caused by a jolt to the head, which produces trauma to the brain (Kirkwood et al., 2006).

The primary cause of this injury is the rotational acceleration of the brain in relation to its cranial setting. It has been suggested that increasing the muscle strength and improving the tone of the muscles around the cervical spine can reduce the impact of acceleration on the brain due to the injury (Meehan et al., 2011).

Prevalence of concussion in children's sport is relatively constant. In the United States alone, there are approximately 300,000 sports-related traumatic brain injuries, of which almost a third of the cases are seen in children and adolescents (Kirkwood et al., 2006).

Traumatic brain injuries vary between youths and adults due to the development of the brain and demands of a child's brain to engage and retain information and motor skills. It has been found that diffuse brain swelling is more common in younger patients and results from the differing impact from that of an adult (Meehan et al., 2011).

The difference between adults and children has been explained by the change in neural depolarisation, release of excitatory neurotransmitters, ionic shifts, altered glucose metabolism, cerebral blood flow, and the brain water content. The incidence of brain swelling and cerebral oedema after moderate brain trauma can partially explain the difference between concussion in youths and adults. Children have been found more susceptible to second impact syndrome, where a child suffers a second trauma to the head while still symptomatic from a previous concussion. The fundamental aspect behind this syndrome is the disruption to the autoregulation of the brain's blood supply (Collins, 2009).

Signs and symptoms of concussion are divided in physical, cognitive, sleep, and emotional impacts (US Department of Health and Human Services, 2010). The most common symptom reported by youths with concussion is the headache sensation (Blinman et al., 2009). Mental fogginess can also be present with concussion, as well as similar signs to anxiety and depression (Collins, 2009). Symptoms must be monitored after the trauma to assess improvement or regression.

Most concussions will recover in the initial phase of hours, days, or a week. However, traumatic brain injuries vary hugely regardless of any patient's characteristics and factors affecting injury. As each subject is different, treatment and management methods will be diverse and specific to the individual. There is little definitive diagnosis for concussion. Clinical reasoning is the most common diagnostic measure for concussion, along with the use of questioning, awareness analysis, and balance and coordination testing.

There is little treatment or management of concussion, other than observation of the child and rest from physical activity. Therefore, there is also little rehabilitation that can be done in relation to traumatic brain injuries.

Ligament injuries

Ligament injuries, in particular tears, were once considered rare among younger children. However, they have become much more frequent particularly with MCL injuries. Ligament injuries are the damage or tear of the ligament fibres, altering the structure and integrity of the ligament. A study showed that of the athletes around the age 12 with ligament disruptions, 90% had intrasubstance tears (Kellenberger & von Laer, 1990). This type of injury becomes increasingly common as children develop further.

Ligament injuries most commonly occur with a twisting motion whilst weight bearing in the lower limb or stretching the ligaments beyond their anatomical capabilities. The fibres of the ligaments stretch until the point of tearing, and the structure is compromised. An injured ligament shows signs of instability, and the patient will report swelling, pain, and possible discolouration. When testing, the ligament will also show laxity and further pain, along with a reduction in range of motion.

An MRI scan may be performed to ascertain whether an ACL tear has occurred. Although MRI has a good ability to predict ACL disruption, with a specificity of 95%, clinical examination is still principal in reasoning the depth of disruption (Lee et al., 1999). Tests will include drawer tests, varus/valgus stress tests, and Lachman's special test.

Conservative treatment of an ACL tear can lead to severe instability and poor knee function, and the patient risks sustaining secondary injuries, such as meniscal problems. Conservative treatment will aim to reduce pain and swelling and regain range of motion stability. However, operative reconstruction of the ACL in skeletally immature patients has the potential to cause growth issues.

In the later stage of rehabilitation, the aim is to achieve hypertrophy and neuromuscular control of the affected area. In order to achieve this, the subject will partake in a combination of balance and stability exercises with strength aspects, such as squats and lunging. This will allow the child to return to physical activity with a reduced chance of re-injury.

Cardiopulmonary Disease

The prevalence of cardiovascular disease in the young athlete population remains low; however, once their level of participation increases from non-competitive to competitive, some individuals are at an increased risk of cardiopulmonary problems (Wier et al., 2011).

Congenital heart disease occurs in 10% per 1000 young infants. Supraventricular tachycardia is the most common paediatric arrhythmia. It is idiopathic, or associated with a congenital heart defect, and is categorised by a fixed heart rate greater than 200 beats per minute. It presents itself in 3 different forms: firstly, atrioventricular (AV) nodal or junctional tachycardia caused by dual AV node pathways; secondly, ectopic atrial tachycardia; or thirdly, the most common cause of non-sinus tachycardia in children, which is AV rentrant tachycardia from the occurrence of an accessory bypass pathway (bundle of Kent).

The development of clinical symptoms for children with supraventricular tachycardia can take several hours or even days. Treatment such as vagal manoeuvres, including unilateral carotid massage or the Valsava manoeuvre, can be used to convert the rhythm. Also, crushed ice in a plastic bag can be applied to the face for up to 30 seconds. If this treatment is unsuccessful or if the patient is haemodynamically unstable, pharmacological interventions may be used, including administration of adenosine (0.05 mg per kg; up to 4 mg) as a rapid intravenous bolus. Further treatment includes digoxin, beta blockers, or oesophageal overdrive pacing, with cardiology consultation (Birrer et al., 2002).

Myocarditis results from a viral or bacterial illness. Enlargement of the heart chambers and impairment of the left ventrical function are viewed from a echocardiograph. Bed rest, diuretics, inotropes, digoxin, gamma globulin, and steroids can be used as treatment alongside a cardiology consultation (Wier et al., 2011).

There is a decline in physical activity participation in the adolescent population. Therefore, an increase in encouragement of participation should take place, once a child reaches adolescence. Thorough pre-participation examinations should identify specific health risks associated with an athlete taking part in physical activity, in particular any underlying cardiovascular or pulmonary disease.

Sudden Death Syndrome

Sudden athletic death has been defined as non-traumatic death. The onset of symptoms occurs during or within an hour of participation. Prevalence is low, ranging from 1 death per 280,000 to 1 death 735,000 persons per year. Van Camp et al. from the National Centre for Catastrophic Sports Injury

Research found that males have a fivefold higher risk than females, and college athletes had a twofold higher risk than high school athletes.

The most common cause of non-traumatic sports deaths in younger athletes is related to congenital cardiovascular structural abnormalities. The most prevalent of which is hypertrophic cardiomyopathy (HCM) followed by coronary artery anomaly and myocarditis. HCM can predispose an individual to malignant ventricular arrhythmias leading to syncope or sudden death. A systolic crescendo-decrescendo murmur may be heard upon a physical examination. It increases in intensity with Valsava or on standing, and decreases when squatting or with isometric hand–gripping exercises. However, the best form of diagnosis is through a two-dimensional and *M*-mode echocardiogram. Congenital coronary anomalies may also cause sudden death in athletes, the most common of which is anomalous origin of the left main coronary from the right sinus of Valsava.

Early referral to a cardiologist for risk assessment and treatment is recommended due to the high risk of sudden death in athletes. Treatment includes a calcium channel blockade, A-V sequential pacing, and/or septal ablation with intra-cardiac alcohol infusion.

Due to the rarity and lack of symptoms of sudden cardiac death, the development of screening strategies remains limited. A focused periodic approach with emphasis on medical history is the current consensus in literature. Further research and refinement of current screening techniques will result in more effective and efficient diagnosis.

Seizures

Seizures can be classified as partial, general, or unclassified. It is a common neurologic disorder affecting more than 1 million people. Seizures should be managed with oxygen to ensure prevention of hypoxia and rolling to one side to avoid oral blockage. Because the seizure will be of unknown cause, an immediate emergency referral should be made.

A regular exercise programme has been found to be beneficial in controlling seizures. Seizures themselves are not seen to be a hazard of epilepsy, but the associated emotional irregularity is of concern. If all relevant precautions, protocols, and specific limitations are followed, there is no reason why participation in sport should be denied.

Conclusion

Common injuries are found in children's sport, resulting in admission to emergency centres and hospitals. The most common emergency in children's sports is fractures to the extremities due to the under development of bone in children and its porous structure. Treatment of each injury is similar as the most important factor is the psychological impact on the child after injury and the demands of the clinician to adapt exercises to suit them. Due to the developmental stages of children, each injury will differ from that of adults in relation to typical anatomical knowledge of each injury in the older population.

Key Points

- Cardiopulmonary injuries increase dramatically with eliteness in children.

- Supraventricular hypertrophy is the most common arrthymia in children

- Sudden death is rare; it is 5 times more likely in males.

References

Birrer, R., Griesemer, B., & Cataletto, M. (2002). *Pediatric sports medicine for primary care* (2nd ed.). Lippincott: Willians and Wilkins.

Blinman, T. A., Houseknecht, E., Snyder, C., Wiebe, D. J. & Nance, M. L. (2009). Post concussive symptoms in hospitalized pediatric patients after mild traumatic brain injury. *Journal of Pediatric Surgery, 44*(6),1223–1228.

Collins, M. W. (2009, July). Update: concussion. *American Orthopaedic Society for Sports Medicine.*

Habelt, S., & Hasler, C. (2011). Sports injuries in adolescents. *Orthopaedic Reviews 2011, 3*, e18.

Hedstrom, E. & Svensson, O. (2010). Epidemiology of fractures in children and adolescents. *Acta orthopaedica, 81*(1),148–153.

Kellenberger, R., & von Laer, L. (1990). Nonosseous lesions of the anterior cruciate ligaments in childhood and adolescence. *Progress Pediatric Surgery, 25*, 123–131.

Kirkwood, M., Yeates, K., & Wilson, P. (2006). Pediatric sport-related concussion: A review of the clinical management of an oft-neglected population. *Paediatrics, 17*(4), 466-469.

Kraus, R., & Wessel, L. (2010). The treatment of upper limb fractures in children and adolescents. *Deutsches Arzteblatt international, 107*(51–52) 903–910.

Lee, K., Siegel, M. J., & Lau, D. M. (1999). Anterior cruciate ligament tears: MR imaging-based diagnosis in a pediatric population. *Radiology, 213*, 697–704.

Meehan, W., Taylor, A., & Proctor, M. (2011). The paediatric athlete: Athletes with sport related concussion. *Clinics in Sports Medicine, 30*(1),133.

Rennie, L., & Court-Brown, C. (2007). The epidemiology of fractures in children. *Injury,38*(8), pp. 913–922.

Shanmugam, C., & Maffulli, N. (2008). Sports injuries in children. *British Medical Bulletin, 86*(1), 33–57.

Simon, T., Bublitz, C., & Hambidge, S. (2004). External causes of pediatric injury-related emergency department visits in the United States. *Academic Emergency Medicine, 11*(10), pp. 1042–1048.

US Department of Health and Human Services, Public Health Service, CDC. (2010). DeWitt DS. Atlanta, GA: Centers for Disease Control and Prevention, National Center for Injury Prevention and Control; 2010

Wier, L., Miller, A., & Steiner, C. (2011). Sports injuries in children requiring hospital emergency care. *Agency for Healthcare Research and Quality, 54*, 3, 203-206.

CHAPTER 16

Common Medical Problems in Children and Adolescent Sport

Richard Seah and Solomon Abrahams

Introduction

Unlike the older athlete, whose medical problems tend to be degenerative in nature (e.g. osteoarthritis, ischaemic heart disease, cerebrovascular disease, dementia), the younger athlete is more likely to be troubled by issues arising from congenital and environmental causes.

As traumatic and overuse musculoskeletal issues are dealt with in other chapters in this book, these are not discussed in great detail within this chapter.

The following diseases and conditions are discussed in this chapter:

- Asthma

- Diabetes mellitus

- Epilepsy

- Infections

- Limping in the child

- Gastrointestinal pathologies

- Dermatological pathologies

Some of these conditions can present as medical emergencies. Acute exacerbations of asthma can give rise to status asthmaticus, infections can fulminate and cause severe sepsis, and epilepsy can lead on to status epilepticus.

Treatment in the context discussed below relates to non-life-threatening situations and addresses prevention strategies.

Asthma

This is a chronic respiratory disorder, characterised by recurrent attacks of shortness of breath and difficult breathing, especially on exhalation, that is related to increased airflow resistance through the bronchioles. There is associated allergic inflammation to the airways. In the context of sport with exercise behaving as a major precipitant, this is termed 'exercise-induced asthma' (Asthma UK, 2012).

Prevalence

During childhood, asthma is more common in boys than in girls. At puberty, this trend reverses as more girls develop asthma for the first time. By the age of 18 years, asthma is seen more commonly in women.

The prevalence in the United Kingdom of a 14-year-old ever having been given a diagnosis of asthma is around 20%. The United Kingdom has one of the highest prevalence for childhood asthma internationally, with about 15% affected (Brukner et al., 2010).

Symptoms and Signs

Asthma can present itself through an audible wheeze, shortness of breath, or chest tightness. The patient will complain of a breathing difficulty, particularly when exhaling. Exercise can induce these responses due to airway hyperactivity, typically between 5 and 10 minutes of strenuous exertion. There is an underlying inflammatory process described as an asthmatic response. Both heat and water losses in the airway are believed to trigger symptoms (Birrer, Griesemer, & Cataletto, 2002).

Differential Diagnosis

The following conditions should be considered amongst the differential diagnosis: allergic rhinitis, bronchiolitis, cystic fibrosis, disordered breathing, foreign body in airway, and gastroesophageal reflux disease (GORD).

Investigations

Investigations like peak expiratory flow rate (PEFR) may be used in the diagnosis of asthma. However, this diagnostic tool can possibly misdiagnose a patient with poor fitness levels who may also have low PEFR rate confusing them with Asthmatics. The other elements of diagnosis include history, physical examination, response to therapy, pulmonary function tests, exercise challenge tests, and X-rays and CT scans of the thorax.

Allergy testing can be carried out to identify the allergens (triggers) that may precipitate asthma symptoms.

Management

Medications, often in the form of inhalers, are the mainstay of treatment. Beta$_2$ agonists (e.g. Salbutamol) are used as 'relievers' to treat the acute symptoms. Inhaled corticosteroids and long-acting beta agonists (LABA) are used to prevent deterioration of symptoms and need to be used regularly. More recently, leukotriene antagonists have also had a role to play for patients with brittle asthma.

Seeing the asthma nurse to receive patient education about the condition is vital to understanding the condition and controlling the symptoms. It is important to try to minimise exposure to possible allergens and precipitants.

Regular asthma monitoring and review with a general practitioner or an asthma specialist is recommended.

Diabetes Mellitus

This in an endocrine disease and a disorder of carbohydrate metabolism characterised by an increased blood glucose level (also known as hyperglycaemia) and glucose in the urine (glycosuria).

Traditionally, this has been classified into two types: *type 1 diabetes*, which is also known as insulin-dependent diabetes mellitus (IDDM) or juvenile-onset diabetes; and *type 2 diabetes*, also known as non-insulin-dependent diabetes mellitus (NIDDM) or adult-onset diabetes.

315

Type 1 diabetes mellitus is caused by the progressive destruction of the pancreatic beta cells, by either an autoimmune or an idiopathic process. Type 2 diabetes mellitus is a defect in both insulin secretion and its action upon the liver and peripheral muscle and is most common in patients aged 40 years or more; however, obesity in adolescence is leading to a higher incidence of type 2 diabetes in youths (Diabetes UK).

Prevalence

In the paediatric and adolescent population, type 1 diabetes is more common with approximately 90% of young people with diabetes suffering from it (Diabetes UK).

Due to increasing levels of inactivity and childhood obesity, levels of type 2 diabetes are rising in the paediatric population, both within the United Kingdom and in the world. Previously, this was very rare.

Symptoms and Signs

The initial presenting symptoms of the disease include excessive thirst, fatigue, frequent urination, irritability, and marked unintentional weight loss.

More specifically, type 1 diabetes mellitus leads to a decrease in insulin production, which predisposes young athletes to hyperglycaemia, weight loss, and ketoacidosis. Over the long term, this can lead to retinopathy, nephropathy, and neuropathy, coronary, and peripheral atherosclerosis. Type 2 diabetes mellitus presents with elevated blood glucose levels and the absence of ketosis (Birrer et al., 2002).

Differential Diagnosis

It is important to distinguish between type 1 and type 2 diabetes. Other causes of hyperglycaemia (raised blood sugar), including physiological stresses caused by acute infection and trauma, need to be considered.

Blood tests (blood glucose, HBA1c, which is a long-term marker of diabetes control) and urine dipstick (for the presence of ketones and glucose) should be done.

Management

Management of type 1 diabetes involves the regular administration of insulin medication, usually by subcutaneous injections.

Patient education by the diabetes nurse and dietary advice by a nutritionist help to address the preventative aspects of the condition.

There should be a regular review by a general practitioner and /or diabetes specialist to ensure that diabetic control is adequate and that secondary complications of diabetes (e.g. hypertension, renal disease, peripheral neuropathy) do not develop subsequently (Diabetes UK).

Epilepsy

This is a common neurologic disorder that is characterised as recurrent seizures that are unrelated to fever or acute cerebral insult. Most people who develop epilepsy have their first seizure when they are young. Young athletes may experience limitations or restrictions to exercise because of their epilepsy. However, a regular exercise programme has been found to be beneficial in controlling seizures (Brukner et al., 2010).

Prevalence

Seizures and epilepsy affect infants and children more than any other age group. Epilepsy is about twice as common in children compared with adults (about 700 per 100,000 children).

Symptoms and Signs

In *idiopathic epilepsy*, the cause is unclear and is not associated with structural damage to the brain. This presents as *generalised epilepsy*, which can take the form of either *grand mal* or *petit mal seizures* (see below). In contrast, *Partial epilepsy* is a symptom of structural disease of the brain. The nature of the symptoms depends on the area of brain affected.

In *grand mal seizures*, also known as major or tonic-clonic seizures, the patient becomes unconscious with muscles in a state of spasm. This tonic phase fades to give way to a clonic phase, in which convulsive movements, including tongue biting and urinary incontinence, can occur.

In *petit mal seizures*, also known as minor or absence seizures, there are brief spells of unconsciousness that last only for a few seconds, but balance and posture is often maintained. There are associated fluttering eyelid movements and twitching of the mouth and fingers. As there are no convulsive elements to this, appearances are often much less dramatic than *grand mal seizures* (Brukner et al., 2010).

Differential Diagnosis

There are several other causes of seizures. These include both acute and chronic pathologies: alcohol intoxication, cerebral abscess, electrolyte abnormality, encephalitis, febrile convulsions, hypoglycaemia, hypoxia, medication induced, meningitis, trauma, and brain tumours.

Investigations

The following investigations can be carried out to make the diagnosis: MRI brain scan, CT brain scan, and EEG (electroencephalography) to look at brain activity; blood tests to look for electrolyte abnormalities and prolactin levels; lumbar puncture and cerebrospinal fluid analysis to look for infection; and urine dipstick to look for signs of diabetes.

Management

Early management of convulsions should be paramount in the prevention of further seizures.

Anticonvulsant medication is the mainstay of epilepsy treatment. These need to be taken regularly.

Avoidance of precipitants (e.g. loud noises, flashing lights, excessive fatigue, use of illicit drugs) and regular reviews by a general practitioner and/or epilepsy specialist are essential (Birrer et al., 2002).

Infections

There can be an invasion of the body by pathogens such as bacteria, viruses, fungi, and protozoa. The infective agent can be acquired by different modes of transmission. Examples include droplet spread (influenza, infectious mononucleosis), direct skin contact (tinea pedis or athlete's foot, herpes gladiatorum or scrum pox), faecal–oral spread (gastroenteritis or food poisoning), insect-borne (malaria), and sexual intercourse (gonorrhoea, chlamydia, HIV).

The incubation period varies, after which time symptoms often appear. Symptoms can be localised or systemic, affecting the entire body.

Systemic symptoms often involve pain, fatigue, fever, and a general feeling of illness.

Investigations

Blood tests (full blood count, inflammatory markers CRP and ESR, monospot test, immunoglobulin counts, viral loads) are usually carried out. Imaging (chest X-rays and CT scan of thorax for pneumonia, ultrasound scan of the liver for amoebic abscesses) can also be helpful.

It is also worth considering procedures like a urine dipstick (for urinary tract infections or UTIs), specimen swabs (for infected wounds and sexually transmitted diseases) and joint aspiration (for suspected joint infections).

Management

Prevention (simple lifestyle measures such as adequate rest and hydration, hand gel, isolation for highly contagious infections to prevent rest of team being affected) can be very effective.

Consider immunisations (e.g. the 'flu jab'), particularly if an athlete is travelling to a susceptible area/ country to train or to compete.

Medication options include topical antibiotics for local bacterial infections (e.g. skin, eye) and oral or intravenous antibiotics for systemic bacterial infections. Antiviral medications are reserved for severe cases.

Both antibiotics and antiviral agents should be used prudently to prevent the development of antimicrobial resistance.

Limping in the Child

A child who presents with a limp for any prolonged period of time must always be taken seriously. There are several causes for a limping child.

Prevalence

The age of the child can be very helpful for determining what the likely diagnosis will be (see below). Gender can also be a helpful pointer. For example, Perthes disease is seen more commonly in males.

Symptoms and Signs

Look for systemic signs of ill health, which include fever, irritability, and drowsiness. Other findings include an antalgic gait, leg length discrepancy, swelling, fixed flexion deformity of the hip, and warmth and tenderness on palpation.

Differential Diagnosis

Causes of a limp include transient synovitis, giving rise to an irritable hip (typically infant: 1–3 years), a developmental dysplasia of the hip (DDH) (typically infant: 1–3 years), Perthes disease (typically childhood: 3–11 years), a slipped upper femoral epiphysis (SUFE) (childhood or adolescence: 12–16 years), trauma, osteomyelitis, septic arthritis (any age), juvenile idiopathic arthritis (any age), and malignancy.

Investigations

These include blood tests (white cell count for infection and leukaemia and ESR and CRP for inflammation and infection), X-rays of the pelvis and the hip (this can reveal a dislocated hip, fracture, Perthes diseases, and SUFE), and ultrasound scans of the hip (hip effusion can be demonstrated in septic arthritis, transient synovitis, hip dislocation, and Perthes disease).

Joint aspiration for microscopy, culture, and sensitivity can be undertaken under ultrasound guidance if infection or inflammatory arthritis is suspected.

MRI scan (soft-tissue pathology, soft-tissue and bone tumours, osteomyelitis, transient synovitis) and isotope bone scan (for suspected malignancy and osteomyelitis) can also be utilised.

Management

Remember to examine the knee as referred pain from the knee can present as hip pain (e.g. Osgood–Schlatter disease, fracture involving the knee).

Analgesia is often required.

Treat the underlying cause; often the involvement of the general practitioner, paediatrician, and other hospital specialists (e.g. radiologists, orthopaedic surgeons) will be required.

Common Gastrointestinal Pathologies in Children and Teens

Gastrointestinal (GI) pathologies in children and teens are common due to changes in diet, stress-related factors (including sports-related factors), and genetics (Birrer et al., 2002). They can be prevalent in 1 in 4 children who participate in sport (Worobetz & Gerrad, 1985).

They are more common in girls and seem to worsen with extreme exercise and sport, even though some research suggests that sport can actually help reduce symptoms (Riddoch & Trinnick, 1988).

The most common childhood pathologies of the upper gastrointestinal tract include gastric emptying pathology, gastric reflux, and gastric bleeding (Birrer et al., 2002).

Gastric emptying occurs naturally after ingestion and digestion of food and drink. However, this can be delayed in some children who are nervous or under enormous emotional stress. This can cause vomiting and nausea during and after the sport. It is exacerbated by highly concentrated food and drinks, dehydration, and extreme exercise (Moses, 1990).

Gastric reflux and heartburn can occur in 10% of teen runners and quite simply is an increase in acidity in the oesophagus, possibly caused by poor sphincter control and swallowing excessive air in sport. This was observed in runners in a study in recreational runners, but the subject numbers were low (Krauss et al., 1990).

Gastrointestinal bleeds are less common in children, but can occur in adolescent runners. Possible mechanisms can be the constant vibration and shuddering of the stomach against other organs that cause bruising and hence, small amounts of bleeding. This can be compounded by acidic foods and drinks and the use of strong non-steroidal anti-inflammatory medication (Birrer et al., 2002).

Lower gastrointestinal pathologies in children and teens include cramps, diarrhoea, the need for a toilet, and faecal bleeding. These pathologies tend to be common in children and adolescent runners.

No conclusive evidence is available, but some authors suggest that running, in particular in a growing athlete, can cause intra-abdominal trauma as the organs rub on each other, causing irritation and pain/cramps. It can be further exacerbated by certain foods/drinks, dehydration or excessive hydration, certain medications, autonomic nervous system and a genetic predispotion to gastro intestinal (GI) problems (Sullivan, 1992).

Management of GI problems in young athletes includes advice on diet; preparation for sport; changes in duration, intensity, and frequency in sport; medications (including stimulants); and conditioning for sport.

If gastric complaints persist, further investigations may be required in the unlikely event that a sinister pathology could be underlying.

Dermatological Pathologies in Children and Teens

Dermatological problems in children are normally not serious, but can be psychologically damaging as well as irritable. For this age group, appearance is everything, and having a skin disorder can create problems with other children teasing them, especially in the changing rooms or when having a shower.

Acne

Acne is common in teen sports. A combination of hormonal changes, excessive activity which can block sebaceous glands of the skin, and possible bacterial influences can create spots on the body (including the face) with pus or blackheads. This can be very irritable and unattractive to the very conscious teen, who is going through enormous bodily changes (Goldstein & Goldstein, 1997).

Normally asymptomatic, they can be irritable, especially in adolescents who perspire or sweat during their sport, or are wearing clothing (and possibly braces or headgear) which can create extra heat.

Management normally involves dermatological preparations including low-dose steroid cream and, in some instances, antibiotics.

Bruising

Bruising is common in children and teens, especially in sports. They can develop from direct trauma and indirect trauma. For example, runners can develop a black heel where the epidermis of the skin rubs against the shoewear, causing an irritation and shearing of the capillary beds, and hence a bruise develops. This can also occur under toenails, in particular the first toe. This again is caused by repeated microtrauma and friction of the toenail against the shoewear. Bruising can be painful, and in extreme cases, analgesics can be used and the potential cause should be investigated and addressed (Birrer et al., 2002).

Eczema

Eczema in children is common, affecting mostly the knees and elbows. It is caused by an irritant or allergen, and usually, a family history of eczema is possible. Other allergies such as asthma and hay fever could be present in the family.

Eczema causes an itching and a dry rash in the joints of the body; it can occur on the body but is less common. Redness of the skin and bumpy spots can develop. It can be managed with low-dose steroidal creams, regular washing, and education (Goldstein & Goldstein, 1997).

Blisters

Blisters in children and teens in sport is common. Caused by an irritation and friction of the skin against clothing, the skin develops a localised fluid formation under the skin to cushion the area of friction. This can be very sore in a child or a teen, especially if the cause is not addressed. Commonly seen on the extremities of the body, it's more prevalent in stop-start sports or sports where there is continuous pounding. In some cases, bleeding can also occur which forms a blood blister, but this is no different in symptomology compared with a normal blister.

Blisters can be managed in various ways, including extra cushioning around the painful site, hydrogel dressings, and use of creams, plasters, and, in some cases, antibiotics if the blister becomes infected. Addressing the cause is important to avoid further development of blisters (Pharis et al., 1997).

Dermatitis

Childhood dermatitis is not common in children or teens, but it can certainly affect some children, especially in sport. It is an inflammation of the skin, normally caused by an irritant, including sweat, excessive heat, creams, taping, and some braces. It can cause itching of the skin, redness of the skin, and heat, and can be sore. It can be managed in various ways, including medication and investigation of the irritant (Goldstein & Goldstein, 1997).

Milliaria (Heat Rash)

Heat rash affects children and teens. Caused by excessive heat which causes blockage of the skin surface, it irritates the skin (Habif, 1996). Redness of the skin is common, and itchiness can be a symptom. It is self-limiting and can be controlled by avoiding tight clothes in the vicinity of the rash. Regular washing with normal soap and water can help.

Tinea Pedis

Tinea pedis is a common skin infection in children, commonly found on the feet. It is caused by moisture, friction, and an unclean surface. it is common in children and adolescents who do not wear shoewear on unclean surfaces and children who do not clean their feet on a regular basis. It can cause mild erythema, or white scales around the side of the foot and between the toes. It can cause a burning pain and itching (Pharis et al., 1997).

Management includes regular washing and drying of feet, wearing shoewear, and using antibacterial or antifungal powder preparations. Normally, education is enough to prevent it from returning.

Impetigo

This is a contagious skin infection caused by bacteria (either staphylococcus or streptococcus). It appears as patches of tiny, red, itchy blisters, often around the mouth and nose, though it can also occur elsewhere.

These blisters break open, oozing a yellow liquid, and then form yellowy-brown scabs. New blisters can form by touching existing sores and then transferring the bacteria to other parts of the body. The blisters usually appear 1–10 days after infection, depending on the type of bacteria present. Impetigo is highly contagious, being spread through touching someone with infected skin or sharing their personal items (i.e. bedsheets or clothing). It is more likely to develop on skin that has already been broken, through a cut or bite, for example (Habif, 1996).

Impetigo is usually treated with oral antibiotics or by washing the sores twice a day and applying a bactericidal cream. The infection can take 1 week to 10 days to cease, in which time the sores should be dressed to prevent its spread. Furthermore, the child's clothing and linen needs to be washed each day in this period. Encourage the child not to scratch and to wear gloves. Regularly wash your hands when treating impetigo (Birrer et al., 2002).

Moles

Moles are benign spots or marks on the skin and are of different shapes and sizes. Moles can jut out or lie flush with the skin, and their colour can range from beige or light pink to dark brown and even black. Some children are born with a few moles, though most develop the mole during their lifetime (Pharis et al., 1997).

Sun exposure can increase the number of moles on a child's skin; however, most of the time they are harmless and no treatment is required. Occasionally, melanoma, the most dangerous type of skin cancer, can arise from moles, though this is very rare in childhood. Nonetheless, it is wise to monitor your child's moles for any changes and speak to your doctor if you notice anything of concern.

Things to look for include moles which are uneven in shape, larger than 0.5 cm in size, have a blend of colours, are irregular or have blurred edges, or appear to be growing (Birrer et al., 2002).

Molluscum Contagiosum

This is a viral infection of the skin caused by a poxvirus. It is a contagious disease particularly common in young children. After approximately 2–3 months of the virus incubating, small, round growths begin to emerge. These are light pink or tan coloured and can look similar to warts. They can sometimes become red and irritated or have a tiny white spot in the centre.

Though they can develop anywhere, mollusca in children commonly appear on the face, arms, legs, or torso. They often arise in clusters in skin folds such as the armpits, behind the knees, or in the groin. Molluscum contagiosum is spread through touching infected skin or objects, and a child can extend them across their own body by touching or scratching the growths (Pharis et al., 1997).

While molluscum contagiosum usually resolves on its own over many months, treatment is recommended to stop its spread. Treatments include cryotherapy (freezing – usually with liquid nitrogen), curettage (removing with sharp instrument under local anaesthetic), laser therapy, use of astringents (substances which destroy the top layers of skin), and applying topical medications to the skin (Habif, 1996).

Ringworm

This is an itchy fungal infection of the skin which presents as scaly rings a couple of centimetres wide. Ringworm is contagious and is passed between contact with infected people, pets, and personal items (i.e. towels, hairbrushes, and clothing).

A topical antifungal usually needs to be applied to the affected areas for 3–4 weeks, continuing after the rash has disappeared. Occasionally, ringworm does not respond to treatment and a stronger prescription – topical or oral medication – will be required from your doctor (Habif, 1996).

The following steps can be taken to prevent reinfection: dry your child thoroughly and keep them cool, don't let your child share personal items, wash the child's linen and clothing, have pets with ringworm treated, and have children wear sandals in communal swimming or bathing areas.

Warts

Warts are benign growths or tumours, usually on the feet (plantar warts) or hands, caused by infection of the human papilloma virus. Warts will occasionally resolve without treatment; however, this can take months, and in the interim the virus within existing warts can proliferate and generate fresh ones. Thus, prompt professional treatment with salicylic acid, canthardin, or liquid nitrogen is recommended.

Key Points

- Asthma is on the increase and exercise-induced asthma remains undiagnosed in many children.

- Type 1 diabetes is more common in children.

- Type 2 is dramatically on the increase in children and adolescents.

- Abdominal complaints remain high in female athletes.

- Tinea pedia is the most common skin infection of the foot in children due to reduced hygiene.

References

Asthma UK (2012). Retrieved from www.asthma.org.uk.

Birrer, R., Griesemer, B., & Cataletto, M. (2002). *Pediatric sports medicine for primary care* (2nd ed.). Lippincott: Williams and Wilkins.

Brukner, P., & Khan. K., et al. (2010). *Clinical sports medicine* (4th ed.). New York, NY: McGraw Hill.

Diabetes.co.uk. Retrieved from www.diabetes.co.uk.

Goldstein, B., & Goldstein, A. (1997). *Practical dermatology* (2nd ed). St Louis, MO: Mosby.

Habif, T. (1996). *Clinical dermatology* (3rd ed.), St Louis: Mosby.

Krauss, B., Sinclair, J., & Castell, D. (1990). Gastrointestinal reflux in runners. *Annals of internal Medicine, 112,* 428.

Lissauer, T., & Clayden, G. (2007). *Illustrated textbook of paediatrics* (4th ed.). St Louis, MO: Mosby.

Marsland D, Kapoor, S., Coote. A., & Haslam, P. *Crash course: Rheumatology and Orthopaedics* (2nd ed.). St Louis, MO: Mosby.

Moses, F. (1990). The effect of exercise on the gastrointestinal tract. *Sports Medicine, 9,* 159.

Patient.co.uk. Retrieved from www.patient.co.uk.

Pharis, D., Teller, C., & Wolf, J. (1997). Cutaneous manifestations of sports participation. *Journal of Amercian Academy Dermatology, 36,* 448–459.

Riddoch, C., & Trinnick, T. (1988). Gastrointestinal disturbances in marathon runners. *Western Journal of Medicine, 141,* 481.

Sullivan, S. (1992). Overcoming runner's diarrhea. *Physician and Sports Medicine, 20,* 63–65.

Worobetz, I. & Gerrad, D. (1985). Gastrointestinal symptoms during exercise and endurance athletes. *New Zealand Medical Journal, 98,* 644.

CHAPTER 17

The Young Female Athlete in Sport

Solomon Abrahams and Stephanie Morgan

Female child and adolescent participation in sport has dramatically increased within the last 30 years (Lemstra, Nielsen, Rogers, Thompson, & Moraros, 2012). The association between regular physical activity and reductions in morbidity and mortality are well established and remain significant attractions for females to play sport. However, there is evidence that physical fitness levels in children are declining, perhaps due to an increase in sedentary lifestyle. The combination of increased exposure and decreased preparedness for sports participation has led to a rise of both acute and chronic sports-related injuries in this population. There are countless well-known health and social benefits for females who participate in sports and/or regular aerobic activity. However, unique injury patterns and medical conditions have been discovered in female athletes. Conditions usually arise through an athlete overtraining or detrimental psychological influences.

In 1992, the American College of Sports Medicine identified the negative aspects for the female adolescent athletes within sport. An association of disordered eating, amenorrhoea, and osteoporosis in athletes participating in sporting activities that emphasise a lean physique was realised. This condition was recognised as the 'female athlete triad' (see Fig. 17.1) (Thein-Nissenbaum & Carr, 2011).

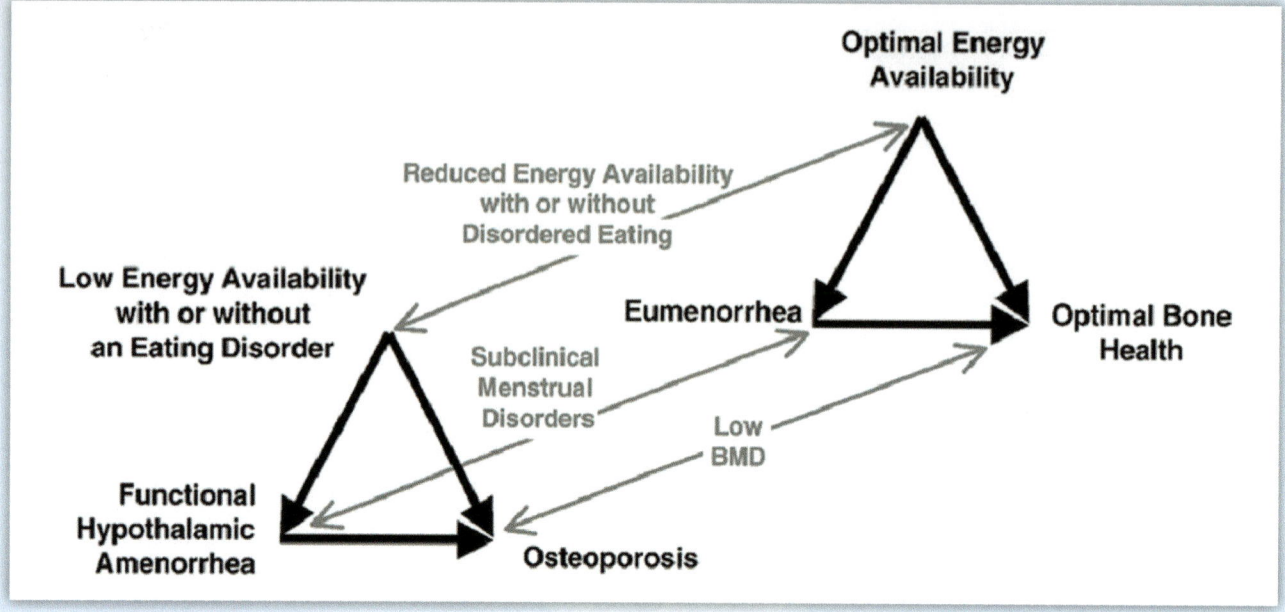

Fig. 17.1 Female athlete triad

The adolescent female athlete triad comprises 3 related disorders: disordered eating, menstrual disorders, and eventual osteoporosis. Performance is greatly determined upon the health state of these combined disorders. Early awareness and structured management can help prevent and/or treat such conditions. The detrimental combination of the physiological aspects of the triad in young adolescent girls can lead to optimal performance pressure.

Psychological stress releases cortisol which changes the endocrinologic control of the menstrual cycle and results in the risk of developing primary or secondary amenorrhoea. This is due to the dysfunction of the hypothalamus and pituitary gland, resulting in a decrease in the follicle-stimulating hormone (FSH) and luteinising hormone (LH). FSH and LH cause production of oestrogen and progesterone from the ovaries, which are responsible for regular menstruation. Oestrogen is also a highly influential hormone in maintaining sufficient bone mineral density. Hypoestrogenism is, therefore, associated with low bone mineral density and increased risk of osteoporosis (Birch, 2005).

Bone

MacKelvie, Khan, and McKay (2002) found that 26% of final bone mass is attained between ages 11.5 and 13.5 years in females. The researchers concluded that early puberty may represent the most critical time to participate in sports that emphasise weight-bearing and high-impact exercises, such as soccer, basketball, racquet games, step-aerobics, and speed skating. Therefore, exercising during growth could represent a primary prevention against the effects of ageing on bone (Ferry, Lespessaillesc, Rochcongard, Duclose, & Courteixa, 2012). An overall review of the influence of sports participation on bone health by Tenforde and Fredericson (2011) concluded that high-impact and odd-impact exercises promote and may help maintain peak bone mass and geometry.

Wolff's law states that in a healthy individual, bone strength increases in response to environmental stressors. Studies by Ferry et al. (2012) and Prelack, Dwyer, Ziegler, and Kehayias (2012) have shown that high-impact or odd-impact loading and weight-bearing activities enhance bone density and bone geometry in females, whereas non-impact sports such as cycling and swimming are not associated with improvements in bone health. Muscles generate the largest mechanical load and strain on bone. Further research by Ferry et al. (2012) has shown that sports involving high acceleration which produced larger loads on bones increases bone strength, compared with sports requiring submaximal forces, such as long-distance running.

Rauh, Nichols, and Barrack (2010) found that the overall causes of low bone mineral density are multifactorial; menstrual dysfunction and disordered eating are also factors that have been found to be associated with low bone mineral density. Reductions in bone mineral density have also been reported in retired female soccer players and female gymnasts. This seems to suggest that sport-specific gains in bone mass may decrease with de-training, and the continual encouragement for female sports participation should be encouraged.

However, adolescent participation in sport has shown to increase bone mineral composition and bone mineral density (Tenforde & Fredericson, 2011). Overall, this suggests that an increase in bone strength provides an athlete with greater resistance against fractures in the future.

Menses (Menstrual cycle)

Roupas and Georgopoulos (2011) described that the main factors relating to menstrual disturbances in athletes included weight, body composition, stress (physical and psychological), energy imbalance, diet, type of sport, and the state of reproductive maturity. They also found that female athletic performance had been associated with a broad spectrum of menstrual dysfunction. Adolescent menstrual dysfunction is extremely common during the first few years following menarche. However, after the first 1–2 years, the capacity for oestrogen positive feedback on the anterior pituitary gland develops with the subsequent mid-cycle luteinising hormone surge and ovulation, resulting in regulation of the menstrual cycle.

Hoch, Pajewski, and Moraski (2009) reported an overall much higher prevalence of menstrual irregularity (54%) in the athletic population. Bullen et al. (1985) reported that untrained, regularly menstruating females developed menstrual disorders when exposed to strenuous exercise and sport.

Soleimany, Dadgostar, Lotfian, Moradi-Lakeh, Dadgostar, and Movaseghi (2012) also found that negative changes in cardiovascular biomarkers can occur in female athletes with functional hypothalamic menstrual dysfunction. Abnormal menstrual function may manifest from other aspects of the female athlete triad. For example, decreased energy availability through disordered eating behaviours, such as anorexia and bulimia nervosa, can lead to menstrual dysfunction. They stated that therapeutic intervention including assessment of the athletes' diet, potentially increasing their calorie intake, or decreasing their exercise load may prevent further damage. Also, medical measures including oral contraceptives or psychological evaluation in order to reverse or prevent menstrual dysfunction could be considered.

Disordered Eating

Disordered eating, another component of the female athlete triad, refers to a group of irregular eating behaviours, including restrictive eating, fasting, frequently skipping meals, overeating, binge eating, self-induced vomiting, and the use of diet pills, laxatives, diuretics, and enemas, (Costa et al., 2013). They found that in many cases, female adolescents with disordered eating develop a clinical mental disorder recognised as an eating disorder (anorexia nervosa and bulimia nervosa).

Adolescent female athletes may be at a greater risk of inadequate energy intake. Costa et al. (2013) found that the prevalence of eating disorders was higher in athletes than in controls, and higher in female athletes than in male athletes. Sundgot-Borgen and Torstveit (2004) also found that eating disorders are more common among those competing in 'leanness-dependent and weight-dependent sports' than in other sports. Schaal et al. (2011) found that the highest rates of eating disorders were found in young females involved in racing sports and fine motor skills sports, while those playing team ball sports had the lowest occurrence of such problems.

In endurance sports such as long-distance running, for physiological reasons, leanness is related to performance. Runners who are several kilogrammes over their optimum-performance weight will not be able perform at their peak. In weight-category sports such as judo (AAU Judo 2013) and boxing (IBO 2012), athletes are unable to compete if they fail to make the prescribed weight for their category. Also, in sports such as gymnastics and high board diving, an aesthetic evaluation is attached to performance. All of these weight-related and body-image-related issues can create considerable pressures and stresses to achieve the necessary or the desired weight loss. Major studies have consistently reported higher prevalence rates in these groups of sports (Schaal et al., 2011). Despite the need for awareness of such disorders, due to the different criteria applied in studies with athletes, it can be challenging to accurately compare findings (Sundgot-Borgen & Torstveit, 2004).

A substantial percentage of young female athletes may be at risk of long-term health consequences associated with disordered eating. Nichols, Rauh, Lawson, Ji, and Barkai (2006) suggested that pre-participation screening to identify these components should be encouraged as a preventive approach to identify athletes who may be at high risk. A collaborative effort among coaches, athletic trainers, parents, physicians, and athletes is optimal for recognising, preventing, and treating eating disorders in athletes (Sundgot-Borgen & Torstveit, 2004).

Injury

Sex and age are both non-modifiable intrinsic potential risk factors for injury in sport (Habelt, Hasler, Steinbrück, Majewski, 2011). Associations have been made among all the female athlete triad components and musculoskeletal injury in adolescent female sports (Rauh, Nichols, & Barrack 2010). Several studies have identified female athletes as having a higher incidence of knee injury and anterior cruciate ligament (ACL) injury than males (Hewett Lindenfeld, Riccobene, & Noyes, 1999; Scand, Loes, Dahlstedt, Thomee, 2000; Waldén, Huston, Boynton, Spindler, Lindenfeld, 2011; Dugan 2005; Benjaminse, Lemmink, Diercks, and Otten, 2010). Many explanations for this have been debated.

Reasons include that ACL injuries occur with hard and awkward landings on the knee when it is positioned near extension (Renstrom et al., 2008). The female knee is in more extension, has greater knee valgus, and has higher quadriceps activation than the male knee at initial contact with the ground; therefore, it has to deal with a greater ground reaction force (Lephart, Abt, Ferris, Sell, Nagai, Myers, and Irrgang, 2005). The straighter knee and the higher quadriceps activation can combine to produce more strain in the ACL (Renstrom et al., 2008).

Hewett et al. (1999) presented electromyograph studies showing sex-related differences in the timing of muscle activation during athletic movement, such as increased peak quadriceps activity in female subjects during the pre-contact phase of landing. They found that greater rectus femoris activity was observed in female subjects than in male subjects, possibly increasing the strain on the ACL during landing. Increased quadriceps activity combined with decreased hamstring activity may decrease kinetic energy absorption during landing and may also increase ground reaction forces and torques associated with ACL injuries.

Variances in the pelvic size and shape, intercondylar notch width, size of the ACL, ligamentous laxity, and Q angle could also be contributing factors (Renstrom et al., 2008).

Lephart et al. (2005) stated that female athletes have also demonstrated decreased hamstrings and quadriceps strength. Renstrom et al. (2008) also found that female athletes presented disparity in knee proprioception and neuromuscular control compared with their male counterparts. However, numerous injury prevention programmes have been developed to modify such neuromuscular and biomechanical characteristics and have successfully reduced the number of ACL injuries in female athletes. Typically, these programmes incorporate a combination of balance, plyometric, agility, resistance, and flexibility exercises (Lephart et al., 2005).

In spite of this, Habelt et al. (2011) have stated that males participating in sport may be at greater risk of injury as they tend to be more aggressive, have larger body mass, and experience greater contact compared with females in the same sport. They are also more involved in contact sports such as rugby and soccer. However, these are all non-modifiable and potentially modifiable extrinsic risk factors

In relation to the female athlete triad, Wojtys, Huston, Boynton, Spindler, and Lindenfeld (2002) found that the phase of the menstrual cycle was significantly associated with female athletes' susceptibility to ACL injury. Results have found that women have a significantly greater risk of ACL injury during the pre-ovulatory phase of the menstrual cycle than during the post-ovulatory phase. Another interesting association found by Wojtys et al. (2002) was a significant association between the distribution of ACL injuries and the phase of the menstrual cycle in relation to oral contraceptives. Hormone profiles vary widely among females with regard to the timing, phasing, and amplitude of hormone changes across the cycle. This variability suggests that some females may experience greater effects of sex hormones on ligament biology than others, potentially exposing those individuals to greater changes in structural integrity and risk of injury (Renstrom et al., 2008).

Some high school athletes experience more than 1 component of the female athlete triad. Athletes with 1 triad component are at greater risk of other conditions, such as musculoskeletal injuries. Barrow and Saha (1988) found an association between menstrual dysfunction and stress factors occurring in the tibia in the collegiate population.

Other musculoskeletal injuries common in young females include overuse injuries, such as patellofemoral pain syndrome (Lankhorst, Bierma-Zeinstra, & Middlekoop, 2012) and rotator cuff tendinitis. The impact of these injuries can also lead to psychological distress.

Conclusion

The female adolescent athlete can encounter the problems described in the female athlete triad as well as many other detrimental factors that may affect their overall sporting performance.

Due to the long-term health risks resulting from the disorders of the female athlete triad, regular and close monitoring of adolescent female athletes in order to recognise and manage potential problems is advised (Rauh, Nichols, & Barrack 2010). All these findings lead to the conclusion that there is a greater need for more education of such risks for athletes. This education, will help parents, coaches, athletic trainers, other sports health care professionals, and the athlete themselves to be more aware of the dangers and hold the necessary skills to identify and prevent the development of the possible conditions.

Key Points

- The female athletic triad consists of disordered eating, amenorrhoea and osteoporosis.

- Excessive sport in females increases cortisol, affecting menstruation.

- Injuries are common in gymnastics, ballet, long-distance running, and boxing.

- Ligaments are 5 times weaker in females than males

References

Barrow, G. W., & Saha, S. (1988). Menstrual irregularity and stress fractures in collegiate female distance runners. *American Journal of Sports Medicine, 16*(3), 209–216.

Benjaminse. A., Lemmink, K. A. P. M., Diercks, R. L. & Otten, B. (2010). An investigation of motor learning during side-step cutting, design of a randomised controlled trial. *BMC Musculoskeletal Disorders, 11*(235), 1–8.

Birch, K. (2005). Female athlete triad. *British Medical Journal, 330*(7485), 244–246.

Bullen, B. A., Skrinar, G. S., & Beitins, I. Z. (1985). Induction of menstrual disorders by strenuous exercise in untrained women. *New England Journal of Medicine, 312*(21), 1349–1353.

Carter, C. W., Micheli, L. J. (2011). Training the child athlete: physical fitness, health and Injury. *British Journal of Sports Medicine, 45*(11), 880–885.

Costa, N. F., Schtscherbyna, A., & Scaber T. (2013). Disordered eating among adolescent female swimmers: Dietary, biochemical, and body composition factors. *Nutrition, 29*(1), 172–177.

Dugan, S. A. (2005). Sports-related knee injuries in female athletes: What gives? *American Journal of Physics Medicine & Rehabilitation, 84*(2), 122–130.

Ferry, B., Lespessaillesc, E., Rochcongard, P., Duclose, M., & Courteixa, D. (2012). Bone health during late adolescence: Effects of an 8-month training program on bone geometry in female athletes. *Bone Joint Spine, 3627*, 1–7.

Habelt, S., Hasler, C. C., Steinbrück, K., & Majewski, M. (2011). Sport injuries in adolescents. *Orthopedic Reviews, 3*(18), 82–86.

Hewett, T. E., Lindenfeld, T. N., Riccobene, J. V., & Noyes, F. R. (1999). The effect of neuromuscular training on the incidence of knee injury in female athletes: A prospective study. *American Journal of Physics Medicine, 27*(6), 699–706.

Hewett, T. E., Zazulak, B. T., Myer, G. D., & Ford, K. D. (2005). A review of electromyographic activation levels, timing differences, and increased anterior cruciate ligament injury incidence in female athletes. *British Journal of Sports Medicine, 39*(6), 347–350.

Hoch, A. Z., Pajewski, N. M., & Moraski, L. (2009). Prevalence of the female athlete triad in high school athletes and sedentary students. *Clinic of Journal Sport Medicine, 19*(5), 421–428.

Lankhorst, N. E., Bierma-Zeinstra, S. M. A., & Middlekoop, M. V. (2012). Risk factors for patellofemoral pain syndrome: A systematic review. *Journal of Orthopaedic & Sports Physical Therapy, 42*(2), 81–95.

Lemstra, M., Nielsen, G., Rogers, M., Thompson, A., & Moraros, J. (2012). Physical activity in youth: prevalence risk indicators, and solutions. *Canadian Family Physician, 58*(1), 54–61.

Lephart, S. M., Abt, J. P., Ferris, C. M., Sell, T. C., Nagai, T., Myers, J. B., & Irrgang, J. J. (2005). Neuromuscular and biomechanical characteristic changes in high school athletes: a plyometric versus basic resistance program. *British Journal of Sports Medicine, 39*(12), 932–938.

MacKelvie, K. J., Khan, K. M., & McKay, H. A. (2002). Is there a critical period for bone response to weight-bearing exercise in children and adolescents? A systematic review. *British Journal of Sports Medicine, 36*(4), 250–257.

Nichols, J. F., Rauh, M. J., Lawson, M. J., Ji, M., & Barkai, H. S. (2006). Prevalence of the female athlete triad syndrome among high school athletes. *Archives of Pediatrics Adolescent Medicine, 160*(2), 137–142.

Prelack, K., Dwyer, J., Ziegler, P., & Kehayias, J. J. (2012). Bone mineral density in elite adolescent female figure skaters. Journal of the International Society of Sports Nutr*ition, 9*(1), 57–63.

Rauh, M. J., Nichols, J. F., & Barrack, M. T. (2010). Relationships among injury and disordered eating, menstrual dysfunction, and low bone mineral density in high school athletes: A prospective study. *Journal of Athletic Training, 45*(3), 243–252.

Renstrom, P., Peterson, M., & Helger, Z. (2008). Non-contact ACL injuries in female athletes: An international olympic committee current concepts statement. *British Journal of Sports Medicine, 42*(6), 394–412.

Roupas, N. D., & Georgopoulos, N. A. (2011). Menstrual function in sports. *Hormones (Athens), 10*(2), 104–116.

Scand, J., Loes, M., Dahlstedt, L. J., & Thomee, R. (2000). A 7-year study on risks and costs of knee injuries in male and female youth participants in 12 sports. *Medicine & Science in Sports, 10*(2), 90–97.

Schaal, K., Tafflet M., & Nassif H. (2011). Psychological balance in high level athletes: Gender-based differences and sport-specific patterns. *PLoS ONE, 6*(5), 1–9.

Soleimany, G., Dadgostar, H., Lotfian, S., Moradi-Lakeh, M., Dadgostar, E., & Movaseghi, S. (2012). Bone mineral changes and cardiovascular effects among female athletes with chronic menstrual dysfunction. *Asian Journal of Sports Medicine, 3(1), 53–58.*

Sundgot-Borgen, J., Torstveit, M. K. (2004). Prevalence of eating disorders in elite athletes is higher than in the general population. *Clinical Journal of Sport Medicine, 14*(1), 25–32.

Tenforde, A. S., & Fredericson, M. (2011). Influence of sports participation on bone health in the young athlete: A review of the literature. *American Academy of Physical Medicine and Rehabilitation, 3*(9), 861–867.

Thein-Nissenbaum, J. M., & Carr, K. E. (2011). Female athlete triad syndrome in school athlete. *Physical Therapy in Sport, 12*(3), 108–116.

Waldén, M., Hagglund, M., Magnusson, H., & Ekstrand, J. (2011). Anterior cruciate ligament injury in elite football: A prospective three-cohort study. *Knee Surgery Sports Traumatology Arthroscopy, 19*(1), 11–19.

Wojtys, E. M., Huston, L. J., Boynton, D., Spindler, K. P., & Lindenfeld, T. N. (2002). The effect of the menstrual cycle on anterior cruciate ligament injuries in women as determined by hormone levels. *American Journal of Sports Medicine, 30*(2), 182–188.

CHAPTER 18

Hypermobility in Children and Adolescent Sport

Jane Simmonds

General joint hypermobility (GJH) is defined as a condition in which most of an individual's joints move beyond the normal limits, taking into consideration their age, gender, and ethnic background (Grahame, 2003). Many people with generalised joint hypermobility are asymptomatic, and indeed, their hypermobility may be considered an asset (Simmonds & Keer, 2007; Simpson, 2006). However, for others, it may predispose them to a sequala of injury, pain, and other complex systemic health issues.

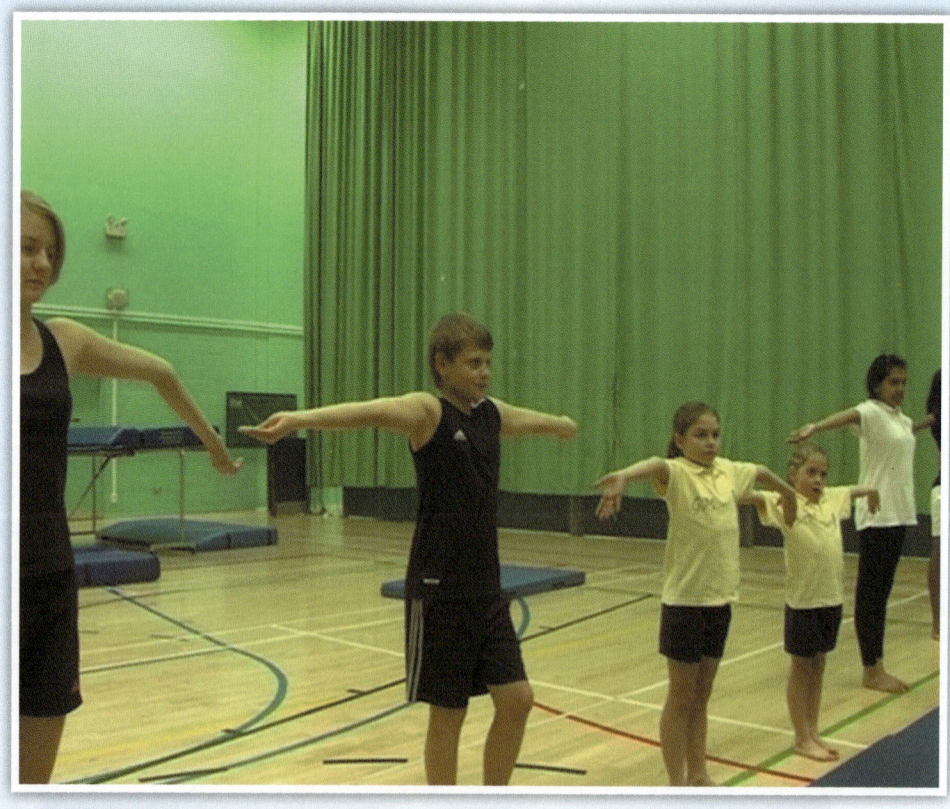

Fig. 18.1 Demonstrating hypermobile elbows

Joint hypermobility syndrome (JHS) is the term which has been used to describe a condition in which joint hypermobility is associated with the occurrence of symptoms in the absence of another defined rheumatological disease (Grahame, 2003). The syndrome was first described by Kirk, Ansell, and Bywater in 1967, providing recognition of the relationship between GJH and pain. JHS is now considered, by many, to be indistinguishable from the hypermobility type of Ehlers–Danlos syndrome (EDS type III) (Grahame, 1999; Tinkle, Bird, Grahame, Lavallee, Levy, & Sillence, 2009). Although, on first appearance JHS/EDSHT may appear to be a chronic musculoskeletal disorder, it is also associated with non-musculoskeletal problems such as fatigue, orthostatic intolerance, and gastrointestinal complaints (Castori, Morleno, Celletti, Celli, Morrone, Colombi, Camerota, & Grammatico, 2011). These systemic complaints have not been extensively studied and often receive little attention in clinical practice. However, because JHS/EDSHT is a connective tissue disorder rather than a musculoskeletal disorder, the clinician working with children should be aware that patients may present with a large variety of symptoms ranging from the musculoskeletal system to far beyond (Castori et al., 2011).

There are a number of contributing factors to joint laxity, including the shape of the joint and joint surfaces, collagen elasticity, neuromuscular tone, and neurological motor control (Bird, 2011). Joint hypermobility Syndrome is thought to be a genetically inherited disorder of the connective tissues with an autosomal dominant pattern (Malfait, Hakim, De Paepe, & Grahame, 2006; Simpson, 2006). The underlying pathophysiology is attributed to an abnormality in the properties and proportions of collagen, whereby there is an abnormally high proportion of type III to type I collagen within the soft-tissue matrix (Russek, 1999). Type III collagen is thinner, disorganised, and more elastic, which results in increased tissue extendibility and fragility (Russek, 1999). Mutations in genes encoding collagen type V have also recently been implicated (Malfait, Symoens, Coucke, Nunes, De Almeida, & De Paepe, 2005; Malfait, Hakim, De Paepe, and Grahame, 2006), with type V collagen under normal control interacting with type I collagen during fibrillogenesis and having a role in regulation of fibril diameter. Moreover, a mutation in tenascin X, a non-collagenous molecule has also been suggested as contributing to joint hypermobility (Zweers, Dean, van Kuppevelt, Bristow, & Schalkwijk, 2005). An alteration in this process may potentially lead to thinner, finer, and more disorganised collagen fibres. Malfait et al. (2005), hypothesise that it is the interference with the processing of the N-propeptide of either -chain (1 or 2) of type I collagen that is responsible for Ehlers–Danlos-like symptoms of skin laxity, joint subluxation, and dislocation. Finally, it is proposed that hormonal influences also contribute towards the pathophysiology, particularly in women (Bird, 2005).

Joint hypermobility is more common in females than in males (Larsson, Baum, & Mudholkar, 1987). The incidence has been shown to decrease with age (Larsson, Baum, Mudholkar, & Srivastava, 1993; Remvig, Jensen, & Ward, 2007a). There is a notable association with ethnic background, with a considerably higher occurrence in those of Asian and African descent than in Caucasian groups (Beighton, Solomon, & Soskolne, 1973; Seow et al., 1999). There is a paucity of epidemiological data for JHS/EDSHT in the general population; thus the true prevalence of the syndrome remains unknown (Ross & Grahame, 2011).

Hypermobility and Sport

As suggested earlier, GJH can be an asset for selected sports and performance activities, particularly those which require a high degree of flexibility. The prevalence of GJH differs in different sporting populations, although reported estimates also vary considerably due to differences in diagnostic criteria (Russek, 1999; Simmonds & Keer, 2007). In a UK-based epidemiological study of teenagers, girls who performed moderate to vigorous physical activity for more than 60 minutes per day were found to be 3 times more likely to be distinctly hypermobile than their inactive counterparts (Clinch, Deere, Sayers, Palmer, Riddoch, Tobias, & Clark, 2011).

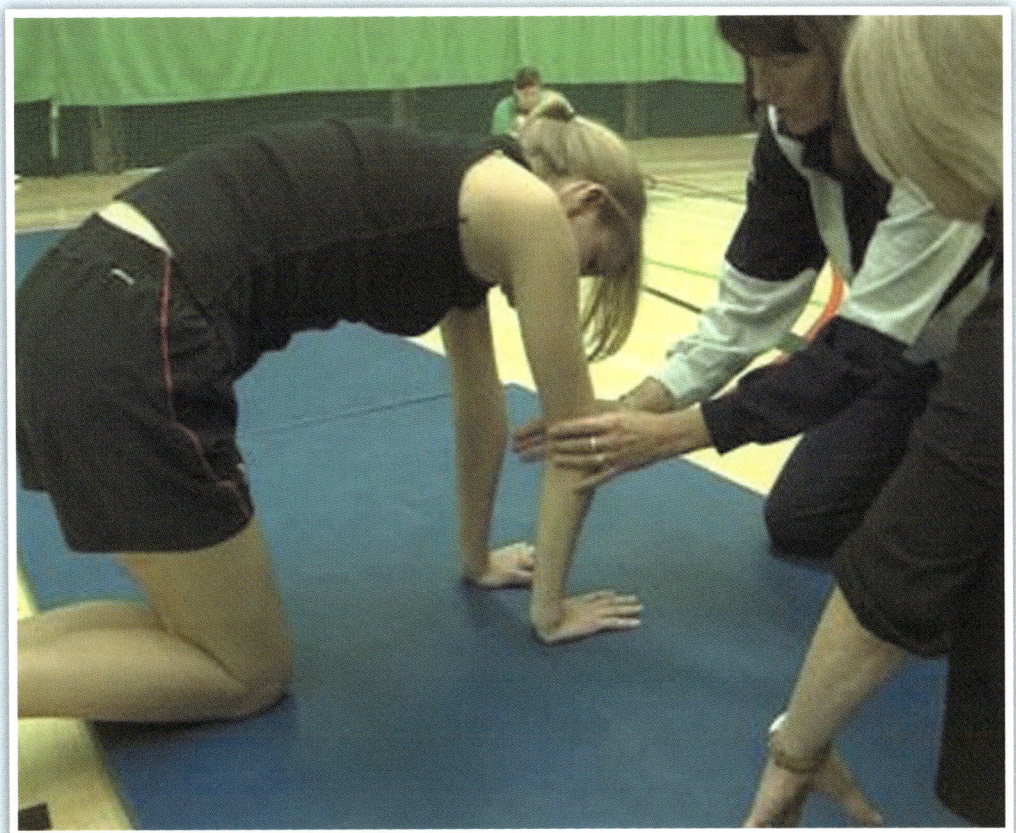

Fig. 18.2 Demonstrating 4-point kneeling in a hypermobile adolescent

Generalised joint hypermobility is very common in ballet dancers, and the prevalence of JHS/EDSHT is also known to be very high in this population (Briggs, McCormack, & Hakim, 2009; McCormack, Briggs, Hakim, & Grahame, 2004). In team sports, the prevalence of GJH has been reported as 33–42% in professional football (Collinge & Simmonds, 2009) and 24% in amateur rugby (Stewart & Burden, 2004). A study of Australian youth netballers reported that 40% were distinctly hypermobile, and a further 26% were moderately hypermobile (Smith, Damodaran, Swaminathan, Campbell, & Barnsley, 2005). Moreover, in a recent study of 32 elite squad netball players, the prevalence of GJH has been reported to be a massive 63%. Common to most epidemiological research, this study used the Beighton score to measure hypermobility (Beighton et al., 1973). However, a different system of scoring classification was used, which makes the results difficult to compare with other studies. There is no published research specifying the prevalence of JHS/EDSHT within sport.

Hypermobility and Injury Risk in Sport

Individuals with JHS/EDSHT are characteristically observed to incur injuries such as joint dislocations, tendinopathies, and ligament ruptures (Keer, 2003;

Russek, 1999; Simmonds & Keer, 2007; Simpson, 2006). Early research in this field proposed that athletes with GJH were at significantly higher risk of sustaining a sporting injury, particularly at the knee (Lichtor, 1972; Nicholas, 1970). The seminal paper by James Nicholas (1970) advocated that athletes should be screened for hypermobility, and those who were found to be hypermobile should be prescribed specific strengthening exercises to decrease their risk of injury. Joseph Lichtor (1972) proposed that the risk of injury to hypermobile participants in contact sports is so high that they should be actively discouraged from participation.

More recent research investigating the association between injury risk and hypermobility has shown mixed results. No additional risk of injury was observed for hypermobile individuals in samples of lacrosse players (Decoster, Bernier, Lindsay, & Vailas, 1999), American collegiate athletes, high school wrestlers (Pasque & Hewett, 2000), or professional footballers (Collinge & Simmonds, 2009). Interestingly, in a study of male professional football players, an increased absence from play following injury was observed in the hypermobile footballers compared with their non-hypermobile counterparts. A similar observation has been made in professional ballet dancers, whereby dancers with JHS / EDSHTmissed more time from dancing due to injury than those without the syndrome (Briggs et al., 2009). In other studies, GJH has been identified as an independent risk factor in professional male football (Konopinski et al., 2012), amateur rugby (Stewart & Burden, 2004), female football (Söderman, Alfredson, Pietilä, & Werner, 2001), and netball (Smith et al., 2005). Inconsistency within the results of these studies can be attributed to several factors, such as inherent different physiological demands within each of the sports which arguably plays an important role in the risk and type of injuries incurred and also affects the relative importance of intrinsic versus extrinsic risk factors for injury. Additionally, in the range of studies presented, there are considerable differences in study design, including method of classification of hypermobility, method of classification of injury, and methods of injury reporting. Interestingly a recent award-winning systematic review with meta-analysis across all sports was able to convincingly conclude that hypermobile individuals have an increased risk of injury at the knee, but not the ankle (Pacey, Nicholson, Adams, Munn, & Munns, 2010).

Neurophysiological Influences

It is recognised that the peripheral and central nervous systems have a profound influence in JHS/EDSHT, both with regards to pain and neuromuscular control

(Bird, 2011). An abnormal musculoskeletal reflex function has been identified in some individuals with JHS/EDSHT (Ferrell, Tennant, Baxendale, Kusel, & Sturrock, 2007). This is proposed to result from a neurophysiological deficit. Interestingly, reflex function was observed to normalise after an 8-week course of exercise, which is attributed to facilitation of interneuronal pathways (Ferrell et al., 2007). Differences in tendon stiffness and passive muscle tension have been also been observed in patients with JHS/EDS type III. This observation may also be attributable to differences in neural excitability.

Autonomic Dysfunction and Hypermobility

There is evidence to suggest that a degree of autonomic dysregulation may afflict individuals with joint hypermobility (Bird, 2011). In an important study conducted by Gazit and colleagues, individuals with JHS, all reported orthostatic symptoms such as palpitations, light-headedness, dizziness, presyncope and syncope (Gazit, Nahir, Grahame, & Jacob, 2003). Some potential explanations for this sympathetic dysregulation include blood pooling in the lower limbs, deconditioning due to inactivity, and impaired central sympathetic control (Gazit et al., 2003). Researchers have observed high incidence of slow transit constipation in hypermobile children, and pan-intestinal dysmotility gives rise to symptoms usually attributed to irritable bowel syndrome.

Beighton Scale		
Individuals are scored on their ability to	Right	Left
Passively dorsiflex the fifth metacarpophalangeal joint to ≥ 90 degrees Oppose the thumb to the volar aspect of the ipsilateral forearm Hyperextend the elbow to ≥10 degrees. Hyperextend the knee to ≥ 10 degrees Place hands flat on the floor without bending the knees	1 1 1 1 Total	1 1 1 1 1 9
One point is gained for each side for each manoeuvre 1–4, with a total possible score of 9 points. A score of 4 or more is considered hypermobile in adult populations.		

Box 1

Assessing and Diagnosing Hypermobility and JHS/EDSHT

Diagnosis of GJH and JHS/EDSHT is entirely clinical as there are no biochemical or imagining markers available currently(Ross & Grahame, 2011). The Beighton Scale (Box 1) is an internationally accepted screening test for GJH and is the most widely used test both clinically and within research literature (Russek, 1999). It has been shown to have good to excellent reliability for screening for GJH (Boyle, Witt, & Riegger-Krugh, 2003; Remvig, Jensen, & Ward, 2007b) and high reproducibility (Juul-Kristensen et al., 2007). It has been used in both adults and children (Beighton et al., 1973; Smits-Engelsman, Klerks, & Kirby, 2011; van der Giessen, Liekens, Rutgers, Hartman, Mulder, & Oranje, 2001). It is generally accepted that a score of 4 or more on the Beighton test indicates GJH, and this is the most widely used criteria within the literature (Remvig et al., 2007b; Simmonds & Keer, 2007; Simpson, 2006). Boyle et al (2003) suggest using criteria of 0–2/9 indicating not hypermobile, 3–4/9 indicating moderate hypermobility, and 5–9/9 indicating distinct hypermobility. This system has also been used within the research literature (Collinge & Simmonds, 2009; Smith et al., 2005). The Beighton score has been widely used with sports people and performing artists, but it has not been formally validated with this population (Collinge & Simmonds, 2009; Konopinski et al., 2012; McCormack et al., 2004; Stewart & Burden, 2004). Despite the universal use of the Beighton scale, it has been criticised for being an all-or-nothing scoring system and biased towards the upper limb (Simmonds & Keer, 2007; Remvig et al., 2007b). In addition, a cut-off score of 4 has been proposed to be too low in children and adolescents (Clinch et al., 2011).

The 1998 Brighton criteria were devised as a diagnostic indicator for JHS (Grahame, Bird, & Child, 2000) (Box 2). They have been shown to be highly reproducible (Juul-Kristensen et al., 2007). The Brighton criteria have also been used consistently within the research literature to classify JHS. However, it should be noted they have not been validated in children. These criteria combine the Beighton score with several 'minor' diagnostic indicators collected from clinical evaluation and history (Tinkle et al., 2009). The Brighton criteria are also under scrutiny amongst rheumatologists and therapists for failing to provide a scientific and objective basis for the minor criteria and failing to acknowledge the predominance of dysautonomic or psychological symptoms in females (Juul-Kristensen et al., 2007; Remvig et al., 2011). Consequently, the Brighton criteria is currently under review by an international panel (Ross & Grahame, 2011).

Brighton Criteria
Major criteria
1. A Beighton score of 4/9 or greater (current of historical) 2. Arthralgia for longer than 3 months in 4 or more joints
Minor criteria
1. A Beighton score of 1, 2 or 3/9 (0–3 if aged 50 or more) 2. Arthralgia in 1–3 joints or back pain or spondylosis, spondylolysis/spondylolisthesis 3. Dislocation in more than one joint, or in one joint on more than one occasion 4. 3or more soft-tissue lesions (epicondylitis, tenosynovitis, bursitis) 5. Marfanoid habitus (tall, slim, arm span >height; upper segment: lower segment ratio less than 0.89 arachnodactily) 6. Skin striae, hyperextensibility, thin skin, or abnormal scarring 7. Eye signs: drooping eyelids or myopia or antimongoloid slant 8. Varicose veins or hernia or uterine/rectal prolapse
Hypermobility syndrome is diagnosed in the presence of 2 major criteria or 1 minor major and 2 minor criteria or 4 minor criteria. 2 minor criteria will suffice where there is an unequivocally affected first-degree relative. Hypermobility syndrome is excluded in the presence of Marfan's syndrome and Ehler–Danlos syndrome, with the exception of the hypermobility type, formerly EDS III.

Box 2

Finally, a five-point questionnaire was developed and validated as a quick screening tool for GJH, whereby the authors found that 2 or more positive responses detect hypermobility with a sensitivity and specificity of 84% (Hakim & Grahame, 2003). Clinicians should be mindful that this questionnaire has only been validated in adults and therefore, should be used with discretion in paediatric populations.

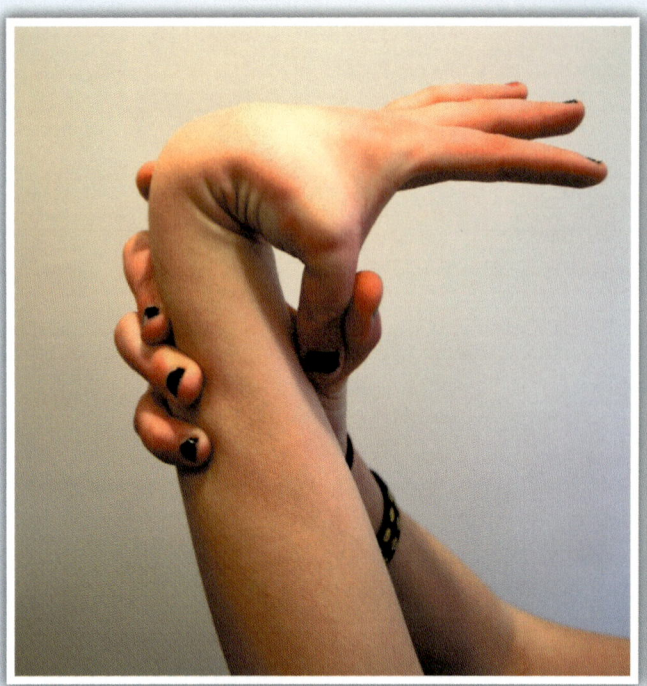
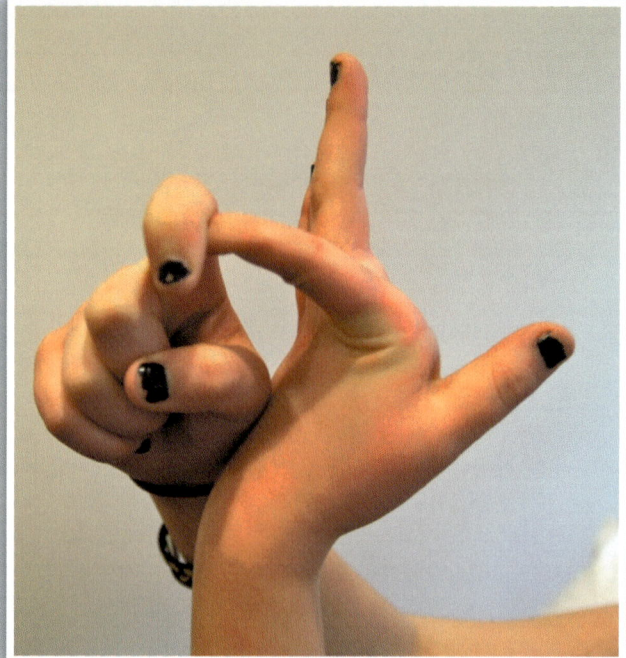

Fig. 18.3 Hypermobile tests

Considerations for Screening and Management

In light of the evidence to date, it seems prudent for sport and dance clinicians to screen for generalised laxity and the more serious connective tissue disorders and autonomic dysfunction. Specific prehabilitation strength and conditioning programmes for individuals with hypermobility should be directed towards strengthening supporting musculature and improving proprioception, particularly in the vulnerable joints. This is particularly relevant for adolescents, who are more vulnerable to injury because of the rapid physiological, biomechanical, and emotional changes associated with this time of life. Some sports and performance activities may be more of an injury risk than others, particularly contact sports and where sharp cutting, acceleration and deceleration, and change of directions are involved.

The use of strapping and supports to augment mechanical support and proprioception would seem reasonable for susceptible players. Finally, rehabilitation following injury may take longer in individuals with GJH, JHS/ EDSHT due to slower healing times relating to altered collagen and reduced proprioception. Sports medicine physicians, coaches, athletic trainers, physiotherapists, sports therapists, sport rehabilitators, choreographers, sport scientists, parents, and PE teachers need to be aware of the issues relating to hypermobility, sport, performance and to consider ways to optimise performance, prevent injury, and facilitate optimal recovery.

5-Part Questionnaire

1. Can you now or could you ever place your hands flat on the floor without bending your knees?

2. Can you now or could you ever bend your thumb to touch your forearm?

3. As a child did you amuse your friends by contorting your body into strange shapes, *or* could you do the splits?

4. As a child or a teenager, did your shoulder ever dislocate on more than one occasion?

5. Do you consider yourself double-jointed?

Answer in the affirmative to 2 or more questions suggests hypermobility with sensitivity 80–85% and specificity 80–90%.

Key Points

- Hypermobility is common in ballet, gymnastics.

- 42% of professional footballers can be hypermobile; 24% rugby players can be hypermobile.

- Hypermobility decreases with age.

- Asians and Africans exhibit more hypermobility than Caucasians.

- No reliable evidence that injury risk is more.

References

Beighton, P., De Paepe, A., Steinmann, B., Tsipouras, P., & Wenstrup, R. J. (1998). Ehlers-danlos syndromes: Revised nosology, Villefranche, 1997. Ehlers-danlos national foundation (USA) and ehlers-danlos support group (UK). *American Journal of Medical Genetics, 77*(1), 31–37.

Beighton, P., Solomon, L. & Soskolnem C. L. (1973). Articular mobility in an African population. *Annals of Rheumatic Disease, 32*, 413–418.

Bird, H. (2005). Joint hypermobility in children. *Rheumatology (Oxford), 44*(6), 703–704.

Bird, H. (2011). Hypermobility: Does it cause joint symptoms? *European Musculoskeletal Review, 6*(1), 34–37.

Bird, H. & Foley, E. C. (2012). Hypermobility in dancers. *Rheumatology* (Oxford). In Press.

Boyle, K. L., Witt, P., & Riegger-Krugh, C. (2003). Intrarater and interrater reliability of the Beighton and Horan joint mobility index. *Journal of Athletic Training, 38*(4), 281–285.

Briggs, J., Mc Cormack, M., Hakim, A., & Grahame, R. (2009). Injury and joint hypermobility syndrome in ballet dancers: A 5 year follow-up. *Rheumatology. 48*, 1613–1620.

Castori, M., Morleno, S., Celletti, C., Celli, M., Morrone, M., Colombi, M., Camerota, F., & Grammatico, P. (2011). Management of pain and fatigue in the joint hypermobility syndrome (a.k.a. Ehlers–Danlos syndrome, hypermobility type): Principles and proposal for a multidisciplinary approach. *American Journal of Medical Genetics, 158a*, 2055–2070.

Child, A. H. (1986). Joint hypermobility syndrome: Inherited disorder of collagen synthesis. *Journal of Rheumatology, 13*, 239–243.

Clinch, J., Deere, K., Sayers, A., Palmer, S., Riddoch, C., Tobias, J. H., & Clark, E. M. (2011). Epidemiology of generalized joint laxity (hypermobility) in fourteen-year-old children from the UK: A population-based evaluation. *Arthritis & Rheumatism, 63*(9), 2819–2827.

Collinge, R., & Simmonds, J. V. (2009). Hypermobility, injury rate and rehabilitation in a professional football squad: A preliminary study. *Physical Therapy in Sport, 10*(3), 91–96.

Decoster, L. C., Bernier, J. N., Lindsay, R. H., & Vailas, J. C. (1999). Generalized joint hypermobility and its relationship to injury patterns among NCAA lacrosse players. *Journal of Athletic Training, 34*(2), 99–105.

Ferrell, W. R., Tennant, N., Sturrock, R. D., Ashton, L., Creed, G. & Brydson, G. (2004). Amelioration of symptoms by enhancement of proprioception in patients with joint hypermobility syndrome. *Arthritis & Rheumatism, 50*, 3323–3328.

Ferrell, W. R., Tennant, N., Baxendale, R. H., Kusel, M., & Sturrock, R. D. (2007). Musculoskeletal reflex function in the joint hypermobility syndrome. *Arthritis Care and Rheumatism, 57*(7), 1329–1333.

Gazit, Y., Nahir, A. M., Grahame, R., & Jacob, G. (2003). Dysautonomia in the joint hypermobility syndrome. *American Journal of Medicine, 115*(1), 33–40.

Grahame, R., Bird, H. A., & Child, A. (2000). The revised (Brighton 1998) criteria for the diagnosis of benign joint hypermobility syndrome (BJHS). *Journal of Rheumatology, 27*(7), 1777–1779.

Grahame, R. (2003). Hypermobility and hypermobility syndrome. In R. Keer & R. Grahame (Eds.), *Hypermobility syndrome, recognition and management for physiotherapists* (pp. 1–14). Edinburgh: Butterworth Heinemann.

Grahame, R. (2007). The need to take a fresh look at criteria for hypermobility. *Journal of Rheumatology, 34*(4), 664–665.

Grahame, R. (2009). Joint hypermobility syndrome pain. *Current Pain and Headache Reports, 13*(6), 427–433.

Grahame, R. (1999). Joint hypermobility and genetic collagen disorders: are they related? *Archives of Disease in Childhood, 80*(2), 188–191.

Greenwood, N. L., Duffell, L. D., Alexander, C. M., & McGregor, A. H. (2011). Electromyographic activity of pelvic and lower limb muscles during postural tasks in people with benign joint hypermobility syndrome and non hypermobile people: A pilot study. *Manual Therapy, 16*(6), 623–662.

Hakim, A. J., & Grahame, R. (2003a). A simple questionnaire to detect hypermobility: An adjunct to the assessment of patients with diffuse musculoskeletal pain. *International Journal of Clinical Practice, 57*(3), 163–166.

Hakim, A., & Grahame, R. (2003b). Joint hypermobility. *Best Practice & Research Clinical Rheumatology, 17*(6), 989–1004.

Hakim, A. J., & Grahame, R. (2004). Non-musculoskeletal symptoms in joint hypermobility syndrome: Indirect evidence for autonomic dysfunction? *Rheumatology (Oxford), 43*(9), 1194–1195.

Hakim, A. J., Malfait, F., & De Paepe, A. (2010). The heritable disorders of connective tissue: epidemiology, nosology & clinical features. In A. Hakim & R. Grahame (Eds.), *Hypermobility, fibromyalgia and chronic pain* (p. 10). London: Churchill Livingstone.

Keer, R. (2003). Physiotherapy assessment of the hypermobile adult. In R. Keer & R. Grahame (Eds.), Hypermobility syndrome, recognition and management for physiotherapists (pp. 67–86). Edinburgh: Butterworth Heinemann.

Kirby, A., & Sugden, D. A. (2007). Children with developmental co-ordination disorders. *Journal of the Royal Society of Medicine, 100*(4), 82–186.

Kirk, J. A., Ansell, B. M. & Bywaters, A. G. L. (1967). The hypermobility syndrome: Musculoskeletal complaints associated with generalized joint hypermobility. *Annals of Rheumatic Diseases, 26,* 419–425.

Larsson, L. G., Baum, J., & Mudholkar, G. S. (1987). Hypermobility: features and differential incidence between the sexes. *Arthritis & Rheumatism, 30*(12), 1426–1430.

Larsson, L. G., Baum, J., Mudholkar, G. S., & Srivastava, D. K. (1993). Hypermobility: prevalence and features in a Swedish population. *British Journal of Rheumatology, 32*(2), 116–119.

Lichtor, J. (1972). The loose-jointed young athlete: Recognition and treatment. *Journal of Sports Medicine, 1*(1), 22–23.

Loeys, B. L., Dietz, H. C., Braverman, A. C., Callewaert, B. L., De Backer, J., Devereux, R. B., & De Paepe, A. M. (2010). The revised Ghent nosology for the marfan syndrome. *Journal of Medical Genetics, 47*(7), 476–485.

Logerstedt, D., Grindem, H., Lynch, A., Eitzen, I., Engebretsen, L., Risberg, M. A. (2012). Single-legged hop tests as predictors of self-reported knee function after anterior cruciate ligament reconstruction: The Delaware-Oslo ACL cohort study. *American Journal of Sports Medicine, 40*(10), 2348–2356.

Malfait, F., Hakim, A. J., De Paepe, A., & Grahame, R. (2006). The genetic basis of the joint hypermobility syndromes. *Rheumatology (Oxford), 45*(5), 502–507.

αMalfait, F., Symoens, S., Coucke, P., Nunes, L., De Almeida, S., & De Paepe, A. (2005). A total absence of the 2(I) chain of collagen type I causes a rare form of Ehlers-Danlos syndrome with hypermobility and propensity to cardiac valvular problems. *Journal of Medical Genetics, 25,* 28–37.

Mallik, A. K., Ferrell, W. R., McDonald, A. G., & Sturrock, R. D. (1994). Impaired proprioceptive acuity at the proximal interphalangeal joint in patients with the hypermobility syndrome. *British Journal of Rheumatology, 33*(7), 631–637.

Mathias, C. J., Low, D. A., Iodice, V., Owens, A. P., Kirbis, M., & Grahame, R. (2012). Postural tachycardia syndrome: Current experience and concepts. *Nature Reviews Neurology, 8*(1), 22–34.

McCormack, M., Briggs, J., Hakim, A. & Grahame, R. (2004). Joint laxity and the benign joint hypermobility syndrome in student and professional ballet dancers. *Journal of Rheumatology, 3,* 173–178.

αMurray, K. J. (2006). Hypermobility disorders in children and adolescents. *Best Practice& Research Clinical Rheumatology, 20*(2), 329–351.

Myer, G. D., Ford, K. R., Paterno, M. V., Nick, T. G., & Hewett, T. E. (2008). The effects of generalized joint laxity on risk of anterior cruciate ligament injury in young female athletes. *American Journal of Sports Medicine, 36*(6), 1073–1080.

Nicholas, J. A. (1970). Injuries to knee ligaments: Relationship to looseness and tightness in football players. *Journal of the American Medical Association, 212,* 2236–2239.

Pacey, V., Nicholson, L. L., Adams, R. D., Munn, J., & Munns, C. F. (2010). Generalized joint hypermobility and risk of lower limb joint injury during sport: a systematic review with meta-analysis. *American Journal of Sports Medicine, 38*(7), 1487–1497.

Pasque, C. B., & Hewett, T. E. (2000). A prospective study of high school wrestling injuries. *American Journal of Sports Medicine, 28*(4), 509–515.

Ramesh, R., Von Arx, O., Azzopardi, T., & Schranz, P. J. (2005). The risk of anterior cruciate ligament rupture with generalised joint laxity. *Journal of Bone & Joint Surgery (British), 87*(6), 800–803.

Rauh, M. J., Koepsell, T. D., Rivara, F. P., Rice, S. G., & Margherita, A. J. (2007). Quadriceps angle and risk of injury among high school cross-country runners. *Journal of Orthopaedic & Sportst Physical Therapy, 37*(12), 725–733.

Remvig, L., Engelbert, R. H., Berglund, B., Bulbena, A., Byers, P. H., Grahame, R., et al. (2011). Need for a consensus on the methods by which to measure joint mobility and the definition of norms for hypermobility that reflect age, gender and ethnic-dependent variation: Is revision of criteria for joint hypermobility syndrome and Ehlers-Danlos syndrome hypermobility type indicated? *Rheumatology (Oxford), 50*(6), 1169–1171.

Remvig, L., Jensen, D. V., & Ward, R. C. (2007a). Are diagnostic criteria for general joint hypermobility and benign joint hypermobility syndrome based on reproducible and valid tests? A review of the literature. *Journal of Rheumatology, 34*(4), 798–803.

Remvig, L., Jensen, D. V., & Ward, R. C. (2007b). Epidemiology of general joint hypermobility and basis for the proposed criteria for benign joint hypermobility syndrome: Review of the literature. *Journal of Rheumatology, 34*(4), 804–809.

Rombaut, L., De Paepe, A., Malfait, F., Cools, A., & Calders, P. (2010). Joint position sense and vibratory perception sense in patients with Ehlers-Danlos syndrome type III (hypermobility type). *Clinical Rheumatology, 29*(3), 289–295.

Rombaut, L., Malfait, F., De Wandele, I., Thijs, Y., Palmans, T., De Paepe, A., et al. (2011). Balance, gait, falls, and fear of falling in women with the hypermobility type of Ehlers-Danlos syndrome. *Arthritis Care & Research, 63*(10), 1432–1439.

Ross, J., & Grahame, R. (2011). Joint hypermobility syndrome. *British Medical Journal, 342*, c7167.

Russek, L. N. (1999). Hypermobility syndrome. *Physical Therapy, 79*(6), 591–599.

Sahin, N., Baskent, A., Cakmak, A., Salli, A., Ugurlu, H., & Berker, E. (2008). Evaluation of knee proprioception and effects of proprioception exercise in patients with benign joint hypermobility syndrome. *Rheumatology International, 28*(10), 995–1000.

Scheper, M. C., de Vries, J. E., de Vos, R., Verbunt, J., Nollet, F., & Engelbert, R. H. (2012). Generalized joint hypermobility in professional dancers: a sign of talent or vulnerability? *Rheumatology (Oxford).* In Press.

Simmonds, J. V., & Keer, R. (2007). Hypermobility and the Hypermobility Syndrome. Masterclass. *Manual Therapy, 13*, 492–495.

Simpson, M. R. (2006). Benign joint hypermobility syndrome: evaluation, diagnosis, and management. *Journal of the American Osteopathic Association, 106*(9), 531–536.

Smith, R., Damodaran, A. K., Swaminathan, S., Campbell, R., & Barnsley, L. (2005). Hypermobility and sports injuries in junior netball players. *British Journal of Sports Medicine, 39*(9), 628–631.

Smits-Engelsman, B., Klerks, M., & Kirby, A. (2011). Beighton score: A valid measure for generalized hypermobility in children. *Journal of Paediatrics, 158*(1), 119–123.

Söderman, K., Alfredson, H., Pietilä, T., & Werner, S. (2001). Risk factors for leg injuries in female soccer players: A prospective investigation during one out-door season. *Knee Surgery, Sports Traumatology, Arthroscopy, 9*(5), 313–321.

Stewart, D. R., & Burden, S. B. (2004). Does generalised ligamentous laxity increase seasonal incidence of injuries in male first division club rugby players? *British Journal of Sports Medicine, 38*, 457–460.

Subramanyam, V., & Janaki, K. V. (1996). Joint hypermobility in South Indian children. *Indian Pediatrics, 33*(9), 771–2.

Tinkle, B. T., Bird, H. A., Grahame, R., Lavallee, M., Levy, H. & Sillence, D. (2009). The lack of clinical distinction between the hypermobility type of Ehlers–Danlos Sundrome and Joint Hypermobility Syndrome. *American Journal of Medical Genetics Part A*, 99991–99993.

Van de Putte, E. M., Uiterwaal, C. S., Bots, M. L. Kimpel, J. L. & Engelbert, R. H. (2005). Is chronic fatigue syndrome a connective tissue disorder? A cross-sectional study in adolescents. *Pediatrics, 115*, e415–e422.

van der Giessen, L. J., Liekens, D., Rutgers, K. J., Hartman, A., Mulder, P. G., & Oranje, A. P. (2001). Validation of beighton score and prevalence of connective tissue signs in 773 Dutch children. *Journal of Rheumatology, 28*(12), 2726–2730.

Wolf, J. M., Cameron, K. L., & Owens, B. D. (2011). Impact of joint laxity and hypermobility on the musculoskeletal system. *Journal of the American Academy of Orthopaedic Surgeons*, 19(8), 463–471.

Zarate, N., Farmer, A. D., Grahame, R., Mohammed, S. D., Knowles, C. H., Scott, S. M., & Aziz, Q. (2010). Unexplained gastrointestinal symptoms and joint hypermobility: Is connective tissue the missing link? *Neurogastroenterology and Motility, 22*(3), 252–e78.

Zweers, M. C., Dean, W. B., van Kuppevelt, T. H. Bristow, J., & Schalkwijk, J. (2005). Elastic fibre abnormalities in hypermobile type Ehlers–Danlos syndrome patients with tenascin-X mutations. *Clinical Genetics, 6*, 330–334.

CHAPTER 19

Strength and Conditioning in Children and Adolescent in Sport

Adam Kerr

Introduction

Paediatric strength and conditioning is an area of sport performance training that is often misunderstood and surrounded by many myths. A compelling body of evidence suggests that both strength and resistance training and conditioning is not only safe but can also elicit significant performance improvements (Behringer, vom Heede, Yue, & Mester, 2010; Faigenbaum, Kraemer, Blimkie, Jeffreys, Micheli, Nitka, & Rowland, 2009; Mikkola, Rusko, Nummela, Pollari, & Häkkinen, 2007; Thomas, French & Hayes, 2009; Williams & Bond, 2012;) and help reduce the risk of injury (Baker, Mitchell, Boyle, Currell, Wilson, Bird, O'Connor, & Jones, 2007; Behm, Faigenbaum, Falk, & Klentrou, 2008; Behringer, vom Heede, Matthews, & Mester, 2011; Faigenbaum et al., 2009; Lloyd, Faigenbaum, Myer, Stone, Oliver, Jeffreys, Moody, Brewer, & Pierce, 2012; Myer, Faigenbaum, Chu, Falkel, Ford, & Best, 2011; Pierce, Brewer, Ramsey, Byrd, Sands, Stone, & Stone, 2008).

Three of the biggest strength and conditioning associations around the world, the National Strength and Conditioning Association (NSCA), the Australian Strength and Conditioning Association (ASCA), and the United Kingdom Strength and Conditioning Association (UKSCA) provide position statements highlighting that proper supervised and progressed resistance training can improve the health, fitness, and sporting performance of young athletes (Baker et al., 2007; Faigenbaum et al., 2009; Lloyd et al., 2012).

Although it has been recommended that strength and conditioning for young athletes has many benefits, implementing a strength and conditioning programme should be considered alongside the growth and maturation status

355

of the anatomical, neurological, hormonal, and musculoskeletal structure and function (Ford, De Ste Croix, Lloyd, Meyers, Moosavi, Oliver, Till, & Williams, 2011; Oliver & Lloyd, 2012;). It has been suggested that basing training around chronological age is considerably flawed (Ford et al., 2011; Oliver & Lloyd, 2012;) and that programme prescription should be based on the status of each individual athlete, looking at biological maturity, training age, motor skill development, technical proficiency, and current strength levels, rather than using age-determined protocols (Lloyd et al., 2012).

This chapter will aim to discuss and give recommendations on all areas of strength and conditioning for both performance improvements and injury reduction across the different growth and maturity stages.

Strength Training
Effects of Strength Training during Childhood

The development of strength in youth athletes is influenced by muscular, neural, and biomechanical factors (De Ste Croix, 2008) and can be greatly influenced by the physiological and biological elements of growth and maturation (Lloyd et al., 2012), as healthy children can be expected to achieve noticeable gains in muscular strength without using any form of strength development training (Rowland, 2005). However, by performing a strength-based training programme that has sufficient training load, intensity, and volume over a continued period of time, youth athletes can increase their strength levels beyond that of normal growth and development (Faigenbaum, 2000; Kraemer, Fry, Frykman, Conroy, & Hoffman, 1989; Malina, 2006).

During the early stages of childhood, before puberty, the training-induced strength increases for both boys and girls are seen to be mostly due to improvements of the central nervous system through motor unit recruitment and synchronisation (Ramsay, Blimkie, Smith, Garner, MacDougall, & Sale, 1990). As the athletes proceed to go through puberty, which is generally around the age of 11 for girls and 13 for boys, the increased changes in strength, after a period of training, are seen to relate to structural and hormonal changes (Tonson, Ratel, Le Fur, Cozzone, & Bendahan, 2008) in addition to the continued development of the central nervous system (Malina, Bouchard, & Bar-Or, 2004). If strength work is implemented in the early stages of childhood, very little hypertrophy will be evident; however, an increase in motor coordination, strength, power production, change of direction speed, and running velocity can all be seen during this time (Behringer et al., 2010; Faigenbaum et al., 2009; Thomas, French, & Hayes, 2009).

Throughout childhood, very little difference is seen in strength levels between girls and boys (Faigenbaum, Milliken, & Westcott, 2003). However as puberty is reached, we start to see that males demonstrate greater changes in training-induced muscular strength and hypertrophy, mostly due to the increase in testosterone levels (Kraemer et al., 1989), whereas training induced changes in females is thought to be limited by the reduced amount of testosterone at this stage of their development (Rowland, 2005).

Despite all the research that suggests the safe nature of strength training for athletes as young as 6 years old (Faigenbaum, Westcott, Loud, & Long, 1999), coaches should be aware of the maturation status of the athlete, as any training programme should ensure that each athlete is trained according to the biological status rather than their chronological age (Lloyd et al., 2012). Emotional maturity should also be a key factor for deciding when to initiate a strength-training programme (Baker et al., 2007). The athletes must be ready not only physically but also mentally so that they can understand and follow their coach's instructions and also be able to cope with the stresses of such training (Faigenbaum et al., 2009).

Training Recommendations

Any training programme design and implementation for young athletes should be fully supervised by qualified strength and conditioning coaches (Baker et al., 2007; Faigenbaum et al., 2009; Lloyd et al., 2012). The programme should be carried out using appropriate equipment, with logical progressions based on technical proficiency, biological status, motor skill competency and existing strength levels (Baker et al., 2007; Faigenbaum et al., 2009; Lloyd et al., 2012). The training programme should be developed based on the individual athlete in order to reflect variance in training age and technical ability. Children who demonstrate greater training age and strength levels would be able to use advanced progressions in comparison to children displaying a low training age.

Exercise selection can vary greatly, though it is important for each strand of exercises selected to have a continuum of progressions and regressions so that

357

each athlete can be provided with appropriate levels of intensity based on their individual needs. All equipment used for any selected exercise should be the appropriate size and weight for the athlete (De Ste Croix, 2007; Stratton & Williams, 2007). Weights should be selected based on technical competency and existing strength levels (Lloyd et al., 2012), as all performed repetitions should be completed with perfect technique. In addition, athletes should not be held back due to age if technical competency and strength is demonstrated; there can be an increase in resistance, or more complex progressions can be added when needed.

It is also suggested that resistance training with free weights is more beneficial than machine-based resistance on muscle activation levels and increasing more functional movements related to sporting performance (Granacher, Goeseles, Roggo, Wischer, Fischer, Zuerny, Gollhofers, & Kriemler 2011; Jones, Fry, Weiss, Kinzey, & Moore, 2008; Schick et al., 2010; Schwanbeck, Chilibeck and Binsted, 2009). Athletes with a very low training age should be performing exercises that improve overall fundamental movement patterns and competency before moving on to more advanced progressions of strength training (Lloyd et al., 2012). In contrast, athletes that have a higher training age can progress to greater intensities using percentages of the athletes' one repetition-maximum (1RM) to determine training weights. It has been suggested that the relative strength levels in the parallel squat for young elite athletes with long-term training experience could be seen to be a minimum of 2.0 for 16–19 year-olds, 1.5 for 13–15 year-olds, and 0.7 for 11–12-year-olds (Keiner, Sander, Wirth, Caruso, Immesberger, & Zawieja, 2013).

The UKSCA Position Statement suggests that beginners may be prescribed 1–2 sets of 8–10 repetitions with around 50–70% 1RM. Then once training has been maintained and the athletes' technical competency and strength levels improve, it can be increased to 2–4 sets of 3–6 repetitions of 60–80% 1RM, with further progress allowing more advanced training modalities of 2–5 sets of 2–8 repetitions with 70–100% 1RM for more experienced and advanced lifters (Lloyd et al., 2012).

Ideally, strength training should be completed 2–3 times a week on non-consecutive days to develop muscular strength (Lloyd et al., 2012), as it has been found that an increase in training frequency is correlated to an increase in training effect (Behringer et al., 2010; Lloyd et al., 2012). The UKSCA also highlights that the recommendations for training prescription should be seen only as a guideline, making sure to take into account each athlete as an individual, with an understanding of maturation status, training age, movement competency, technical understanding, and existing strength levels (Lloyd et al., 2012).

Aerobic Conditioning

Effects of Aerobic Conditioning during Childhood

The development of aerobic fitness during growth occurs due to changes of the peripheral and central cardiovascular system, muscle function, and cellular capacity (Oliver & Lloyd, 2012), all of which can be influenced by training (Rowland, 1985). However, there is much conflicting evidence around the trainability of the endurance system during childhood (Oliver &Lloyd, 2012), and although it is felt that all children can make training-induced gains during growth and maturation, the mechanism for these adaptations may vary depending on biological status (Oliver & Lloyd, 2012).

Performing a period of endurance training with sufficient overload of intensity can cause an increase in VO_2 peak beyond that of normal growth and development in young athletes (LeMura, von Dullivard, & Carlonas, 1999; Williams & Bond, 2012). It has also been found that young athletes are seen to recover more quickly between high-intensity exercise bouts compared with adults and are, therefore, able to repeat the efforts more consistently, suggesting a shift of focus from steady state training to high-intensity interval training (Williams & Bond, 2012).

Training Recommendations

Specific protocols for the improvement of aerobic capacity during childhood will vary greatly depending on both sport and the individual athlete due to maturity status and existing levels of fitness. Therefore, any training programme should be overseen by suitably qualified coaches that understand the physiological and psychological variations between children of different chronological and biological ages (Williams & Bond, 2012).

The number of various training parameters should be based on a high-intensity intermittent nature, working above 85% max HR (Williams & Bond, 2012), as supplementing with this type of training has shown to be a time-efficient strategy to supplement the technical and tactical elements of training to elicit sufficient improvements of aerobic fitness (Williams & Bond, 2012).

Speed and Power Training
Effects of Speed and Power Training during Childhood

The development of speed and power during growth is seen to occur due to the development of the central nervous system and muscle-tendon size, structure, and function (Oliver & Lloyd, 2012); again, these fitness characteristics have been seen to be influenced by training throughout maturation (Rumpf, Cronin, Oliver, & Hughes, 2012). Although the number of studies is limited, a review paper highlighted the most effective types of training at different stages of biological growth for developing speed and power. Prior to the athlete going through peak height velocity, most benefits come from plyometric activity before speed training (Rumpf et al., 2012). The types of training at the different stages of maturation seem to align with the natural development phases throughout childhood. In the early stages of growth, it is the central nervous system that becomes fully developed, so more neural-type training is needed; then as children go through peak height velocity, changes in the muscular system occur, so training to improve muscle structure and function is needed (Oliver & Lloyd, 2012).

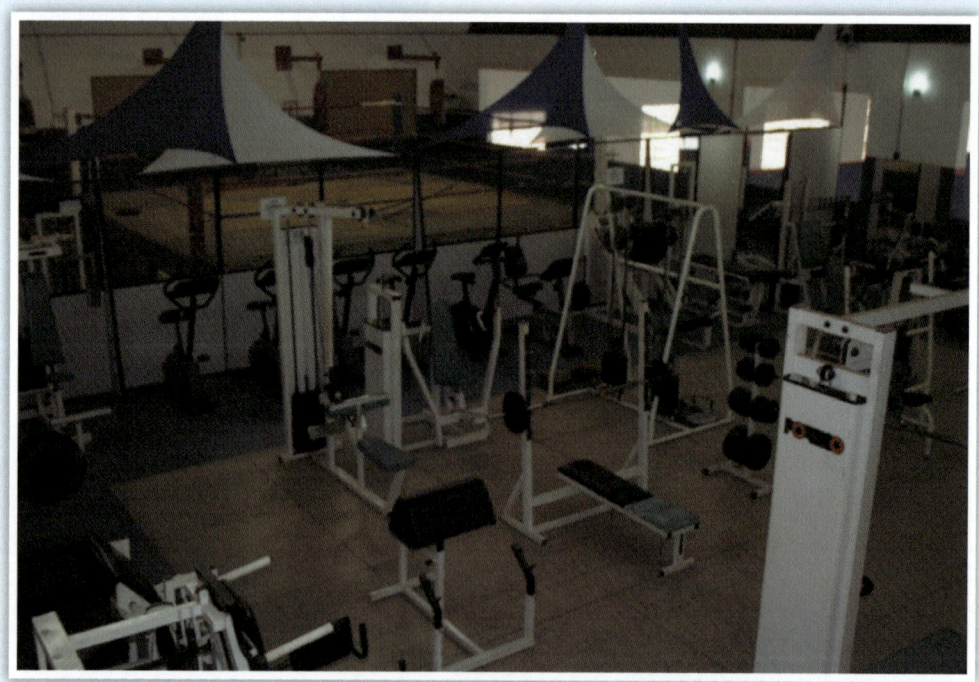

Fig. 19.1 Strength training in the club gym

Training Recommendations

Specific protocols for the improvement of strength and power during childhood will vary greatly depending on both sport and the individual athlete, due to maturity status and existing levels of fitness. So any training programme should be overseen by suitably qualified coaches that understand the physiological and psychological variations between children of different chronological and biological ages (Williams & Bond, 2012).

Many studies have highlighted that adding additional speed and plyometric training to technical and tactical work can help improve markers of functional performance, such as sprint speed, vertical jump height, and change of direction speed (Buchheit, Mendez-Villanueva, Delhomel, Brughelli, & Ahmaidi, 2010; Chelly, Ghenem, Abid, Hermassi, Tabka, & Shephard, 2010; Diallo, Dore, Duche, & Van Praagh, 2001; Mujika, Santisteban and Castagna, 2009). However, these look at various volumes and intensities, so it is difficult to give specific recommendations.

It has also been suggested that reducing training time dedicated to aerobic fitness work by approximately 20% and then supplementing it with explosive strength, jumping, and sprint work, can improve sprinting speed over 30 m without sacrificing aerobic fitness levels (Mikkola et al., 2007).

Overall, the findings for improving speed and power during growth and maturation suggest using some of the training time dedicated to aerobic fitness for more explosive speed and power work, performing this type of work 2–3 times a week, making sure to appreciate the type of work needed to improve these fitness characteristics depending on stages of development, and follow proper progressions and regressions of plyometric training, ensuring that intensity and volume is never prioritised over technical competency (Oliver & Lloyd, 2012; Rumpf et al., 2012; Williams & Bond, 2012).

Conclusion

A compelling body of scientific research suggests that children of all ages and maturation levels can make training-induced improvements in strength, power, speed, and aerobic fitness that surpass the improvements from natural growth and development. All types of training covered are considered safe and effective if the strength and conditioning coach understands and appreciates the complex nature of the growing athlete and ensures that any training is properly progressed and monitored. Any training prescription should be based on biological status, training age, technical competency, existing fitness levels, and emotional maturity. Following these guidelines will help young athletes to improve performance levels on the pitch, court, track, or field and help to reduce the risk of injury, and not promote injury or retard growth as is commonly thought by the general public.

Key Points

- Strength and conditioning is safe in children, if applied properly.

- Strength training can help children as young as 6 years old.

- Speed training can help to increase functional speed.

- Training as little as twice a week can make a physical difference.

- Children and adolescents can do free weights (under supervision).

References

Baker, D., Mitchell, J., Boyle, D., Currell, S., Wilson, G., Bird, S. P., O'Connor, D., & Jones, J. (2007). Resistance training for children and youth: a position stand from the Australian Strength and Conditioning Association (ASCA). Retrieved from: www.strengthandconditioning.org [accessed on 2/12/2012].

Behm, D. G., Faigenbaum, A. D., Falk, B., & Klentrou, P. (2008). Canadian society for exercise physiology position paper: Resistance training in children and adolescents. *Applied Physiology Nutrition and Metabolism, 33*, 547–561.

Behringer, M., vom Heede, A., Matthews, M., & Mester, J. (2011). Effects of strength training on motor performance skills in children and adolescents: A meta-analysis. *Pediatric Exercise Science, 23*, 186–206.

Behringer, M., vom Heede, A., Yue, Z. & Mester, J. (2010). Effects of resistance training in children and adolescents: A meta-analysis. *Pediatrics, 126*, 1199–1210.

Buchheit, M., Mendez-Villanueva, A., Delhomel, G., Brughelli, M., & Ahmaidi, S. (2010). Improving repeated sprint ability in young elite soccer players: repeated shuttle sprints vs. explosive strength training. *Journal of strength and Conditioning Research, 24*(10), 2715–2722.

Chelly, M. S., Ghenem, M. A., Abid, K., Hermassi, S., Tabka, Z., & Shephard, R. J. (2010). Effects of in-season short-term plyometric training program on leg power, jump- and sprint performance of soccer players. *Journal of strength and Conditioning Research, 24*(10), 2670–2676.

De Ste Croix, M. (2007). Advances in paediatric strength assessment: Changing our perspective on strength development. *Journal of Sports Science and Medicine, 6*, 292–304.

De Ste Croix, M. (2008). Muscle strength. In N. Armstrong & W. Van Mechlen (Eds.), *Paediatric exercise science and medicine* (pp. 199–211). Oxford: Oxford University Press.

Diallo, O., Dore, E., Duche, P., & Van Praagh, E. (2001). Effects of plyometric training followed by reduced training programme on physical performance in pre-pubescent soccer player. *Journal of Sports Medicine and Physical Fitness, 41*, 342–348.

Faigenbaum, A., Milliken, L., & Westcott, W. (2003). Maximal strength testing in children. *Journal of Strength and Conditioning Research, 17*, 162–166.

Faigenbaum, A., Westcott, W., Loud, R., & Long, C. (1999). The effects of different resistance training protocols on muscular strength and endurance development in children. *Pediatrics, 104*, e5.

Faigenbaum, A. (2000). Strength training for children and adolescents. *Clinical Sports Medicine, 19*, 593–619.

Faigenbaum, A. D., Kraemer, W. J., Blimkie, C. J., Jeffreys, I., Micheli, L. J., Nitka, M., & Rowland, T. W. (2009). Youth resistance training: updated position statement paper from the

National Strength and Conditioning Association. *Journal of Strength and Conditioning Research, 23,* S60–S79.

Faigenbaum, A. D., McFarland, J. E., Keiper, F. B., Tevlin, W., Ratamess, N. A., Kang, J., & Hoffman, J. R. (2010). Effects of a short-term plyometric and resistance training program on fitness performance in boys age 12 to 15 years. *Journal of Sports Science and Medicine, 6,* 519–525.

Ford, P., De Ste Croix, M., Lloyd, R., Meyers, R., Moosavi, M., Oliver, J., Till, K., & Williams, C. (2011). The long-term athlete development model: Physiological evidence and application. *Journal of Sports Science, 29,* 389–402.

Granacher, U., Goeseles, A., Roggo, K., Wischer, T., Fischer, S., Zuerny, C., Gollhofers, A., & Kriemler, S. (2011). Effects and mechanisms of strength training in children. *International Journal of Sports Medicine, 32,* 357–364.

Jones, R. M., Fry, A. C., Weiss, L. W., Kinzey, S. J., & Moore, C. A. (2008). Kinetic comparison of free weight and machine power cleans. *Journal of Strength and Conditioning Research, 22,* 1785–1789.

Keiner, M., Sander, A., Wirth, K., Caruso, O., Immesberger, P., & Zawieja, M. (2013). Strength performance in youth: Trainability of adolescents and children in the back and front squats. *Journal of Strength and Conditioning Research, 27*(2), 357–362.

Kraemer, W., Fry, A., Frykman, P., Conroy, B., & Hoffman, J. (1989). Resistance training and youth. *Pediatric Exercise Science, 1,* 336–350.

LeMura, L. M., von Dullivard, S. P., & Carlonas, R. (1999). Can exercise training improve maximal aerobic power (VO2 max) in children: A meta-analytic review. *Journal of Exercise Physiology, 2*(3), 1–14.

Lloyd, R. S., Faigenbaum, A. D., Myer, G. D., Stone, M. H., Oliver, J. L., Jeffreys, I., Moody, J., Brewer, C., & Pierce, K. (2012). UKSCA position statement: Youth resistance training. *Professional Strength and Conditioning Journal, 26,* 26–39.

Lloyd, R. S., Oliver, J. L., Meyers, R. W., Moody, J. A., & Stone, M. H. (2012). Long-term athletic development and its application to youth weightlifting. *Strength and Conditioning Journal, 34*(4), 55–66.

Malina, R. (2006). Weight training in youth-growth, maturation and safety: An evidenced based review. *Clinical Journal of Sports Medicine, 16,* 478–487.

Malina, R. M., Bouchard, C., & Bar-Or, O. (2004). *Growth, maturation, and physical activity* (pp. 3–20). Champaign, IL: Human Kinetics.

Mikkola, J., Rusko, H., Nummela, A., Pollari, T. and Häkkinen, K. (2007). Concurrent endurance and explosive type strength training improves nueromuscular and anaerobic characteristics in young distance runners. *International Journal of Sports Medicine, 28,* 602–611.

Mujika, I., Santisteban, J., & Castagna, C. (2009). In-season effect of short-term sprint and power training programs on elite junior soccer players. *Journal of Strength and Conditioning Research, 23*(9), 2581–2587.

Myer, G. D., Faigenbaum, A. D., Chu, D., Falkel, J., Ford, K., & Best, T. (2011). Integrative training for children and adolescents: Techniques and practices for reducing sports related injuries and enhancing athletic performance. *Physician and Sports Medicine, 39,* 74–84.

Oliver, J. L. & Lloyd, R. S. (2012). Long-term athlete development and trainability during childhood: A brief review. *Professional Strength and Conditioning Journal, 26,* 19–24.

Pierce, K. C., Brewer C., Ramsey, M. W., Byrd, R., Sands, W. A., Stone, M. E., & Stone, M. H. (2008). Youth resistance training. *Professional Strength and Conditioning Journal, 10,* 9–23.

Ramsay, J. A., Blimkie, C. J. R., Smith, K., Garner, S., MacDougall, J. D., & Sale, D. G. (1990). Strength training effects in prepubescent boys. *Medicine and Science in Sports and Exercise, 22,* 605–614.

Rowland, T. (2005). *Children's exercise physiology* (2nd ed., pp. 181–195). Champaign, IL: Human Kinetics.

Rowland, T. (1985). Aerobic response to endurance training in prepubescent children: a critical analysis. *Medicine and Science in Sports and Exercise, 17,* 493–497.

Rumpf, M. C., Cronin, J. B., Oliver, J. L. & Hughes, M. G. (2012). Effect of different training methods on running sprint times in male youth. *Pediatric Exercise Science, 24,* 170–186.

Schick, E. E., Coburn, J. W., Brown, L. E., Judelson, D. A., Khamoui, A. V., Tran, T. T., & Uribe, B. P. (2010). A comparison of muscle activation between a Smith machine and free weight bench press. *Journal of Strength and Conditioning Research, 24,* 779–784.

Schwanbeck, S., Chilibeck, P. D., & Binsted, G. (2009). A comparison of free weight squat to Smith machine squat using electromyography. *Journal of Strength and Conditioning Research, 23,* 2588–2591.

Stratton, G., & Williams, C. A. (2007). Children and fitness testing. In E. M. Winter, A. M. Jones, R. C. R. Davison, P. D. Bromley, & T. H. Mercer (Eds.), *Sport and exercise physiology testing guidelines: The British Association of Sport and Exercise Sciences guide* (pp. 211–223). Oxon: Routledge.

Thomas, K., French, D., & Hayes, P. R. (2009). The effect of plyometric training techniques on muscular power and agility in youth soccer players. *Journal of Strength and Conditioning Research, 23,* 332–335.

Tonson, A., Ratel, S., Le Fur, Y., Cozzone, P., & Bendahan, D. (2008). Effect of maturation on the relationship between muscle size and force production. *Medicine and Science in Sports and Exercise, 40,* 918–925.

Williams, C., & Bond, B. (2012). High intensity training in young athletes. *Professional Strength and Conditioning Journal, 26,* 3–8.

CHAPTER 20

Nutrition in Children and Adolescent Sport

Richard Goddard and Solomon Abrahams

Nutrition is extremely important during the developmental stages of adolescence to aid both health and growth. The education of sport (via physical education) and a balanced diet at a young age not only encourages a healthy, active lifestyle in childhood but further develops an understanding of the importance of a balanced lifestyle in later life, thus discouraging the development of health-related diseases such as coronary heart disease and other degenerative diseases. (Nevin-Folino, 2005).

These athletes are more exposed to high-intensity training regimes, and inadequate nutrition may cause growth delay (Demorest & Landry, 2004).

To optimise growth, health, and performance, the young adolescent needs to consume a balanced and appropriate diet. Elite athletes' nutritional intake is an essential factor in their performance and capacity to compete both mentally and physically (Economos, Bortz, & Nelson, 1993). A more common practice among these subjects, however, is to follow popular trends and not necessarily sports nutritional recommendations. In some sports where a low body weight and fat percentage is required, the pursuit of optimal performance may lead to increasing the risk of delayed growth and maturation, amenorrhoea, associated eating disorders, and reduced bone density (Meyer, O'Connor, & Shirreffs, 2007).

Energy requirements differ largely between various age groups during development of the child and the adolescent and in conjunction with assorted levels of participation in physical activity. (Black Prentice, Goldberg, Jebb, Bingham, Livingstone, Coward, 1993). Therefore, the greater the energy expenditure of the child, the larger the energy requirements would be.

It is suggested that the energy requirement of young children is far greater than that of adolescents in their late teens. This is primarily due to the presumption that during the early years, children tend to explore and 'play' in their environment, thus calculating a greater energy expenditure than that of a larger being with larger and more developed bones and muscles who lead a fairly sedentary lifestyle. Energy requirements would also be greater in the earlier years as development and growth are both at a rapid rate (Torun, 2005); therefore, the energy requirements of children are far larger than those of adolescents.

The stages in which obesity develops in children and adolescents are generally the pre-teen and teenage years. Here the demands for energy required for growth in the earlier years are diminished, generally along with the desire to explore the environment, thus decreasing the amount of physical activity completed. Energy intake must also be reduced in this period of development, as the previous energy requirements needed in the earlier years of development do not meet the current energy expenditure, thus increasing the amount of energy being stored in the body as fat when it is not needed for increased physical activity (Goran & Treuth, 2001). In addition, there can be an opposite effect, whereby pre-teens and adolescents can experience rapid weight loss when the uptake of physical activity is vast and they do not meet the energy requirements that their larger and stronger muscles demand, along with the maintainenance of enough energy required to complete the final stages of development and growth.

The occurrence of various developmental diseases, such as osteoporosis, can, therefore, occur at a young age as the growing bones do not receive enough nutrition to maintain their development, thus weakening the structures within. There may also be a delay in puberty (particularly in girls having an irregular or non-existent menstrual cycle in late teenage years) when energy requirements do not meet the demands of the energy expenditure (Herbold & Frates, 2000).

During exercise, children and teens have a higher metabolic cost in movement and preferential fat oxidation. In addition, children and younger athletes are at a 'thermoregulatory disadvantage due to a higher surface area to weight ratio, a slower acclimatization, and lower sweating rate' (Meyer et al., 2007).

Younger athletes primarily depend on more on fat as a fuel and have smaller glycogen stores and reduced glycolytic capacity. This suggests a diminished requirement of carbohydrate but a greater capacity to oxidise fat. Currently, the advice given to elite young athletes is derived from that given to adults, and further research is required to provide appropriate evidence-based guidelines (Jeukendrup & Cronin, 2011).

Fat intake is necessary to provide fat-soluble vitamins and essential fatty acids for energy requirements and weight sustainment. In addition, fat intake should provide 20–25% of energy intake, and an intake of less than 15% shows no performance or health advantage. The association aforementioned also advised against daily weigh-ins and 'adequate food and fluid should be consumed before, during, and after exercise to help maintain blood glucose concentration during exercise, maximize exercise performance, and improve recovery time'.

During competitive events, it is essential that the correct dietary requirements are met so that the body can match the demands placed upon it during physical activity. It is also essential that the correct amount of energy is stored running up to these events to meet these demands. Carbohydrates are a large provider of energy that can be stored to provide a quick release of energy when it is required (Stubbs, Prentice, & James, 1997). 'Carb loading' is the term generally used by athletes and nutritionists to determine the intake of large amounts of carbohydrates from a few days to a few hours before a competitive sporting activity. These carbohydrates are then stored in the body as glycogen to provide the working muscles with the energy they require during physical activity.

Carbohydrates and fats are, therefore, generally recommended to source training requirements and is the main fuel for muscle performance. Approximately 60–70% of carbohydrates are advised for total calorific intake for adult athletes (Economos et al., 1993) and, logically, for adolescents and young athletes, but again further research is required for this specific group (Petrie, Stover, & Horswill, 2004).

Therefore, in theory, the more carbohydrates and fat consumed prior to activity, the more glycogen stores there are. Children may also follow this pattern of carb loading, but not to such an extreme as professional competitive athletes. Too many carbohydrates would be stored as fat in the body when they are not used for physical activity, as children's competitive sports do not match the intensity and duration of adults' sports. Thereby, a small intake of carbohydrates in children and increasing the intake before physical activity in teens would aid performance if the carbohydrates were consumed in proportion to that of the energy requirements of the activity (Williams & Serratosa 2006).

In conjunction with the uptake of carbohydrates, increased volumes of fluids (such as water or specific sporting drinks) are also required prior to and during competition. The body needs to remain hydrated throughout physical activity to maintain homeostasis; therefore, when undergoing physical activity, fluids are required to keep both a safe core and external body temperature (Lindeman, 1990). Again, this is also true in physical activity for children and, more importantly, for adolescents when their physical activity becomes more vigorous and of a higher intensity. Fluids are required in young children as well due to the amount of time they spend playing and exploring, and therefore, they are in constant need of rehydration and replenishment to prevent themselves from becoming dehydrated throughout the day.

It is important to be well hydrated prior to and post exercise to replenish fluid losses. Hydration has been described as one of the most important ergogenic aids to athletes. Sports drinks are also recommended to provide fuel for muscles, maintain blood glucose concentration, and reduce the risk of dehydration, and the thirst mechanism, hyponatremia (Rodriguez, Di Marco, & Langley, 2007, 2009).

Likewise, in post-event meals, carbohydrates need to be re-consumed, but not in the amount that they were in pre-event meals, to balance out the carbohydrates and, therefore, energy that has been used during the activity. Fluid consumption is also important post event to maintain the healthy balance of water in the body in everyday life.

To conclude, the evidence for dietary recommendations for elite adolescents/ children needs further research. To date, the advice is derived from dietary recommendations for adults. Appropriate nutritional advice and adherence may optimise sports performance. An appropriate balanced dietary intake is recommended as opposed to supplementation (except when clinically advised) (Meyer et al., 2007). Athletes with extreme nutrient requirements, or with nutritional problems, should seek individual assessment and counselling from a sports nutrition expert (Burke, 1995). An important aspect for the diet of elite adolescent athletes is that it should adhere to the principles of the basic guidelines in healthy eating.

Key Points

- Energy requirements in children is higher than in adolescents.

- Obesity develops in the pre-teen years.

- Children are at a thermoregulatory disadvantage, and therefore, they are vulnerable in extreme weather such as humidity or cold.

- Younger athletes depend more on fat than on carbs for energy.

- 25% of a child's diet should be fat, as they cannot store excessive amounts of carbs as glycogen.

References

Black, A. E., Prentice, A. M., Goldberg, G. R., Jebb, S. A., Bingham, S. A., Livingstone, B. E., & Coward, A. (1993). Measurements of total energy expenditure provide insights into the validity of dietary measurements of energy intake. *Journal of the American Dietetic Association, 93*(5), 572–579.

Burke, L. (1995). Practical issues in nutrition for athletes. *Journal of Sports Science, 13,* S83–90.

Cotunga, N., Vickery, C. E., & McBee, S. (2005). Sports nutrition for young athletes. *Journal of School Nursing, 21*(6), 323–328.

Dalton, S. E. (1992). Overuse injuries in adolescent athletes. *Sports Medicine, 13*(1), 58–70.

Demorest, R. A., & Landry, G. L. (2004). Training issues in elite young athletes. *Current Sports Medicine Reports, 3*(3), 167–200.

Economos, C. D., Bortz, S. S., & Nelson, M. E. (1993). Nutritional practices of elite athletes. Practical recommendations. *Sports Medicine, 16*(6), 381–399.

Goran, M. I., & Treuth, M. S. (2001). Energy expenditure, physical activity, and obesity in children. *Pediatric Clinics of North America, 48*(4), 931–953.

Herbold, N. H., & Frates, S. E. (2000). Update of nutrition guidelines for the teen: Trends and concerns. *Current Opinion in Pediatrics, 12*(4), 303–309.

Jeukendrup, A. & Cronin, L. (2011). Nutrition and elite young athletes. *Journal of Sports Science and Medicine, 56,* 47–58.

Lindeman, A. K. (1990). Eating and training habits of triathletes: A balancing act. *Journal of the American Dietetic Association, 90*(7), 993–995.

Maffulli, N. (1990). Intensive training in young athletes. The orthopaedic surgeon's viewpoint. *Sports Medicine, 9*(4), 229–243.

Maffulli, N., Longo, U. G., Spiezia, F., & Denaro, V. (2011). Aetiology and prevention of injuries in elite young athletes. *Journal of Sports Science and Medicine, 56,* 187–200.
Meyer, F., O'Connor H., & Shirreffs, S. M. (2007). Nutrition for the young athlete. *Journal of Sports Science and Medicine, 1,* S73–82.

Nevin-Folino, N. (2005). Sports nutrition for children and adolecents. In P. Q. Samour & K. K. Lelm. *Handbook or pediatric nutrition.* (p. 213, 3rd ed.). London: Jones and Bartlett Publishers International.

Petrie, H. J Stover, E. A & Horswill, C. A. (2004). Nutritional concerns for the child and adolescent competitor. *Nutrition, 20*(7–8), 620–31.

Rodriguez, N. R., Di Marco, N. M., & Langley, S. (2009). American college of sports medicine position stand. Nutrition and athletic performance. American Dietetic Association; Dietitians of Canada. *American College of Sports Medicine, 41*(3), 709–31.

Stubbs, R. J. Prentice, A. M., &James, W. P. T. (1997). Carbohydrates and energy balance. *Annals of the New York Academy of Sciences, 819*(1), 44–69.

Torun, B. (2005). Energy requirements of children and adolescents. *Public Health Nutrition, 8*(7A), 968–993.

Williams, C. Serratosa, L. (2006). Nutrition on match day. *Journal of Sports Sciences, 24*(7), 687–697.

CHAPTER 21

Obesity in Children and Adolescent Sport

Alexandra Chaplin

The World Health Organisation (WHO) defines obesity as a 'disorder of excess body fatness that is associated with an increased risk of disease' (World Health Organisation Technical Consultation, 2007). Obese children and adolescents are presenting for treatment in substantial numbers. The imbalance between energy expenditure and energy intake is the main factor accounting for the progression of obesity (King, Tremblay, & Blundell, 1997).

In America, more than 30% of children and adolescents are overweight or obese and around 20% in Europe (Lobstein, Baur, & Uauy, 2004). Research has shown that in the United Kingdom, approximately one-quarter of children are currently obese by the time they leave primary school (Reilly, 2006).

Body fatness in children and adolescents can be difficult to interpret; body fat content at which disease risks increase substantially is unclear and represents a complex issue that depends on age, sex, ethnicity, and the method of expressing body fatness (Reilly, 2006). There is also a concern that muscular children may be mis-classified as obese as a result of having a high body mass index (BMI) for age – a false positive (Reilly, 2006). Recent evidence from research-based guidelines from the United States and United Kingdom recommends that BMI for age should be interpreted relative to national reference data and percentiles approach for clinical applications of the diagnosis of obesity (NICE, 2006).

In the United Kingdom, BMI for age charts based on BMI of UK children in 1990 show that the 91st and 95th percentile lines have been provided and it has been recommended that they be defined as overweight and obese. However, in the United States the 85th and 95th percentiles have been recommended to define being overweight and obese and an extra 99th percentile has been recommended to define extreme obesity (Barlow & the Expert Committee, 2007; Krebs, Himes, Jacobsen, Nicklas, Guilday, & Styne, 2007).

The Youth Risk Behaviours Surveillance System (YRBSS) in the United States provides self-reported physical activity data on boys and girls in the 9–12th grades (Lobstein et al., 2004). The report suggests that only 40% of boys and girls are meeting the physical activity recommendations of at least 60 minutes of physical activity per day. There are many factors that influence energy balance and therefore, can be identified as a contributor to the current obesity epidemic in children and adolescents. These factors include biological, behavioural, environmental, and social influences. Biological factors affecting weight gain include low resting energy expenditure, low fat oxidation rate, low plasma leptin levels, and low muscle oxidative potential (Leibel, Rosenbaum, & Hirsch, 1995).

Early studies showed that obesity tends to run along family lines. The obesity-promoting environmental factors are sometimes referred to as 'obesogenic'. When individuals live in an 'obesogenic' environment, many will gain weight. A child's genetic make-up 'loads the gun', while the environment 'pulls the trigger' (Lobstein et al., 2004).

Overweight women are more likely to have pregnancy complications due to glucose intolerance and diabetes. This can lead to a high-birth-weight baby and the onset of the transgenerational cycle. A direct relationship between time spent watching television (TV) and obesity has been found in most studies of children and adolescents (Must & Taylor, 2005). Epstien et al. (2000) looked into reducing sedentary time in children in a randomised control study of 9-year-olds in California. Results showed that a reduction of time spent in watching TV was associated with reduced obesity. Among adolescents of age 13–18 years, there is evidence that in males, parental education, self-efficacy, attitude, goal motivation, physiccal education/school sports, family influence, and the support of friends are all positively associated with physical activity levels (Van der Horst, Paw, Twisk, & van Mechelen, 2007).

Most studies on obesity relate to dietary intake and eating patterns. A larger percentage of the US population falls short of meeting certain nutritional recommendation. Many studies have been shown that iron and calcium are deficient in diets of children and adolescents (Wagner & Madison, 2005).

50% of children do not eat adequate amounts of calcium. Calcium-deficient diets have shown to cause obesity, high blood pressure, and type 2 diabetes (Wagner & Madison, 2005).

10% of the world's school-aged children are estimated to be carrying excess body fat. One-quarter of these children are obese with a significant likelihood of developing risk factors for type 2 diabetes and heart disease. Many studies have shown that obese children and adolescents are at a greater risk of a range of medical conditions (Lobstein et al., 2004). It is very important to understand this and avoid obesity as conditions can be potentially serious and carry life-threatening consequences.

There are many physical consequences of obesity in childhood and adolescence. These include sleep-associated breathing disorders such as heavy snoring, hypopnea, as well as Pickwickian syndrome, a serious condition associated with pulmonary embolism and sudden death (Riley, Santiago, & Edelman, 1976).

Silvestri, Weese-Mayer, Bass, Kenny, Hauptmann, and Pearsall (1993) found that abnormal sleep patterns occur in 94% of obese children. A study in the United States of children aged between 2 months and 18 years, showed BMI above 85th centile was linked to increased asthma prevalence.

Yen, Chen, Ho, and Mak (2009) investigated and reported 4 case studies evaluating posterior lumbar apophyseal ring fractures in adolescents (PLAR). The apophyseal ring ossifies between ages 4–6 years and fuses at 18 years. It is also shown that the osteocartilaginous portion between the apophyseal ring and the vertebral body is relatively weak. Individual cases were compared and similar findings were found. In every case, the adolescents were overweight and presented with radiating pain into the lower leg or calf. In each case, their single leg raise (SLR) varied from 20 degrees to 50 degrees, which is below normal. Normal range of motion in a non-injured client should be between 70 degrees and 90 degrees. Each of these children had a narrowed, compressed, or bulging disc space in the lower back. Chronic stress or repeated trauma may account for a proplapsed intervertebral disc and apophyseal ring fractures in adolescents. All the cases showed similar results as these are common symptoms of PLAR, paralumbar muscle spasm and tenderness, restricted back motion, tight hamstrings, a waddling gait with flexed knees, and neurological deficits caused by compressed nerve roots.

There are many orthopaedic complications in overweight or obese adolescents including the tensile strength of bone cartilage, which did not evolve to carry such substantial quantities of excess weight. This excessive weight combined with lower tensile strength of bone can lead to 'bowing' of the tibia and femur. The effect of weight on the growth plate is the overgrowth of the medial aspect of the proximal tibial metaphysis, known as Blount disease (Tibia Vara), which causes the upper epiphysis of the tibia to undergo changes in the critical growth period (Dietz, 1998).

Slipped capital femoral epiphysis arises during adolescent growth spurts and is highly common in obese children. Randall and Loder (1998) suggested that it is the most common hip disorder in adolescents. However, because of the anatomic innervation of the hip, it is often mistaken and presented as referred pain in the thigh or knee and is often associated with groin pain. Obesity in adolescents results in an increased sheer stress across the physeal plate. The stress combined with a weaker physeal plate and the endocrine changes connected with puberty leads to a slippage of the epiphyseal inferiorly and posteriorly in the direction of the weight-bearing force (Randall & Loder, 1998).

Perthes disease, also known as Legg–Calvé–Perthes disease, is a childhood disorder which affects the head of the femur. Perthes disease has an unknown aetiology. The blood supply to the growth plate and to the femoral epiphysis of the femur becomes inadequate, and as a result, avascular necrosis occurs. It may be concluded that the prognosis of Perthes disease is proportional to the degree of infarction present within the epiphysis (Silvestri, Weese-Mayer, Bass, Kenny, Hauptmann, and Pearsall, 1993).

Conclusion

It is seen from numerous studies that obesity is increasing in the young, and this may be largely due to the decrease in physical activity and a nutritionally poor diet. This can lead to deteriorating health, including skeletal damage. So obesity in children and adolescents should be reduced and eliminated in order that subsequent generations remain fit and healthy.

Key Points

- 30% of children in the United States are obese or overweight.

- 20% of children in Europe are obese or overweight.

- BMI is unreliable for the assessment of obesity.

- Obesity in children runs in families most of the time.

- 50% of children lack the right amounts of daily calcium and iron.

- Obesity in children increases risk of vertebral fractures.

References

Barlow, S. E., & the Expert Committee. (2007). Expert Committee recommendations regarding the prevention, assessment, and treatment of child and adolescent overweight and obesity: Summary report. *Pediatrics, 120,* s124–s192.

Bouchard, C., Blair, S. N., & Haskell, W. (2007). Why study physical activity and health? In physical activity and health. *Applied Physiology Nutrition & Metabolism, 33,* 3–19.

Dietz. H. W. (1998). Health consequences in obesity in youth. *Childhood Predictors of Adult Disease,* 5, 21, 518–524.

Jebb, S. A., Rennie, K. L., & Cole, T. J. (2004). Prevalence of overweight and obesity among young people in Great Britain. *Public Health Nutrition, 7,* 461–465.

Katzmarzyk, P. T., Baur, L. A., Blair, S. N., Lambert, E. V., Oppert, J-M., & Riddoch, C. (2008). International conference on physical activity and obesity in children: Summary statement and recommendations. *Applied Physiology Nutrition Metabolism. 33,* 371–388.

King, N. A., Tremblay, A., & Blundell, J. E. (1997). Effects of exercise on appetite control: Implications for energy balance. *Medicine & Science in Sports & Exercise, 29*(8), 1076–1089.

Krebs, N. F., Himes, J. H., Jacobsen, D., Nicklas, T. A., Guilday, P., & Styne, D. (2007). Assessment of child and adolescent overweight and obesity. *Pediatrics, 120,* s193–s228.

Leibel, R. L., Rosenbaum, M., & Hirsch, J. (1995). Changes in energy expenditure resulting from altered body weight. *New England Journal of Medicine, 332,* 621–628.

Lobstein, T., Baur, L., & Uauy, R. (2004). Obesity in children and young people: A crisis in public health. *Obesity Reviews 5*(Suppl 1), 4–104.

Must, A., & Tybor, D. J. (2005). Physical activity and sedentary behavior: A review of longitudinal studies of weight and adiposity in youth. *International Journal of Obesity,* 4, 10.

National Institute for Health and Clinical Excellence (NICE) (2006). Obesity: The prevention, identification, assessment, and management of overweight and obesity in adults and children. NICE Clinical Guideline Number 43.

Randall, T., & Loder M. D. (1998). Slipped capital femoral epiphysis. *American Family Physician,* 14, 43, 2135–2142.

Reilly, J. J. (2006a). Diagnostic accuracy of the BMI for age in paediatrics. *International Journal of Obesity, 30,* 595–597.

Reilly, J. J. (2006b). Tackling the obesity epidemic: New approaches. *Archives of Disease in Childhood, 91,* 724–725.

Reilly. J. J (2010). Assessment of obesity in children and adolescents: Synthesis of recent systematic reviews and clinical guidelines. *Journal of Human Nutrition and Dietetics*, 6, 7, 205–209.

Riley, D. J., Santiago, T, & Edelman, N. H. (1976). Complications of obesity-hypoventilation syndrome in childhood. *American Journal of Diseases of Children, 130*, 671–674.

Rodriguez, M. A., Winkleby, M. A., Ahn, D., Sundquist, J., & Kraemer, H. C. (2000). Identification of population subgroups of children and adolescents with high asthma prevalence: Findings from the Third National Health and Nutrition Examination Survey. *Archives of Pediatric Adolescence in Medicine, 156*, 269–275.

Scottish Intercollegiate Guidelines Network (SIGN). (2010). Management of obesity: A national clinical guideline. SIGN clinical guideline. Retrieved from http://www.sign.ac.uk [accessed on 14/2/2013].

Silvestri, J. M., Weese-Mayer, D. E., Bass, M. T., Kenny, A. S., Hauptmann, S. A., & Pearsall, S. M. (1993) Polysomnography in obese children with a history of sleep-associated breathing disorders. *Pediatric Pulmonology, 16*, 124–129.

Stenius-Aarniala, B., Poussa, T., Kvarnstrom, J., Gronlund, E. L., Ylikahri, M., & Mustajoki, P. (2000). Immediate and long term effects of weight reduction in obese people with asthma: Randomised controlled study. *BMJ, 320*, 827–832.

Van der Horst, K., Paw, M. J. C. A., Twisk, J. W. R., & van Mechelen, W. (2007). A brief review on correlates of physical activity and sedentariness in youth. *Medicine and Science in Sports Exercise, 39*, 1241–1250.

Wagner, T., & Madison, J. (2005). Fortified food intake of school aged children: What should health professionals be recommending? *Illinois Journal, 12*, 3, 21–23.

World Health Organization (WHO) (2007). WHO Growth Reference BMI for age 2–5 years. WHO. Retrieved from http://www.who.int/childgrowth/standards/en [accessed on 15/2/2013].

Yen, C. H., Chan, S. K., Ho, Y. F., & Mak, K. H. (2009). Posterior lumbar apophyseal ring fractures in adolescents: a report of four cases. *Journal of Orthopaedic Surgery, 17*, 85–89.

Zadeh. H. G, & Monsell. F. (1998). The painful hip. *Current Paediatricians, 8*, 11–18.

CHAPTER 22

The Physically Challenged in Children and Adolescent Sport

Solomon Abrahams

Those who suffer from physical impairments are often viewed as disadvantaged individuals in various areas of our society. Whether it be in the workforce, at home, or on the sports field it is no shock that people often fail to understand what it's like to be less able-bodied.

Although disabilities limit people in certain ways, it does not limit them nearly as much as people perceive. Physical activity is often one of the many things that is overlooked in relation to children with disabilities in sport. The advantage of exercise and physical activity for anyone, whether they be a child or an adult, is extremely significant to one's health, both mentally and physically. Although children with disabilities might have lower levels of fitness than children who do not have physical disabilities, their participation in sport and physical activity is just as beneficial and is something that should not be overlooked. If anything, sport is the one focus they have to prove a point. Physical fitness at any level can make a huge difference in the life of someone who suffers from a physical impairment, and all endeavours should be made to ensure they can be helped where possible.

A physical impairment certainly holds a person back from being completely functional in some sports. A child who has Down's syndrome, for example, will have a tough time competing in a full basketball game against other children who are without impairment. However, does this mean that this child should refrain from becoming a part of a team, shooting hoops, or taking part in practices?

Participation in these recreational activities is a way of promoting such things as inclusion and teamwork, both of which promote positive thinking and higher levels of self-esteem that can change a child's life in some cases (McConachie,

Colver, Forsyth, Jarvis, & Parkinson, 2006). Participation and acceptance among other children will give such children a feeling of belonging and encourage them to continue partaking in physical activities, regardless of their individual skill level.

Some restrictions will exist for some children suffering from a chronic condition or disability. They cannot support the same amount of exercise as someone who does not suffer from an illness. Paediatricians and parents can overestimate the risk of a child who takes part in these activities; however, big strides have been made for promoting this type of physical fitness (Murphy & Carbone, 2008). In 1968, the Special Olympics was established in an effort to allow children with disabilities to compete in athletic events with other children who suffer from similar illnesses (Murphy et al., 2008). The organisation has grown to over 1 million athletes in 125 countries (Murphy et al., 2008). These children possess impairments that include lower levels of cardiorespiratory fitness, lower levels of muscular endurance, and higher levels of obesity.

However, the physical activities that they can take part in help in controlling or slowing down the progression of their physical disabilities, which improves their overall health and function (McConachie et al., 2006). The establishment and continued growth of the Special Olympics also helps these children and their families with the psychological part of their disabilities (Murphy et al., 2008). This is an impact that holds tremendous value in the life of a child with a disability.

Participating in activities means just as much for children who do not suffer from a disability as it does for those impaired children. They still seek the same benefits from playing team sports and exercising as other children. These activities help children to form friendships and encourage creativity, imagination, competitiveness, and a feeling of being a member of a team, while continuing to build mental and physical health (McConachie et al., 2006). Allowing these children to grow up in a less restrictive environment than what they are used to will help them to deal with the physical exhaustion that comes from other aspects of their lives.

When exploring the physical benefits of participating in physical activities, one must understand that just because the physical ability of an impaired child is not equal to a child who is fully functional, it doesn't mean that they are not bettering their physical welfare by participating in athletic events and exercise (McConachie et al., 2006).

By participating and improving fitness, a child can reverse the deconditioning secondary to impaired mobility, optimise physical functioning, and enhance their overall well-being (Murphy et al., 2008). These exercises will help to strengthen muscles, increase flexibility, and improve joint structure. This will help to decrease the rate at which their bodies' ability to function declines. A child with Down's syndrome, for example, who does not possess the same physical strength as an able-bodied child, can increase exercise endurance and work capacity after participating in these aerobic training workouts.

Children with disabilities are also at a higher risk of obesity due to limited endurance and stamina. Their impairments that result in inactivity can have consequences that include reduced cardiovascular fitness, osteoporosis, and impaired circulation (Murphy et al., 2008). These effects also translate into psychological dangers, as children will suffer from self-esteem issues caused by social acceptance problems. They have lower levels of independence when it comes to daily living – an issue that will continue to damage their mental well-being as they get older. Their participation in athletic events will help them to deal with the issues they face and also decrease problems with immobility and physical inability (McConachie et al., 2006).

Children take part in athletics at a young age for numerous reasons other than their attraction to the specific sport. They join a team as a way of being sociable with classmates and with the idea of being included in the group. A child with impairment is at a higher risk of falling victim to exclusion; therefore, it is vital to promote their participation in these athletic events (McConachie et al., 2006). That is the reason the Special Olympics or Paralympics has grown in popularity since its establishment. It allows these children opportunities that they would not have, like competing with typical young athletes. For children with physical impairments, exercising and being on athletic teams is just as much advantageous for their mental well-being as it is for their physical well-being. One cannot undervalue the way a child feels when he is a part of a team and performing the same activities as children who do not suffer as they do. Promoting this fitness can help to slow the effects of their illnesses, while increasing their physical ability (McConachie et al., 2006). Sports help children in so many different ways, and even more so a child suffering from a disability. It can change their lives.

Key Points

- Sport can be hugely beneficial physically, emotionally, and mentally.

- Sport can improve functionality in the physically challenged.

- Sport can recondition a child with obesity secondary to physical disability.

References

McConachie, H., Colver, A. F., Forsyth, R. J., Jarvis S. N., & Parkinson. K. N. (2006). Participation of disabled children: how should it be characterised and measured? *Disability and Rehabilitation, 28*(18), 1157–1164.

Murphy, N. A., & Carbone, P. S. (2008). Promoting the participation of children with disabilities in sports, recreation, and physical activities. *American Academy of Pediatrics, 121*(5), 1057–1061.

CHAPTER 23

Psychology Principles in Children and Adolescent Sport

Daniel Manzi and Solomon Abrahams

Psychology has many effects on children's participation in sporting activities along with involvement of parents, peers, past injuries, stresses, and illnesses. As well as many of these factors encourage and enhance a child's desire to participate in sport, some likewise, diminish the desire to participate in physical activity altogether.

The psychology of the child athlete and their response to an injury depends on many factors, including age, gender, severity, type of injury, pain tolerance, ability to cope, confidence in the medical management, seasonal timing, context of injury, and support from family and friends (Patel, Greydanus, & Baker, 2009).

The majority of children understand their injury, especially as they get older, and, more importantly, the implications of the injury. Some enjoy the special attention they get, and depending on how good they are, they can enjoy the relative rest, if, for example, they are not playing too well.

Family Influences

The environment in which a child is brought up can heavily influence their participation in sports and other physical activities. Generally, if a child's parents enjoy sports, frequently participate in sports themselves and encourage the child to do so, the child will most likely participate in physical activity. A parent's praise towards a child for participating in physical activities with them or a parent going to watch their child play sports would further encourage the child to continue their participation in physical activities, as this is seen as positive reinforcement for the participation in physical activity (Dowda, Ainsworth, Addy, Saunders, & Riner, 2001). Likewise, if a child is raised around a family that lead a primarily sedentary lifestyle and do not participate in any physical activities in their leisure time, a child would be discouraged to participate in sports as well.

Parents who don't participate in activities themselves will also be less likely to travel to observe their child participate in activities, thus leading to further negative reinforcement towards the child who is willing to participate in sport. This can often lead to an increase in child obesity, and it is common for the children of obese parents to carry the same trait.

Friends and Peers

Peers can have a psychological effect on a child's participation during school years or in classes outside of the school environment. For example, a child who is friends with a group of children who enjoy sports at school and who partake in extra-curricular sporting activities is more likely to participate and enjoy those activities with their friends. On top of this, a child who goes to classes outside of schooling hours, such as ballet or karate classes, will be meeting other children away from school who enjoy the sport (the common interest), which will further encourage them to continue participating. Peer groups may also have a negative effect on the participation in physical activities during school years. A child who has become friends with a group of peers who do not enjoy sports and therefore don't take part in any extra-curricular activities is less likely to enjoy participating in physical activities. This is because if they were to participate in any activities without their friends, they may feel out of place and also fear that their friends would no longer enjoy their company as their interests differ.

There are many studies that suggest that participation in sports at a young age aids a child's psychosocial development along with their emotional intelligence which develops beyond that of their peers' (Scanlan, Babkes, Scanlan, 2005).

Importance of Sport

One of the more important factors influencing the emotional response is the relationship between the importance of sport in their lives and their future (Williams, 2009). For example, in contrast to an amateur, if a professional footballer receives a long-term injury or one that is likely to terminate his career, then he will experience a stronger sense of loss in a way that has been well documented in counselling psychology. Reactions include identity loss, fear and anxiety, lack of confidence, and performance detriments. Those who sustain career-ending injuries may require long-term psychological care (Weinberg &and Gould, 2003). In these situations, it is not uncommon for professional trainers to refer the athletes to a sport psychologist (Williams, 2009).

Improving Communication and Social Interaction

Children who participate in sport have a lot more social interaction with various groups of people; therefore, their communicative skills with various age groups would be vastly improved compared with those of children who don't participate in sporting activities. During sports training, a child needs to be able to communicate with not only their teammates (if competing in a team sport) or their classmates (if participating in a solo sport) but also their coach and the referee. This, therefore, develops the child's ability to communicate with adults in a professional and mature manner and form a cohesive relationship with children on their team or in their class. The ability of the sporting child to also construct 'game play' and to understand tactics would further their intellect compared with those who do not take part in team sports.

Psychological Stress

However, there are many psychological stresses that come with participation in sport as a child that children do not experience when they don't participate in sport. For example, a sporting injury can affect the athlete not only by taking them out of the game but also by causing stress and, sometimes, depression (Williams & Andersen 1998). These emotions are more likely to occur in teenage athletes who compete at a high level rather than younger children who play sports at school and during extra-curricular activities (Smith, Smoll, & Barnett, 1995). For example, young athletes who are performing at an exceptional standard for their age may feel stress from their coach, family, and peers to continue to do well and excel. This may, however, have a negative effect on the athletes' performance, resulting in a poor standard during competition. Sometimes, it can lead to an injury if the athletes push themselves to achieve a higher standard that is beyond the capabilities of their bodies. Both of these stresses can lead to a reduced or even complete stop of participation. Due to the feeling of failure or worthlessness, depression can develop in the young athletes (Lanea, & Terrya, 2000).

On the contrary, there are many studies which suggest that participation in sporting activities also aids in recovering from depression (Dishman, Hales, Pfeiffer, Felton, Saunders, Ward, Dowda, Pate (2006) along with improving young people's self-esteem and body confidence. This can also reduce the probability of a person going into depression at a young age or developing it in their later life.

Benefits of Being Injured

There is evidence to suggest that athletes can perceive benefits in being injured (Brewer, 2001). For example, if an athlete feels that they need to work hard to be a part of the team in comparison with a teammate who perhaps is more established or seen as one of the better players, it is likely that the injured athlete will be more sensitive to the coach's needs. If the coach creates an environment that reduces the injured athletes to feel a sense of worthlessness, then they will be more likely to play with an injury or try to return prematurely (Weinberg &and Gould, 2003).

How Can We Help?

Those athletes that remain most positive are the ones that recover most quickly (Brewer, 2001); therefore, it is worth making sure that the rehabilitation experience is a positive one. First impressions and experiences are crucial (Biddle, Hanrahan, & Sellars, 2001). If sport is perceived to be important, it is wise to guard against the potential for a premature return to training. Given the importance of the athlete's first positive experience, care should be taken to ensure that they do not perceive a poor recovery, which may well be the case if an early return results in further setbacks.

It is important to be perceived as helping the injury to recover and dealing with emotional reactions, improving motivation, and increasing the adherence to treatment programmes using techniques such as imagery and relaxation, goal-setting, enhancing self-motivation, positive self-talk, and informing significant others clearly and regularly to elicit important social support (Brewer, 2001; Weinberg & Gould, 2003)

Knowing techniques such as imagery and relaxation with a good goal-setting strategy may help (Williams, 2009). Be aware of applying general principles as each athlete will understand things differently and will need individual attention and help to manage the situation. The importance of understanding the athlete's position from a subcultural perspective cannot be underestimated. However, with more severely injured athletes, the rehabilitation process may take more of a psychological turn. In a qualitative account of a case study by Richard Cox, he outlines a 12-point process for the successful completion of the final activity phase (Cox, 2002).

Conclusion

Both personal and situational circumstances will affect happiness and adherence to programmes that improve health. Creating happy experiences will simply speed up recovery. To improve adherence to health programmes, factors like having good social support and psychological skills like imagery, goal-setting, self-talk, and routines are helpful. By managing emotions and motivation, both these aspects can be used to improve the experience of injury. This, in turn, will help in future injuries.

Key Points

- Family influences can affect a child's mental approach to recovery.

- Strong team sports can help children recover more quickly.

- Sport can increase communication and intelligence in children.

- Sport can help depression.

- Underperforming athletes or those under enormous pressure can benefit from being injured.

References

Biddle, S. J. H., Hanrahan, S. J., Sellars, C. N. (2001). Attributions: Past, present and future. In R. N. Singer, H. A. Hausenblas & C. M. Janelle (Eds.), *Handbook of sport psychology*. New Jersey, NJ: John Wiley.

Brewer, B. W. (2001). Psychology of sport injury rehabiliatation. In R. N. Singer, H. A. Hausenblas & C. M. (Eds.), *Handbook of sport psychology*. New Jersey, NJ: John Wiley.
Brewer, B. W. (2010). The role of psychological factors in sport injury rehabilitation outcomes. *International Review of Sport and Exercise Psychology, 3*, 40–61.

Cox, R. (2002). The psychological rehabilitation of a severly injured rugby player. In I. M. Cockerill (Ed.), *Solutions in sport psychology*. London: Thomson.

Dishman, R. K., Hales, D. P., Pfeiffer, K. A., Felton, G. A., Saunders, R., Ward, D. S., Dowda, M., & Pate, R. R. (2006). Physical self-concept and self-esteem mediate cross-sectional relations of physical activity and sport participation with depression symptoms among adolescent girls. *Health Psychology, 25*(3), 396–407.

Dowda, M., Ainsworth, B. E., Addy, C. L., Saunders, R., & Riner, W. (2001). Environmental influences, physical activity, and weight status in 8 to16-Year-Olds. *Archives of Pediatrics & Adolescent Medicine, 155*(6), 711–717.

Gill, D. L. (2000). *Psychological dynamics of sport and exercise*. Champaign, IL: Human Kinetics.

Heil, J. (2012). Pain on the run: Injury, pain and performance in a distance runner. *Sport Psychologist, 26*, 540.

Horn, T. S. (2002). *Advances in sport psychology*. Champaign, IL: Human Kinetics.

Jowett, S., & Lavallee, D. (2007). *Social psychology in sport*. Champaign, IL: Human Kinetics.

Lanea, A. M. & Terrya, P. C. (2000). The Nature of Mood: Development of a Conceptual Model with a Focus on Depression. *Journal of Applied Sport Psychology*. 12 (1), 16–33.

Mankad, A., Gordon, S., & Wallman, K. (2009a). Psycho-immunological effects of written emotional disclosure during long-term Injury rehabilitation. *Journal of Clinical Sport Psychology, 3*, 205–217.

Mankad, A., Gordon, S., & Wallman, K. (2009b). Perceptions of emotional climate among inured athletes. *Journal of Clinical Sport Psychology, 3*, 3–14.

Patel, D., Greydanus, D., & Baker, R. (2009). *Pedaitricpractice Sports Medicine*, New York, NY: McGraw Medical.

Petitpas, A., & Danish, S. J. (1995). Caring for injured athletes. In S. M. Murphy (Ed.), *Sport Psychology Interventions*. Champaign, IL: Human Kinetics.

Ruddock-Hudson, M., O'Halloran, P., & Murphy, G. (2012). Exploring psychological reactions to injury in the Australian football league (AFL). *Journal of Applied Sport Psychology, 24*, 375–390.

Scanlan, T. K., Babkes, M. L., & Scanlan, L. A. (2005). Participation in sport: A developmental glimpse at emotion. In J. L. Mahoney, R. Larson & J. S. Eccles (Ed.), *Organized Activities as Contexts of dDevelopment: Extracurricular aActivities.* (pp. 275–309). New Jersey, NJ: Laurence Erlbaum Associates, Inc.

Singer, R. N., Hausenblas, H. A., & Janelle, C. M. (Eds.) (2001). *Handbook of sSport pPsychology* (2nd edition.). ed. New Jersey, NJ: John Wiley..

Smith, R. E., Smoll, F. L., & Barnett, N. P. (1995). Reduction of children's sport performance anxiety through social support and stress-reduction training for coaches. *Journal of Applied Developmental Psychology,. 16*(1), 125–142.

Udry, E., & Andersen, M. B. (2002). Athletic injury and sport behaviour. In T. S. Horn (Ed.), *Advances in sport psychology*. Champaign, IL: Human Kinetics.

Wadey, R., Evans, L., Evans, K., & Mitchell, I. (2011). Perceived benefits following sport injury: A qualitative examination of their antecedents and underlying mechanisms. *Journal of Applied Sport Psychology, 23*, 142–158.

Weinberg, R. S., & Gould, D. (2003). *Foundations of sport and exercise psychology*. Champaign, IL: Human Kinetics.

Weiss, M. R. (1995). Children in sport: An education model. In S. M. Murphy (Ed.), *Sport psychology interventions*. Champaign, IL: Human Kinetics.

Williams, J. M., & Andersen, M. B. (1998). Psychosocial antecedents of sport injury: Review and critique of the stress and injury model. *Journal of Applied Sport Psychology, 10*(1), 5–25.

Williams, J. (2009). *Applied sport psychology: Personal growth to peak performance* (6th ed.), New York, NY: McGraw-Hill. Humanities/Social Sciences/Languages.

Wippert, P. M., & Wippert, J. (2010). The effects of involuntary athletic career termination on psychological distress. *Journal of Clinical Sport Psychology, 4*, 133–149.

CHAPTER 24

Functional Rehabilitation in Children's and Adolescent Sport

Alexandra Chaplin and Solomon Abrahams

When designing and executing a functional rehabilitation training programme for adolescent players, the emotional and psychological maturity of the player should also be taken into account (Kraemer & Fleck, 2005; Stratton, Jones, Fox, Tolfrey, Harris, Maffulli, Lee, & Frostick, 2004).

An area that has received little study is that of neuromuscular and functional training in adolescents, which includes sports-specific instruction on the technique and the practice of fundamental movement mechanisms (Gamble, 2008). In most sports, fundamental movements occur in some combination of squatting, lifting, pushing, pulling, jumping, landing, running, and changing direction; therefore, the neuromuscular postural control and movement biomechanics must be installed and established in order to reduce injury (McGill, 2004). There is no point trying to advance specific training in sport if the fundamental movement patterns are flawed.

Specific instructions and training of proper movement mechanisms have been shown to increase the precise movements safely (Myer, Ford, Palumbo, & Hewett, 2005). Continued practice and development of correct techniques equips the young players to react to the challenges in a game situation. Barber-Westin, Galloway, Noyes, Corbett, and Walsh (2005) found that young female athletes showed traits of neuromuscular deficits such as valgus hip, knee, and ankle alignment during jumping and therefore, increasing risk of injury. Myer et al. (2005) found that if specific instructions and repetition of the jump landing movement occurred, this improved vertical jumping technique and the movement biomechanics in high school children. Females have neuromuscular control issues which may contribute to making their ligaments dominant due to inactive muscular stabilisation. Neuromuscular training intervention significantly improves lower limb alignment and reduces knee valgus angles in young female athletes. Working on repetitions and neuromuscular control in training helps to guard against injuries (Gamble, 2008).

Functional Rehabilitation Training

Youth sports players appear to be at a greater risk of injury when there is inadequate physical preparation or poor rehabilitation. Sports rehabilitation of a sprinter should incorporate plyometric and sports-specific sprinting rather than pushing weights in a gym.

Injuries are also more likely to occur when muscle fatigue occurs in the later stages of a game than when they have more energy. Studies have also shown that at the start of the season, more injuries occur due to the players' fitness levels not being adequate (Thacker, Stroup, Branche, Gilchrist, Goodman, & Kelling, 2003). Therefore, physical preparation such as functional strength training, cardiovascular fitness, and developmental skills should be established to help injury prevention (Adirim & Cheng, 2003).

When organising sports and physical training, it is important to remember that adolescents are still growing (Bompa, 2000), as bone, muscles, and connective tissues are not fully developed in adolescents.

Sports-specific and functional resistance training refers to a method of functional physical conditioning which involves the progressive use of resistive loads that mimic movements within the sport, using different movement velocities and a variety of equipment (Faigenbaum & Myer, 2010).

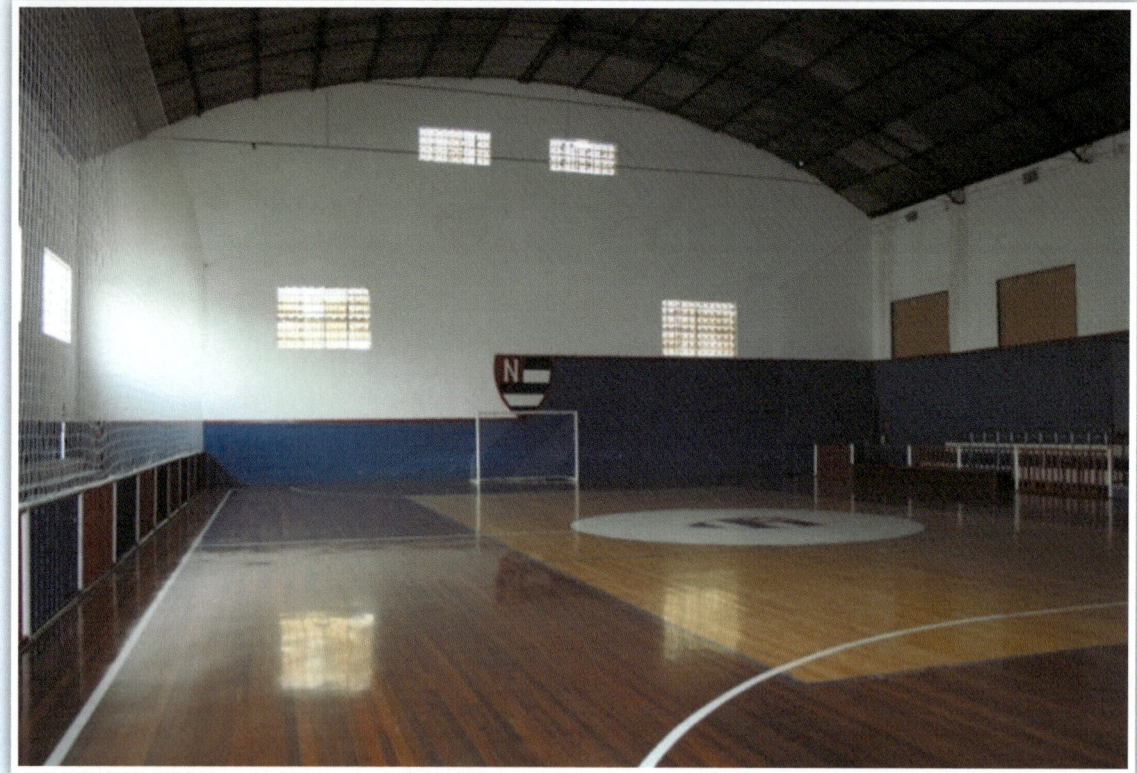

Fig. 24.1 Large gymnasium for rehabilitaiton training

The benefits of sports-specific resistance training are being increasingly recognised and its use is becoming universally accepted among health professionals, particularly in the United States (Goldberg, Moroz, Smith, & Ganley, 2007) and recently within the United Kingdom (Stratton et al., 2004). Professional fitness associations and health organisations are now in agreement that age-appropriate youth functional training is safe and beneficial when performed under supervision (Stratton et al., 2004). Evidence has shown that functional training and rehabilitation along with a healthy diet has the potential to enhance growth at all stages of development (Faigenbaum et al., 1996).

Hormonal response to this type of training in adolescents at the early stages of development can lead to structural changes to the muscle and associated connective tissue (Faigenbaum et al., 1996). Similarly, this kind of training and rehabilitation has been reported to increase bone mineral density while not adversely affecting maturational growth (Sadres, Eliakim, Constantini, Lidor, & Falk, 2001). A correctly designed and supervised functional rehabilitation training programme for young athletes can improve the functional muscular strength and power, enhance the cardiovascular system, increase a young athlete's resistance to sports-related injuries, and help to promote and develop exercise habits during childhood and adolescence that continue into adulthood (Brukner & Khan, 2010).

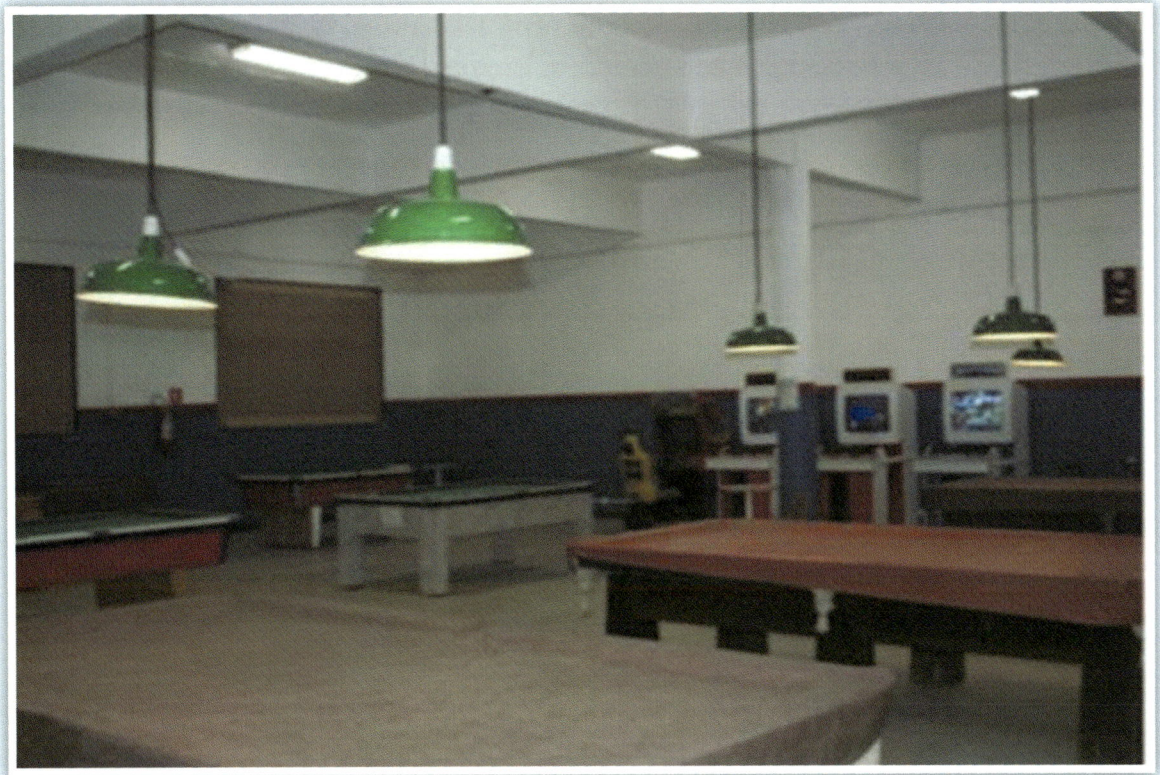

Fig. 24.2 Rehabiliation gym with more relaxing equipment

Speed and Acceleration Training

Plyometric training is a technique which adolescents can use in the later part of training. Plyometric exercises use the natural elastic recoil elements of the human muscle and the neurological stretch reflex to produce a stronger and faster muscle response. This is a form of resistance training that combines rapid eccentric muscle contraction followed by a rapid concentric contraction (Brukner & Khan, 2010).

Plyometric training involves body mass jumping exercises and medicine ball throws that are performed quickly and explosively. With these movements, the neuromuscular system is conditioned to react more quickly to the stretch–shortening cycle, which may enhance a young athlete's ability to increase speed of movement and improve power production safely (Chu, Faigenbaum, & Falkel, 2006). The young athlete should commence plyometric training with less intense drills (double-leg jumps) and gradually progress to more advanced drills (single-leg hops) (Behm, Faigenbaum, Falk, & Klentrou, 2008). This type of exercise can increase a child's speed of movement, improve power production (Diallo, Dore, Duche, & Praagh, 2001), and strengthen the bones (Greene, 2006). Plyometric training programmes have been shown to be effective during puberty for improving running speed and jumping ability (Markovic, 2007) with an increase in strength. Strength training can improve muscle performance and coordination of muscle groups. Therefore, plyometric training may be an appropriate intervention for improving the motor ability of children to run, jump, hop, skip, kick, and throw, but it should be carefully supervised in adolescents as it has a high potential for causing injury. Khlifa, Aouadi, Hermassi, Chelly, Jlid, Hbacha and Castagna (2010) found that using a standard plyometric training protocol, with or without added load, improved the vertical jumping ability in young male basketball players. However, the best effects for jumps were observed in the loaded plyometric group, which showed significantly higher gains than the non-loaded plyometric training group. Thus the correct use of weights may be an advantage, even in the young.

Conclusion

Young athletes' participation in sport can lead to injury if improper training or rehabilitation occurs as the muscles, bones, and connective tissues of their bodies are not yet mature. Specific functional training techniques and the understanding of controlled biomechanical movements reduce the risk of injury.

This has led to the increased safe use of this kind of training to encourage the athletic advancement of the developing body of youngsters, including the recent use of plyometric training programmes. Using the natural elastic recoil of muscle and ensuring that the rehabilitation is as functional as possible allows the neurological reflexes in combination with loading to improve the motor ability in the young.

Key Points

- Sports-specific rehabilitation reduces re-injury in children.
- Plyometric training can increase functional speed.
- Improper rehabilitation in children can cause more injuries.
- Sports-specific rehabilitation improves neuro-adapability.

References

Adirim, T. A., & Cheng, T. L. (2003). Overview of injuries in the young athlete. *Sports Medicine, 33*, 75–81.

Barber-Westin, S. D., Galloway, M., Noyes, F. R., Corbett, G., & Walsh, C. (2005). Assessment of lower limb neuromuscular control in prepubescent athletes. *American Journal of Sports Medicine, 33*, 1853–1860.

Barber-Westin, S. D., Noyes, F. R., & Galloway, M. (2006). Jump-land characteristics and muscle strength development in young athletes. *American Journal of Sports Medicine, 34*, 375–384.

Behm, D. G., Faigenbaum, A. D., Falk, B., & Klentrou, P. (2008). Canadian Society for Exercise Physiology position paper: Resistance training in children and adolescents. *Appllied Physiology, Nutrition, & Metabolism, 33*, 547–561.

Bompa, T. (2000). *Total training for young champions* (pp. 1–20). Champaign, IL: Human Kinetics.

Brukner and Khan (2010). Clinical sports medicine (3rd ed., p. 133). New York, NY: McGraw Hill Medical.

Caine, D., Caine, C., & Maffulli, N. (2006). Incidence and distribution of pediatric sport-related injuries. *Clinical Journal of Sports Medicine, 16*, 500–513.

Chu, D., Faigenbaum, A., & Falkel, J. (2006). *Progressive plyometrics for kids.* Monterey, CA: Healthy Learning.

Diallo, O., Dore, E., Duche, P., & Van Praagh, E. (2001). Effects of plyometric training followed by a reduced training programme on physical performance in prepubescent soccer players. *Journal of Sports Medicine and Physical Fitness, 41*, 342–348.

Faigenbaum, A. D., & Myer, G. D. (2010). Resistance training among athletes: Safety, efficacy and injury prevention effects. *British Journal Sports Medicine, 44*, 56–63.

Faigenbaum, A. D., Kraemer, W. J., Cahill, B., Chandler, J., Dziados, J., Elfrink, L. D., Forman, E., Gaudiose, M., Micheli, L., Nikta, M., & Roberts, S. (1996). Youth resistance training: position statement paper and literature review. *Strength Condition Journal, 18*, 62–75.

Gamble, P. (2008). Approaching physical preparation for youth team-sports players. *Strength and Conditioning Journal, 30*, 29–42.

Goldberg, A. S., Moroz, L., Smith, A., & Ganley, T. (2007). Injury surveillance in young athletes: a clinician's guide to sports injury literature. *Sports Medicine, 37*, 265–278.

Greene, D. A. (2006). Adaptive skeletal responses to mechanical loading during adolescence. *Sports Medicine, 36*, 723–732.

Kelling, E. (2003). Prevention of knee injuries in sports: A systematic review of the literature. *Journal of Sports Medicine and Physical Fitness, 43*, 165–179.

Khlifa, R., Aouadi, R., Hermassi, S., Chelly, M. S., Jlid, M. C., Hbacha, H., & Castagna, C. (2010). Effects of a plyometric training program with and without added load on jumping ability in basketball players. *Journal of Strength and Condition Research.*

Kraemer, W. J., & Fleck, S. J. (2005). Strength training and your child. In *Strength training for young athletes* (2nd ed., pp. 1–17). Champaign, IL: Human Kinetics.

Lubans, D. R., Aguiar, E. J., & Callister, R. (2010). The effects of free weights and elastic tubing resistance training on physical self-perception in adolescents. *Psychology of Sports and Exercise, 11*(6), 497–504.

Maffulli, N. (1992). The growing child in sport. *British Medical Bulletin, 48*, 561–568.

Maffulli, N., & Helms, P. (1988). Controversies about intensive training in young athletes. *Archives of Disease in Childhood, 63*, 1405–1407.

Malina, R. M., Meleski, B. W., & Shoup, R. F. (1982). Anthropometric, body composition, and maturity characteristics of selected school-age athletes. *Pediatric Clinics of North America, 29*, 1305–1323.

Markovic, G. (2007). Does plyometric training improve vertical jump height? A meta analytical review. *British Journal of Sports Medicine, 41*, 349–355.

McGill, S. M. (2004). Developing strength, power, and agility. In Ultimate back fitness and performance (pp. 282–308). Canada: Wabuno.

Myer, G. D., Ford, K. R., Palumbo, J. P., & Hewett, T. E. (2005). Neuromuscular training improves performance and lower-extremity biomechanics in female athletes. *Journal of Strength & Conditioning Research, 19*, 51–60.

Naughton, G., Farpour-Lambert, N. J., Carlson, J., Bradley, M., & Van Praagh, E. (2000). Physiological issues surrounding the performance of adolescent athletes. *Sports Medicine, 30*, 309–32.

Pope, R. P., Herbert, R. D., & Kirwan, J. D. et al. (2000). A randomized trial of preexercise stretching for prevention of lower-limb injury. *Medicine and Science in Sports and Exercise, 32*, 271–277.

Powell, J. W., & Barber-Foss, K. D. (1999). Injury patterns in selected high school sports; A review of the 1995–1997 seasons. *Journal of Athletic Training, 34*, 277–284.

Rowley, S. (1986). *The effect of intensive training in young athletes: A review of the research literature* (pp. 1–115). London: Sports Council.

Rowley, S. (1989). *The effect of intensive training on young athletes* (pp. 6–7). London: Sports Council.

Sadres, E., Eliakim, A., Constantini, N., Lidor, R., & Falk, B. (2001). The effect of longterm resistance training on anthropometric measures, muscle strength, and self concept in prepubertal boys. *Pediatric Exercise Science, 13*, 357–372.

Sahlin, Y. (1990). Sport accidents in childhood. *British Journal of Sports Medicine, 24*, 40–44.

Shrier, I. (2000). Stretching before exercise: an evidence-based approach. *British Journal of Sports Medicine, 34*, 324–325.

Shanmugam, C. & Maffulli, N. (2008). Sports injuries in children. *British Medical Bulletin, 2008*(86), 33–57.

Stratton, G., Jones, M., Fox, K. R., Tolfrey, K., Harris, J., Maffulli, N., Lee, M., & Frostick, S. P. (2004). BASES position statement on guidelines for resistance training in young people. *Journal of Sports Science, 22*, 383–390.

Thacker, S. B., Stroup, D. F., Branche, C. M., Gilchrist, J., Goodman, R. A., & Porter Kelling, E. (2003). Prevention of knee injuries in sports: A systematic review of the literature. *Journal of Sports Medicine and Physical Fitness, 43*, 165–179.

Quatman, C. E., Ford, K. R., Myer, G. D., & Hewett, T. E. (2006). Maturation leads to gender differences in landing force and vertical jump performance. *American Journal of Sports Medicine, 34*, 806–813.

CHAPTER 25

Protection of Children and Adolescents in Sports

Hollie Whitworth

What Is Child Abuse?

The National Commission of Inquiry (UK), which specialises in the prevention of child abuse (1996), defines it as 'anything which individuals, institutions or processes do or fail to do which directly or indirectly harms children or damages their prospects of safe and healthy development into adulthood' (Childhood Matters, 1996).

An abuser can be any individual who comes into contact with a child. As the definition by the National Commission of Inquiry states, abuse can also include a situation where a person knowingly fails to prevent abuse from occurring. The National Society for Prevention of Cruelty to Children (NSPCC) defines 4 categories of abuse as follows:

- **Sexual abuse** involves forcing or enticing a child into sexual activity regardless of whether the child understands what is happening. Within sport, sexual abuse can, for example, occur where there is inappropriate touching of a child (e.g. between a child and the coach). This can be sometimes hard to spot, particularly where the sport is a contact sport and requires physical interaction.

- **Physical abuse** involves, amongst other things, the hitting, punching, strangling, drowning, suffocating, throwing, burning, or poisoning of a child and fabricating illness or inducing illness. Examples of physical abuse in sport can be where a child is forced to undertake physical activity that may be too strenuous for his developing body. Another example could be encouraging a child to take performance-enhancing drugs.

- **Emotional abuse** constitutes any action that causes a child emotional trauma; an example of this could be a child witnessing a domestic violence situation or being persistently made to feel unloved or worthless. Emotional abuse is always harder to recognise because it does not necessarily require a physical action. An example of emotional abuse within sport could be the persistent criticism of a child on his performance or the lack of praise/affirmation when a child performs well.

- **Neglect** is failing to meet the physical and psychological needs of a child, which leads to a serious impairment of that child's health or development. Neglect can include failing to provide adequate food, shelter, and clothing and failing to access adequate medical care when required. Within sport, emotional abuse can occur in situations where a child is not supervised properly, which could result in an accident and/or injury (NSPCC Website).

What Is Child Protection?

'Child protection' is the intervention of an individual or an organisation (such as a local authority) to prevent the abuse or likelihood of abuse of a child. Everyone who comes into contact with children has a responsibility to ensure their safety and welfare. In England and Wales, child protection is the overall responsibility of the Department for Children, Schools, and Families (DCSF). The DCSF issues both statutory and non-statutory guidance to the local authorities on how child protection procedures should be followed.

Within the sporting world, the need for child protection is as important as in any other area of a child's life. With this in mind, the NSPCC and Sport England established and jointly fund the Child Protection in Sport Unit (CPSU). The CPSU works with organisations such as sports councils and national governing bodies to help reduce the risk of a child being subjected to abuse during sporting activities by providing advice to sporting organisations and by developing training procedures. The NSPCC website also provides sporting organisations with guidance on how a sporting organisation should be set up in order to promote child welfare. Examples of this include guidance on how to develop an active child protection policy and what to do if you suspect a child is suffering from abuse.

Signs to Spot a Vulnerable Child

Spotting a child who is being abused is not always easy; however, there are certain signs that a child may exhibit either through their physical appearance or behaviour that may indicate that he is being abused.

- **Signs of emotional abuse:** A child may appear anxious or withdrawn. He may show signs of extreme behaviours such as being exceedingly aggressive or passive. He may act in a manner that is not appropriate to his age, such as acting in an adult-like manner and not appearing to have an attachment to a parent or caregiver (NSPCC Website).

- **Signs of physical abuse:** As well as the physical signs such as bruises, scratch marks, burn, etc., a child may also exhibit signs of physical abuse by flinching at sudden movements, expecting to be chastised if as he has done something wrong, or wearing inappropriate clothing to cover up injuries (such as jumpers on a hot day).

- **Signs of neglect:** Issues with hygiene (soiled clothes, body odour, etc.), ill-fitting clothing, being left alone for long periods of time, continuous complaints of hunger, high absenteeism from school, and untreated illnesses or physical injuries are examples of neglect.

- **Signs of sexual abuse:** As well as the more conclusive signs such as pregnancy or sexually transmitted diseases, a child may also exhibit signs such as having difficulty walking or sitting, acting in a sexualised manner, or being aware of or displaying an interest in sexual acts that are not appropriate to his age (NSPCC Website).

How Abuse Affects a Child

Every child needs stability, security, boundaries, and knowledge that they are loved in order to thrive. Any form of abuse can have damaging effects both short- and long-term. As well as the physical scars that can occur, an abused child can suffer from emotional and psychological scars that can last into adulthood and can have an effect on how that child develops relationships and manages in life later on.

A child being abused by someone he trusts can have a profoundly damaging effect. Without the basis of trust in a child's relationships, a child may develop issues in trusting people and developing healthy relationships later on in life for fear of being subjected to further abuse. Felitti et al. (1998) suggest that there are strong links between child abuse and health issues later on in life, such as heart disease, cancer, and liver disease (Felitti et al., 1998, as cited in Lazenbatt, 2010).

An abused child may have issues in regulating and identifying emotions (Goldsmith & Freyd, 2005). A child can feel confused, ashamed, angry, and scared about what is happening. These feelings can manifest themselves in other ways and particularly later on in life as he attempts to come to terms with what happened as a child. It is not uncommon for adult survivors to suffer from anxiety disorders, depression, and hostility (Brown & Finkelhor, 1986, as cited in Springer et al., 2003).

With emotional abuse, if a child is told over again that he is worthless, inadequate, and unloved, a child can develop low self-esteem and have confidence issues. A child may feel that if the abuser does not love them, then no one can. Later on in life, an adult survivor of abuse may not strive to achieve certain educational or career goals because they feel they are unable and unworthy to attain them. In relationships, adult survivors can become dependent and needy, always seeking reassurance from others in the hope that they will feel deserving of love or attention.

Specifically in relation to the sporting world and physical abuse, if a child is coerced or encouraged to take performance-enhancing drugs, this can have a particularly damaging effect on a child both physically and mentally. The use, for example, of anabolic steroids in pre-pubescent children can cause 'epiphyseal closure following initial growth' (Dawson, 2001).

What to Do When Coming into Contact with an Abused Child and What Not to Do

If there is a suspicion that a child is being abused, there are many ways in which help and advice can be sought. If the person who suspects a child is being abused knows the child on a professional basis (such as a coach within a football team), then that person must discuss his or her concerns with the designated Child Protection Officer within that organisation and should report these concerns in accordance with their national governing body's policy and procedures.

Written records and incident reports should be accurately kept, outlining the concerns and allegations made. Details of those involved should also be recorded, particularly of those who allege to have witnessed any abuse. The Local Authority Designated Officer (LADO) should also be contacted, details of which should be located within the organisation's child protection policy. The LADO will provide guidance and help on whether further action is required and whether a further referral should be made.

If the person who suspects that a child is being abused is not within a professional body or organisation, then that person must contact their Local Authority Children Services team and report their concerns to the Duty Social Worker or to the NSPCC. It is always advisable to report concerns of abuse to an individual who has been trained to handle such allegations. A person must never assume that he or she is able to investigate or handle the situation without informing the appropriate authorities. If a person suspects a child is in immediate and serious danger, then that person must contact the police and report his or her concerns without delay.

In both situations, and where possible, the person or professional who suspects abuse should try to speak with the child and ascertain his wishes and feelings in a manner that is appropriate to his age and understanding. Depending on the nature and seriousness of the allegation, the person may wish to seek the advice of social services or the police before approaching a child in order to ensure that his safety is not compromised. A person must reassure the child but must never promise that he or she will not tell anyone. A person must also never confront a suspected abuser without clear guidance and advice from the relevant authorities or without consent from the relevant authorities that it is appropriate to approach the suspected abuser. Approaching a suspected abuser may lead to further and potentially more serious harm to the child.

Notes

(Endnotes)

1. National Commission of Inquiry into the Prevention of Child Abuse (1996) Childhood Matters, Vols. 1 and 2. London: NSPCC, as cited in *British Medical Journal, 314*, 622.

2. For ease of reference, throughout this chapter, where reference is made to a child, it will be made in the masculine, but it should be noted that all references apply equally to both male and female children.

3. http://www.nspcc.org.uk/Inform/cpsu/helpandadvice/organisations/defining/definingchildabuse_wda60692.html.

4. The Child Protection System in the UK, NSPCC Inform Factsheet (2010): http://www.nspcc.org.uk/Inform/research/questions/child_protection_system_wdf76008.pdf.

5. http://www.nspcc.org.uk/Inform/trainingandconsultancy/learningresources/coreinfo/emotional-neglect-emotional-abuse-PDF_wdf90154.pdf.

6. http://www.nspcc.org.uk/inform/trainingandconsultancy/consultancy/helpandadvice/definitions_and_signs_of_child_abuse_pdf_wdf65412.pdf.

7. Whilst this list is not exhaustive as every child will display different signs depending on the nature or seriousness of the abuse, they do highlight some of the more common and subtle signs that a child may display that every professional or other persons coming in to contact with children should be aware of.

8. Lazenbatt, A. (2010). The impact of abuse and neglect on the health and mental health of children and young people. (p. 2). London: NSPCC. https://www.nspcc.org.uk/Inform/research/briefings/impact_of_abuse_on_health_pdf_wdf73369.pdf.

9. Goldsmith, R., & Freyd, J. (2005), Effects of emotional abuse in family and work environments. *Journal of Emotional Abuse, 5*(1), 96.

10. Brown & Finkelhor. (1986). Impact of child sexual abuse: A review of the research. As cited in Springer et al. (2003), The long term health outcomes of childhood abuse. *Journal of General Internal Medicine, 2003 18*(10), 864–870. http://europepmc.org/articles/PMC1494926/reload=0;jsessionid=pDbthsZqX3xJ2c3nnKDK.2.

11. Dawson, R. T. (2001), Hormones and sport; drugs in sport, the role of the physician. *Journal of Endocrinology, 170,* 55–61.

12. Sometimes also known as the Child Welfare Officer.

13. Information on how to find national governing body in relation to a particular sport can be found at http://www.nspcc.org.uk/Inform/Applications/Search/default.asp.

Index

A

abduction   63-4, 146, 149, 164, 223, 225-7, 229, 234, 243, 261
Achilles tendon   188-91
ACL (anterior cruciate ligament)   157-8, 160, 308, 312, 333-4
ACL injuries   158, 334-5
acromioclavicular joint   63, 219, 222, 230-1
acromion   219, 222-5, 230, 232-4
adduction   63-4, 129, 138, 229, 237
adductor strain   129
aerobic conditioning   359
AIIS (anterior inferior iliac spine)   123, 134
analgesics   90, 92, 107, 113-15, 118, 126, 136, 141, 171, 294, 323
androgens   17, 25, 27, 41
ankle sprains   61, 183, 185, 193
annular ligament   236-7
anterior dislocation   95, 224, 226-7, 229, 246
anterior talofibular ligament   183-4, 186
anterior tibiofibular ligament   183-4
apophysis   24, 68, 70, 130, 188, 190
apophysitis   68, 70-1, 73-5
ASIS (anterior superior iliac spine)   68, 123, 133-4
asthma   56-7, 313-14, 323, 327, 379
  childhood   14, 314
avascular necrosis   77, 105, 138, 145, 155, 204, 214, 247, 265-6, 376

B

bacteria   319, 325
Beighton Scale   345-6
Beighton score   343, 346-7, 354
benchmark   58, 61
bilateral symptoms   88, 97
blisters   324-5
blood tests   120, 149, 316, 318-20
BMI (body mass index)   373, 377-8
body fat   7, 9, 15, 23, 38, 43, 48
bone growth   5, 11-14, 17, 19, 25, 28, 30, 37-8, 276
bone health   18, 331, 337-8
bone mass   15-16, 18, 41, 331
  peak   5, 15-16, 18, 39, 331
bone mineral density   22, 40, 330-1, 338
bone scans   81, 106, 112-15, 132-3, 137, 139, 141, 176-7, 195, 206, 209, 283, 321
bone strength   16, 22, 331
bones   11-16, 19-20, 24, 26-30, 37-41, 68, 76, 86, 98-100, 110-11, 220-1, 240, 256-7, 304-6, 330-1
bracing   81-2, 93, 107-8, 113, 163, 165, 168
brain damage   295, 297-8
brain weight   32

C

calcaneal apophysitis   188-9, 201
calcium   11, 15, 19, 374-5
capitellum   78, 85, 243-4, 247-8
carpal bones   255-6, 263, 271
cartilage   5, 7, 11-12, 28-30, 40, 76, 256, 276, 284
CDH (congenital dislocation of the hip)   151
cervical spine   62, 80, 86, 88, 93-5, 98, 101, 115, 122, 291, 294, 299, 306
child abuse   400-5

testosterone 9, 21, 23, 25, 30, 37-8,
     46, 357
TFCC (Triangular Fibrocartilage
     Complex) 270-1, 279
thigh strains 124-5
thoracic spine 100, 105-6, 116, 120
tibia 157-60, 175-7, 183, 186, 193-5,
     197, 335, 376
tibial tuberosity 24, 69-70, 170-1
traction apophysitis 63-5, 69, 71, 170, 172
trauma 84-5, 96-7, 100, 117, 119, 136,
     140, 145, 166, 177, 204-5, 209, 214,
     285, 305-7
trochlea 199, 243-4, 246

U

ulna 236, 244, 253, 255-7, 267, 271-2
urine dipstick 316, 318-19

V

valgus 162, 168, 202
vertebrae 47, 99, 105, 109, 114, 121, 291

W

water 48, 88, 99-100, 288, 296, 307, 369
World Health Organisation (WHO) 373

X

X-rays 92-4, 99, 105-6, 114-15, 120,
     131-6, 138-9, 145-6, 194-5, 206-9,
     214, 228-30, 239, 241-8, 263-6